EVERY BRANCH OF THE HEALING ART

A History of the Royal College of Surgeons in Ireland

First published 2023 by Eastwood Books
Dublin, Ireland

www.eastwoodbooks.com
www.wordwellbooks.com

First edition

Eastwood Books is an imprint of the Wordwell Group

Eastwood Books
The Wordwell Group
Unit 9, 78 Furze Road
Sandyford
Dublin, Ireland

ISBN: 978-1-913934-54-5 (hardback)

Cover design and layout by Fiachra McCarthy (fiachramccarthy.com)
Copyediting by Neil Burkey (neilburkey.com)
Index by Peigin Doyle
Printed in Northern Ireland by W & G Baird

EVERY BRANCH OF THE HEALING ART

A History of the Royal College of Surgeons in Ireland

RONAN KELLY

To Emilie

CONTENTS

Chancellor's Preface

In 1784, a small group of Irish surgeons broke ranks with the Guild of Barber-Surgeons to form the Royal College of Surgeons in Ireland (RCSI). *Every Branch of the Healing Art* tells the story of RCSI through its contributions to a near-quarter-millennium of surgical, medical and societal change. From nineteenth-century bodysnatchers to the 1916 Rising, through two pandemics and two world wars, with a vivid cast of characters, and reaching right to the present day, the author, Dr Ronan Kelly, has produced here a fast-moving narrative of a great Irish – and, in recent times, global – institution.

As an institutional history, this book is unusual in a number of respects. For a start, it is an entertaining read. It was commissioned not to mark any particular round-numbered anniversary (though 2023 is, as it happens, 250 years since the birth of one of the great figures from the pages herein, Abraham Colles); rather, it was RCSI's achievement of University status in 2019 that inspired the project.

This book is unusual too in that it brings RCSI's story up to the present day. For perspective to emerge with the passage of time, historians generally complete their narratives at a remove of twenty to thirty years. But to do so here would be to miss a remarkable series of accomplishments. Committees don't write books — at least not good ones — so the portrait of RCSI's recent past here is necessarily singular to the author; others might have different perceptions. The Editorial Board felt the risks involved — particularly of names omitted — were outweighed by the gains, and we encouraged Dr Kelly onto terrain where others might justifiably fear to tread. The result, we feel, is an excellent book — one that is worthy of its subject.

For their invaluable contributions to me as Chair, and to Ronan as our author, I would like to thank my fellow members of the Editorial Board: Ms Aíne Gibbons (Director of Development & Alumni Relations), Mr Michael Horgan (former CEO/Registrar), Prof Clive Lee (Prof of Anatomy) and Prof Kevin O'Malley (former CEO/Registrar).

Maurice Manning

Dr Maurice Manning
Chancellor, National University of Ireland
11 February 2023

Chapter 1:
Origins, Before 1784

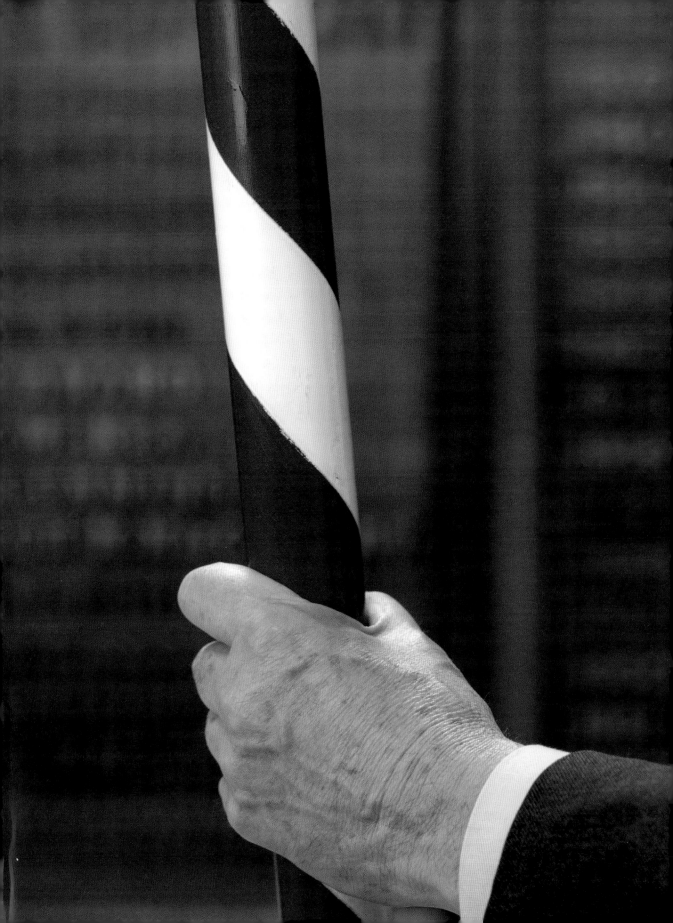

Chapter 1:
Origins, Before 1784

A DECLARATION OF INDEPENDENCE

Dublin has the distinction of being the home of the oldest royally decreed professional body for surgery in these islands. On 18 October 1446, Henry VI established the city's Guild of Barber-Surgeons – ahead of similar corporations in London (1462), Edinburgh (1505) and Glasgow (1599). At this time, religious and civic matters were intertwined, and each guild, or fraternity, was named for its patron saint. The barber-surgeons of Dublin thus constituted the Guild of St Mary Magdalene, and their associated chapel was in Christ Church Cathedral. A second charter, granted by Elizabeth I, copper-fastened the connection in 1577.[1]

For the founders of the Royal College of Surgeons in Ireland (RCSI), however, this distinction of longevity was a dubious honour. The union of barbers and surgeons proved an uneasy one, especially for the surgeons, who were outnumbered – sometimes by as many as ten to one[2] – by their barber brethren. For the best part of 330-plus years, then, whenever the surgeons attempted to reform their practice and institute meaningful standards, they were simply outvoted. (Insult was added to injury in 1687, when a third charter expanded the guild to include apothecaries and periwig-makers.)

At various points, the surgeons of Dublin attempted to extricate themselves from the guild – as their counterparts in Edinburgh and London had managed to do, in 1722 and 1745, respectively[3] – but each attempt was thwarted.

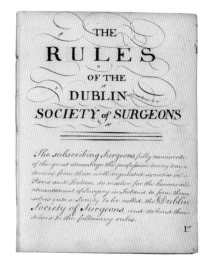

Until, that is, the year 1780, when a group who called themselves the Dublin Society of Surgeons began meeting twice a month – always on a Thursday – in various taverns in the city centre.[4] In a revolutionary era (four years earlier, in 1776, the United States had declared its independence from Britain, while in France, the Bastille would be stormed before the decade was out, ushering in a secular state), these individuals were determined to start a revolution. The minute book of these meetings – now in RCSI Heritage Collections – records that in the King's Arms, Fownes Street, they agreed to the following resolution:

> That it is the opinion of this Committee that a Royal Charter, dissolving the proposterous [sic] and disgraceful union of the Surgeons of Dublin with the Barbers, and incorporating them seperately [sic] and distinctly upon liberal, and scientific principles would highly contribute not only to their own Emolument and the advancement of the profession in Ireland but to the good of Society in general by cultivating and diffusing, surgical knowledge.[5]

In effect, the Dublin surgeons were making their own declaration of independence, both from the barbers' dominance and from all religious influence. (Indeed, even as RCSI has shapeshifted over the ensuing two and a half centuries, these originary ideals – administrative independence and a secular ethos – have endured as constants.) How long the Dublin Society of Surgeons continued to meet is not known: there are no entries in the minute book after 3 May 1781 (by which time fines were being discussed for non-attendance, and the occasional meeting was adjourned for lack of a quorum).

In any case, the major work had been done: the surgeons collected subscriptions to meet the expense of procuring a charter, and they engaged an agent to liaise with the Attorney General. Referring in particular to the precedent in London ('whereof the profession of surgery has been highly cultivated and improved'), their petition to the Lord Lieutenant reads in part:

> ...your petitioners humbly conceive that a similar regulation in this kingdom would be a means of further improving the science of surgery, and of great advantage to the public.
>
> Your petitioners therefore humbly pray your Excellency to recommend to His Majesty, that His Majesty may be graciously pleased to grant his royal letters patent, under the great seal of this kingdom, for dissolving and vacating the union and incorporation of the barbers and surgeons by the said charter of Queen Elizabeth, and for making your petitioners, and such others as may hereafter be elected members, a separate and distinct corporation, by the style and title of 'The Royal College of Surgeons in Ireland;' with such powers and authorities, and under such regulations, as are contained in the annexed draft (which is humbly submitted), or in such manner as to His Majesty in his great wisdom shall seem meet.[6]

Now all they could do was wait.

A BRIEF HISTORY OF PHYSIC AND CHIRURGERIE

All of these divorce proceedings beg the question: why were the surgeons yoked to the barbers in the first place?

Surgery as a profession is defined by its 'authority to cure by means of bodily invasion'.[7] As a practice, there is evidence of rudimentary procedures – such as trepanation – going back to Neolithic times.[8] Any *regulation* of the practice, however, comes much later. By the Middle Ages, most medical 'treatment' in Europe took place under religious auspices, usually at a monastery ('treatment' perhaps overstates what was essentially symptom control and a preparation for death, illness and disease being considered just rewards for sin). Two papal edicts – in 1163 and 1215 – forbade clergy from coming in contact with blood and other bodily fluids, after which they confined themselves to the more intellectual, book-based aspects of healing. Responsibility for bloodletting – by far the favourite response to just about any ailment – and other minor procedures devolved to the *barbitonsores*, those lay servants who already wielded sharp instruments for taking care of the monks' tonsures.

This division of medical labour fostered an already-evolving distinction between medicine, also known as physic (hence 'physicians') – and surgery,

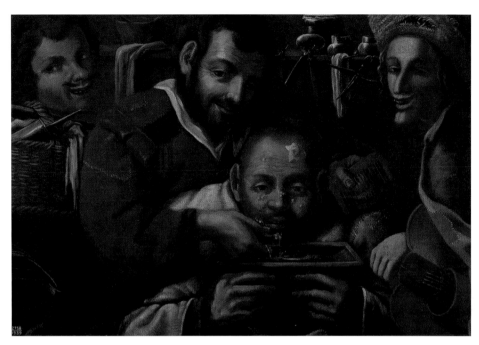

A barber-surgeon attending to a man's forehead. Oil painting. Wellcome Collection.

also known as chirurgerie (etymologically, the word comes from the union of 'hand' and 'work' in ancient Greek). As secularisation continued, the study of medicine found a new home in the early universities at Montpellier, Bologna, Paris, Oxford, Cambridge and elsewhere. In Ireland, the sole university, Trinity College, Dublin (established 1592), opened its 'School of Physic' in 1711. Physicians, then, were learned, literate, obtained medical degrees and called themselves 'doctors'; it was not until the nineteenth century that they even used any instruments in making their diagnoses.

Unfortunately for their patients, their diagnoses were largely based on the second-century teachings of Galen (CE 129–c.216). In his theory, human health depended on an internal balance of four fluids, or humours: blood, phlegm, and black and yellow bile. The physician's task was to interpret external signs –

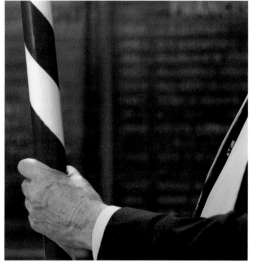

On ceremonial occasions, barbers' poles are carried by the two most junior members of the College Council.

fevers, rashes, spots, diarrhoea – and prescribe a cure. More often than not, this was bloodletting (for which, call the barber-surgeon). Alternatively, he might prescribe the ingestion or application of herbs, purgatives or emetics (for which he sent the patient to the third branch of medieval healthcare, the apothecary). For a millennium and half, until the Renaissance, Western medicine hardly moved on from Galen's theories. Nor did it question his anatomical teachings, which were based on his dissection of cattle, sheep, pigs, goats – even elephants – but not human corpses, which was entirely taboo. In general, physicians did not (physically) intervene into the fabric of the body.

Rightly or wrongly, then, medicine enjoyed high status in medieval Europe. Surgical practice, meanwhile, as it spread beyond the monastic setting, endeared itself to few. Only when a patient had exhausted the expertise of their physician (or, for the poor, the local wise woman or folk healer) was surgical intervention contemplated. The practice inevitably meant pain, sometimes to excruciating degrees; operations had to be performed fast, often mercilessly; and anaesthesia, needless to say, was non-existent, though both patient and surgeon might swig something high-proof to steady nerves and lessen the horror.

Some operators were better than others, but there was little meaningful distinction between a barber and a surgeon; with the necessary sharp blade, one could lance an abscess as easily as shave a beard. As guilds evolved as units of medieval civic society, the hybrid barber-surgeons were considered as one. For the benefit of their largely illiterate customers, they placed a sign above their door: the helical red-and-white pole still familiar in barbershops today (the occasional addition of a blue stripe is a much later American invention).[9] Red and white remain the colours of RCSI's livery.

The surgeons were further separated from the physicians by the range of instruments they carried: saws, knives, hooks, needles and lancets. Having such tools of the trade identified surgeons as practical, hands-on craftsmen. And like other craftsmen – blacksmiths, say, or coopers or tailors – aspirant surgeons were trained by apprenticeship. Training began at age 13 or 14 and lasted about seven to nine years. How competent anyone turned out was a case-by-case affair, entirely dependent on the master's diligence – or lack thereof. (As far as guilds were concerned, regulation was largely about protecting their exclusive rights and prosecuting outsiders, as opposed to overseeing its members.)

Exceptional figures did of course appear, such as Roger Frugardi of Salerno (before 1140–c.1195), Guido Lanfranchi of Milan (c.1250–1315), France's Guy de Chauliac (c.1300–1368) and the Englishman known as John of Arderne (1307–1392). War also advanced surgical knowledge, with barbers retained by armies for their ability to treat wounds. Concomitant with the introduction of the arquebus – basically, the first handgun – military surgery flourished during the Habsburg–Valois Wars of the Italian peninsula (1494–1559), whereas in peaceful Tudor England (1485–1603) surgical practice 'fell back sharply'.[10]

Even so, military surgery itself was limited; at a later date, looking back, an early RCSI President, Clement Archer (1748–1803, PRCSI June–December 1795, first Professor of Surgical Pharmacy, 1789–1803), noted that so-called 'capital' operations were undertaken by 'itinerant empiricks, hardened in butchery, ready to commit such acts of cruelty as the sober regular practitioners would shudder to think of'.[11]

What drove a wedge between some barbers and the surgeons was the Renaissance revolution in anatomical understanding, exemplified in the work of Brussels-born Andries van Wesel (1514–1564) – aka Vesalius. His 1543 publication, *De Humani Corporis Fabrica*, overturned much Galenic thought, not least as Vesalius was a dedicated dissector of human cadavers. Across Europe, the provision of executed criminals for dissection was legalised, albeit in extremely limited circumstances. The first recorded anatomical dissection in Ireland took place in 1676, under the auspices of the Royal College of Physicians (founded twenty years earlier).

The endeavour remained controversial, and on that occasion soldiers had to be posted outside to prevent relatives and sympathisers from seizing the body. (Vesalius, incidentally, was much maligned by his elders for threatening the Galenic system on which they had based their careers; eventually he burnt his unpublished works, abandoned his scientific career and took up private practice in Padua.) From a summary of a treatise of 1630 it is clear that the scope of surgical practice had enlarged significantly:

> The first part of surgery treated wounds, ulcers, fractures, dislocations and also tumours... The second part comprised separating parts of the body for either cosmetic or functional reasons, such as, for instance, those who 'have been brought into the world with the anus and vulva quite shut up'... The third part of surgery removed what was superfluous to the body, such as a dead child in the womb, ruptures or hernias, limbs that had mortified, and parts of the body that had become cancerous; also 'things by their owne nature superfluous', such as wens, cataracts and 'stones in sundry parts of the body'. The fourth part made good 'the defects of the body', for instance 'restoring of the Nose lost or curing of the haire-lip'...[12]

THE FRENCH CONNECTION AND O'HALLORAN'S *PROPOSALS*

In France, the barber-surgeons were less prevalent than elsewhere, and surgery developed differently. In 1268, a group of surgeons succeeded in registering themselves as a *confrérie*, or confraternity, in the *Livre des Mestiers* (Book of Trades). Soon after, Louis IX's surgeon, Jean Pitard, established them as a hierarchically structured guild: surgeons who wore a long robe were entitled to carry out medical procedures; those who wore a short robe were essentially confined to barbering. The *confrérie* was under the invocation of St Cosmas and St Damian – two third-century Arabic doctors who were martyred under the emperor Diocletian – and was variously known as the *Collège de St Côme*, or the *Collège des Chirurgiens* (in both instances, the word *collège* is used in the sense of a collective professional grouping, as opposed to a teaching establishment).

This spiritual dedication bore fruit several centuries later, when Louis XIII (1601–1643) took a special interest in the *Collège* for the simple reason that he had been born on the saints' feast day, 27 September. He was made an honorary member of the *Collège* and, in turn, he give it the right to add the royal fleur-de-lis to its heraldic blazon of three little ointment boxes; he also endowed it with a motto, *Consilioque Manuque* – a shortened form of *consilioque manuque morte artem pellet* (Thanks to his wisdom and his hand, death is kept in check[13]).

When the *Collège* was superseded in 1731 by the *Académie Royale de Chirurgerie* – curiously, one of its founders, Georges Mareschal (1658–1736), was the son of an *émigré* Irishman, John Marshall – the heraldry and motto endured. (Thus, by 1775, when Beaumarchais staged his *Barber of Seville*, audiences would have recognised the surgical reference in the eponymous hero's curtain-lines at the end of Act One: 'My shop is close by – blue paint, lead windows, three little boxes in the air... Consilio Manuque – and the name, Figaro, Figaro, Figaro!') In all other respects, however, the new *Académie* was the most forward-thinking and – crucially – scientifically minded surgical institution of its time.

Someone who admired the innovative spirit of the *Académie Royale de Chirurgerie* was Sylvester O'Halloran (1728–1807).

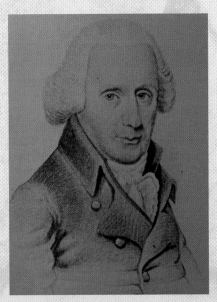

Sylvester O'Halloran. Artist unknown.

This Limerick-born surgeon had a particular interest in ophthalmology, publishing – at age 22 – *A New Treatise on the Glaucoma, or Cataract* (1750), based on his experiments with recently killed calves and living dogs. He also published on amputation (1763), gangrene (1765) and cranial injuries (1793), the last apparently derived from his experience in attending to the aftermaths of local faction-fights.

As a young man, O'Halloran had furthered his training in Paris, London and possibly Leiden. He brought back from the French capital a singular sartorial style – a contemporary remembered him as 'the tall, thin doctor, in his quaint French dress, with

AN

APPENDIX,

CONTAINING

Proposals for the ADVANCEMENT *of* SURGERY *in* IRELAND;

With a retrospective View of the ANTIENT STATE *of* PHYSIC *amongst us.*

PRESENTED

With Great DEFERENCE and high ESTEEM to

LUCIUS O'BRIEN, Esq;

REPRESENTATIVE in PARLIAMENT for the BOROUGH of ENNIS.

THOUGH it be universally admitted, that the profession of surgery is of the greatest utility to the state in time of war, and to the public at all times; and as scarce a man from the prince to the peasant, but must fall under the hands of surgery, at some period or other of his life, it must necessarily

Proposals for the Advancement of Surgery in Ireland (1765).

his goldheaded cane, beautiful Parisian wig, and cocked hat'.[14] In addition, he brought first-hand knowledge of the *Académie Royale*, whose many achievements ('the great advantages of which are universally acknowledged') threw into relief their egregious absence in Ireland. So he published a document called *Proposals for the Advancement of Surgery in Ireland* (1765), laying out, as he saw it, what needed to be done.[15]

After a digressive, historical preamble – O'Halloran was also a popular and prolific, if not entirely reliable, antiquarian and historian – the *Proposals* gets to the heart of the matter: the parlous state of Irish surgical practice, where 'the daily injuries committed by ignorant quacks call loudly for reformation'. To prevent fatal mistakes in the future, he writes, 'and to preserve the vigor of our commonalty, already greatly degenerated: the following proposals for the advancement of surgery, are submitted to public consideration'.

An executive summary of his proposals might read as follows: 'a decent and convenient edifice' should be erected in Dublin; professorships should be founded and prospective candidates should be examined without charge; and a list of reputable surgeons should be published. Or, in the full Georgian flavour:

I.   That a decent and convenient edifice be erected in the capital, and three professorships founded: one for anatomy, a second for the disorders of surgery and midwifry, and the third for the operations of surgery; and that each do give a course of lectures in succession every Winter free to all people.

II. That an exact list be taken through the kingdom of all reputable surgeons, with their names and places of abode: that no other presume to practice surgery, much less perform capital operations; and that all young surgeons for the time to come be interdicted practice, 'till they shall procure a faculty of their abilities, signed by the above professors, or their successors.

III. In order to procure this, the candidate or candidates must by written notice apply for a public examination, and this to be published before the exhibition which should be from twelve to three o'clock. That this hold for three days: the first intirely for anatomy, the second for disorders of surgery, and, if a candidate for midwifry, for this also; and the third to finish, with performing all of the operations of surgery on a body, with their apparatus and bandaging. When a proper faculty, signed by the professors, is given to the candidate, to which if some little honor were annexed, it might add greater stimulus to the young students.

IV. That this course be attended with no kind of expence to the candidate; and that it be free to all Irishmen *only*, without distinction; genius being unconfined to principle or party, and such narrower considerations being worthier a little republic of Ragusa, than the representatives of a powerful kingdom. And that the number be by no means limited, because the more surgeons of eminence, the better the public will be served.

V. That a printed list be published annually of the registered surgeons and men-midwives of the kingdom, with their places of abode, signed by the professors: by which means the public will, as heretofore, know where to apply for certain relief.

ANATOMY OF A NAME

It is likely that the Dublin Society of Surgeons were familiar with these *Proposals*; on 21 September 1780, at a meeting in the Eagle Tavern, O'Halloran had been elected an honorary member of the Society. Indeed, the *Proposals* may be seen as a blueprint for the type of Royal College outlined in the Society's petition. Not everyone saw this as the way to advance Irish surgery, however. Unsurprisingly, the Guild of Barber-Surgeons objected to the Society's petition ('we cannot nor ought we, by any act or concurrence whatsoever, consent that the prayer of the petitioners should be granted'), but this time, finally, they were on the losing side. George III was indeed 'graciously pleased', and on Wednesday, 11 February 1784, the petitioners received their Charter and the Royal College of Surgeons in Ireland was established.

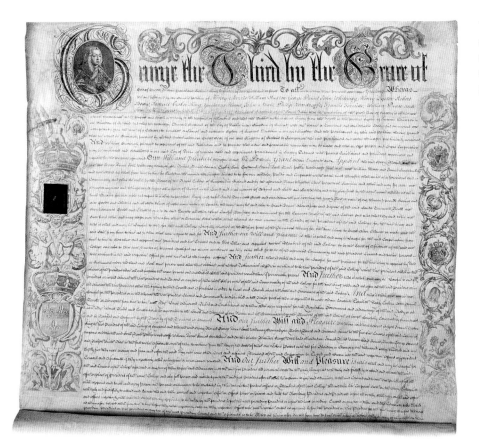

The Charter
of the Royal
College of
Surgeons in
Ireland (1784).

This vellum document, about the size of a small tablecloth, begins with a name, the authority by which all else follows: 'George the Third, By the Grace of God, of Great Britain, France and Ireland, King, Defender of the Faith, and so forth.' Then there are the names of the petitioners, including Henry Morris, President of the Dublin Society of Surgeons; Samuel Croker-King (1728–1817), the first President of RCSI (1784–85); William Dease, first Professor of Surgery (1784–98) and fourth PRCSI (1789); and James Henthorn (1744–1832), long-time Secretary of both bodies and, remarkably, PRCSI in 1822, at the age of 78.

At the very end, there are even the names of the two clerks who enrolled the Charter in the High Court of Chancery. (Did King George himself ever actually see the document? He had enough to be getting on with: there were signs already of the mental illness that blighted his later years, and in 1782 and 1783 he was deeply affected by the deaths of two infant sons; and then there was admission, via the Treaty of Paris (1783), that America was lost... No matter: his Great Seal is the only imprimatur that is needed.) The name of the Royal

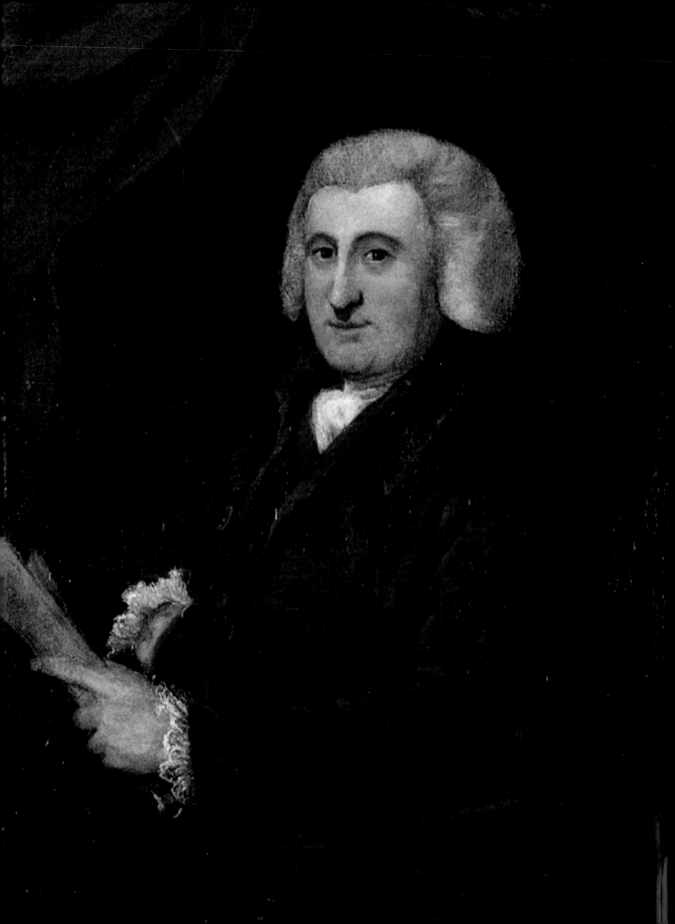

College of Surgeons in Ireland, however, is somewhat buried in the text, amid the legalese of bye-laws, ordinances, rules and constitutions.

But it is a name whose elements are worth unpacking, not least to understand the complications that flow from it in later periods. 'Royal' means the legal status is backed by the ultimate authority in the land; after 1922, this authority transferred to Oireachtas Éireann – that is, the Irish parliament. 'Royal' never meant that the College was in any way sponsored or supported by the Crown. Nor did it imply any particular fealty amongst the original petitioners, as the story of William Dease – of whom more anon – will attest.

Next: 'College'. This indicated a professional grouping, as seen above with the *Collège* in Paris. The word did not designate a school of any sort; in fact, no school is mentioned in the Charter, although it is clear that, in addition to the regulation of surgery, some provision of surgical education, as per O'Halloran's *Proposals*, was envisioned. The relevant lines are:

> ... the regulation of the profession of surgery is of the utmost importance to the publick, and highly necessary to the welfare of mankind, and that the publick sustain great injury from the defects in the present system of surgical education in our Kingdom of Ireland; and that the regularly educated surgeons of the City of Dublin (who are become a numerous and considerable body) find themselves incompetent (from want of a Charter) to establish a liberal and extensive system of surgical education.

What can be considered an undergraduate medical school, or the forerunner of such, had to wait two years, until 1786, to come into being – by which time Professorships in Anatomy and Physiology, and Surgery, had been established. In theory, then, the College and its 'School' are distinct entities – hence the existence of both a President (of the former) and a Registrar (later Vice Chancellor and CEO, of the latter); indeed, in RCSI's first hundred years the idea of separation was occasionally mooted. In practice, however – and in this history – they function largely as two sides of the same coin. And day to day, even from early on, 'College' came to denote whatever aspect of RCSI life was being referred to at any given moment.

Moving on to 'of Surgeons', then. The historical aspect has been dealt with above: the establishment of RCSI was very much part of a wider effort to put surgical practice on a professional footing. But the profession advanced so quickly in the first half of the nineteenth century that it came to encompass

Facing page: Samuel Croker-King, first President of RCSI. Artist unknown.

13

what had traditionally been the physician's closely guarded terrain. As one of RCSI's luminaries, Arthur Jacob (Licentiate of RCSI 1813, Member of RCSI 1816,[16] Prof of Anatomy and Physiology 1827–67, PRCSI 1837, 1864–65), put it in 1844:

> This College [Jacob is using the word in the educational sense], although called a College of Surgeons, is as you all know, just as much a College of Physicians. We have the same corps of professors, or even a larger one; we require the same course of medical studies, or even a more extended one; and we examine as carefully on medical subjects as they do in the schools of medicine. In fact, this is a College of Medicine and Surgery, and the diploma you receive from it is universally accepted as evidence of your fitness to practice every branch of the healing art.[17]

The distinction (not to say discrimination) that Jacob points to essentially would be dissolved in 1886, when a 'triple qualification' – in medicine, surgery and midwifery – became essential requirements for entrance on the Medical Register. At this point, RCSI came to an agreement with the nearby Royal College of Physicians of Ireland, and thereafter RCSI students obtained full 'medical' qualifications. This meant that students from 'Surgeons' – as it was colloquially known – became doctors and, indeed, dentists. (They could become surgeons later, if they pursued that further training.)

For the best part of a century, no one was too confused by this, but later, in a more globalised medical education world, these nomenclatural nuances provoked a little too much puzzlement. As a solution, RCSI embraced the acronymic brand, 'RCSI'. (The potential loss here – the elision of a complex history – was exactly the gain.) In 2019, when RCSI gained the right to call itself 'RCSI University of Medicine and Health Sciences', the name, or the *signifier*, as linguists would say, finally matched the *signified* – that is, the full range of higher educational practice that was carried out inside.

And finally, there is 'in Ireland'. From the Dublin Society of Surgeons' first resolutions, and indeed O'Halloran's *Proposals*, this was always the island-sized remit envisioned. In theory, city limits might have been observed, as the Royal College of Surgeons of Edinburgh (1778) had done, and the Royal College of Surgeons of London (1800) were about to do (only later, in 1843, did it follow the Irish example and restyle itself the Royal College of Surgeons of *England*).

After 1922, this all-Ireland status was a point of pride for many at RCSI, as though surgery were above mere politics. But nothing is ever really above politics, and RCSI's regulatory remit in Northern Ireland ended in 2005. By then, of course, RCSI was also a global medical education institution, even as its identity remained firmly rooted in Ireland.

As to the last preposition, no one else committed to the outlier 'in' (though as late as the 1880s, RCPI was sometimes 'in', sometimes 'of'[18]). Back in 1780, 'of' and 'in' were likely the least of the Society of Surgeons' concerns, and conceptually there is little difference between the two. In any case, RCSI can claim the virtue of prepositional consistency since that time. ∎

Chapter 2:
Foundations, 1784–1820

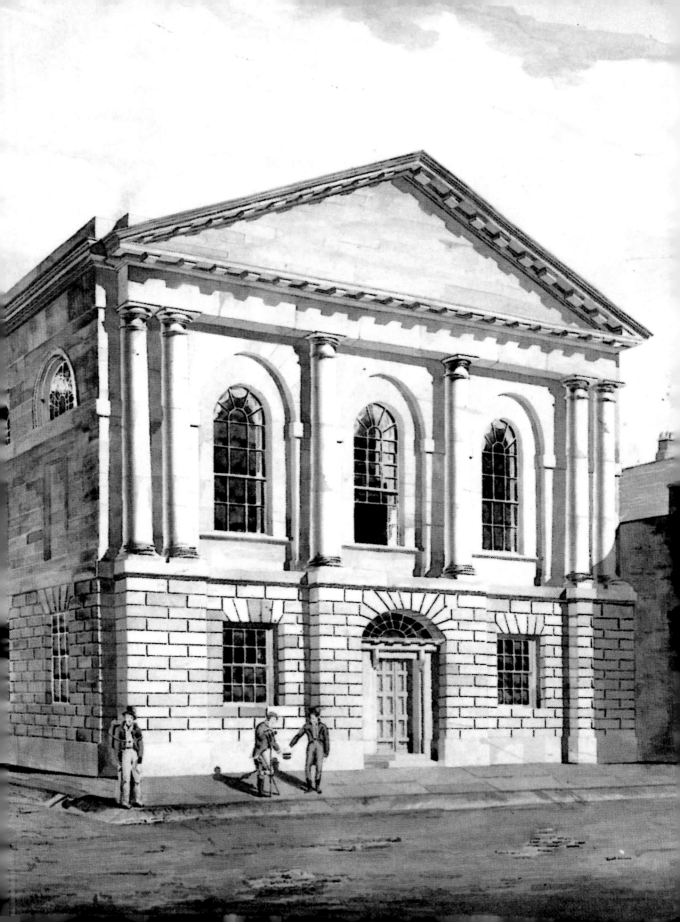

Chapter 2:
Foundations, 1784–1820

THE FIRST LICENTIATES AND MEMBERS

The birth of the Royal College of Surgeons in Ireland – to quote Charles Cameron, RCSI President, Professor of Political Medicine, and first historian – 'fitly took place in the great maternity founded by Surgeon Bartholomew Mosse'.[1]

By this he meant that the inaugural meeting of the newly Chartered College took place on Tuesday, 2 March 1784, in Dublin's Rotunda Hospital, or as it was then known, 'the Lying-In Hospital'. The embossed red leather minute book records the election of Croker-King as first President, Henthorn as Secretary, as well as six 'censors' – that is, examiners – and twelve 'assistants'. An initial cohort of fifty surgeons were granted Letters Testimonial – later called the Licence – by dint of which they were now officially qualified for the practice they were already doing. Forty-nine of these Licentiates were subsequently elected Members of the College (one neglected to pay his fees), meaning they would have voting rights in how the College was governed.

Previous page:
RCSI in 1810.
Watercolour.
Artist unknown. At some point afterwards, the same red leather minute book went missing, only to be rediscovered in time for RCSI's Bicentenary celebrations in 1984. To mark that occasion, the Council of the day convened in the Rotunda's Board

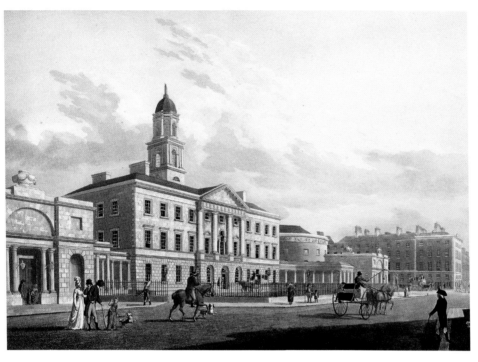

The Lying-In Hospital by James Malton. Reproduced courtesy of the National Library of Ireland (PD 3181 TX 111).

Room, where extracts from the 200-year-old minutes were read. According to one of those present, the general impression in the room was that the more things change, the more they stay the same.

For the first year of its existence, the College continued to meet at the Rotunda. Various committees were formed, including, as a priority, one charged with finding a suitable 'Hall for carrying on the business of the College'.[2] An early bye-law levied one guinea (that is, one pound and one shilling) annually on each Member to defray College expenses and to establish a library. The decision was also made to declare RCSI's raison d'être to the population at large:

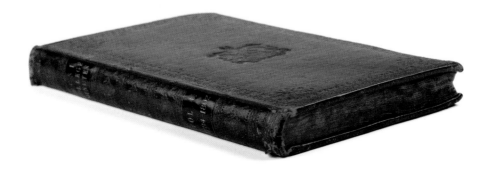

RCSI's first Minute book.

To advertise in the public journals that the President, Vice-President, and Censors were prepared to examine all regularly-educated surgeons, and to grant to those found competent, Letters Testimonial, qualifying the holders thereof to practise surgery and to be eligible for election as members of the College.[3]

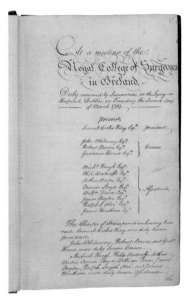

Minutes of the first meeting of the College, 2 March 1784.

The first person to answer that advertisement and present himself for examination was a man called John Birch. He paid his fees (ten guineas) and was examined over two days – 12 and 14 August 1784 – in anatomy, physiology, surgery and surgical pharmacy. He passed, becoming RCSI's first Licentiate by examination.[4] Little else is known about Birch, except that he practised for many years in Roscrea, Co. Tipperary.

By contrast, the second Licentiate by examination, Solomon Richards (c.1760–1819, Lic. 1785) – born in York Street, and trained in London, Edinburgh and Paris – stayed close to the College. He was elected a Member (1785) and four-time President (1794, 1803, 1808, 1818). He was famous in Dublin for his gourmandizing, his generosity to the poor, and for having once performed an emergency tracheotomy in public. (If that is not enough, he also won a lottery prize of £10,000.)

In truth, however, RCSI was not deluged with applicants for the Licence in its early years; fewer than ten were granted by 1789.[5] A far greater number presented themselves for the less strenuous, single-sitting exams for army and naval diplomas. For decades previously, the low bar for ship's surgeons was a subject of satire. In Tobias Smollett's novel *Roderick Random* (1748), this is how the hero is examined:

'If,' continued he, 'during an engagement at sea, a man should be brought to you with his head shot off, how would you behave?' After some hesitation, I owned such a case had never come under my observation, neither did I remember to have seen any method of care proposed for such an accident, in any of the systems of surgery I had perused...[6]

From 1785, the Lord Lieutenant had requested that RCSI take responsibility for examining two military grades, that of 'surgeon' (fee: three guineas) and of 'surgeon's mate' (one guinea).[7] The declaration of war between Britain and France in 1793 saw a further boost in such candidates, and in time RCSI raised the standard of its army and navy exams to that of the Licence.[8]

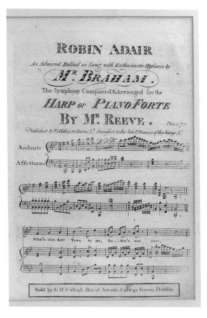

'What's this dull town to me? / Robin's not near…' Sheet music for 'Robin Adair'.

During these years, the fledgling institution also sought to consolidate its credentials by conferring Honorary Membership on various eminent surgeons, the first of whom was Robert Adair (c.1714–1790, Hon MRCSI 1784). The Irish-born Adair was Inspector General of Military Hospitals, Surgeon General, Sergeant Surgeon to George III and Surgeon to Chelsea Hospital, but his best claim to immortality rests on his inspiration for 'Robin Adair', a lovelorn ballad of that name; as well as appearing in Jane Austen's *Emma* (1816), its accompanying tune serves as the processional air for RCSI conferrals.

The College likewise honoured Sylvester O'Halloran (1786), not least for having inspired its very existence. Other early Honorary Members include Benjamin Bell of Edinburgh (1784), Antoine Louis of the Académie Royale de Chirurgerie (1786), and the Londoners Percivall Pott (1788) and John Hunter (1790). And on the subject of reputation management, in 1789 a man named Frederick Drury earned the dubious distinction of being the first Member expelled from the College ('having given false and corrupt testimony'[9]).

THE SCHOOL AND ITS FIRST PROFESSORS

In the case of John Birch, who had been trained by apprenticeship elsewhere, RCSI functioned entirely as an examining and accrediting body. But the College authorities were not slow in acting on the ambition expressed in the Charter, 'to establish a liberal and extensive system of surgical education'. The decision to appoint professors was taken in May 1785: there would be one in surgery (the first such chair in Ireland), one in anatomy and physiology, and one in midwifery (also the first of its kind in the country).

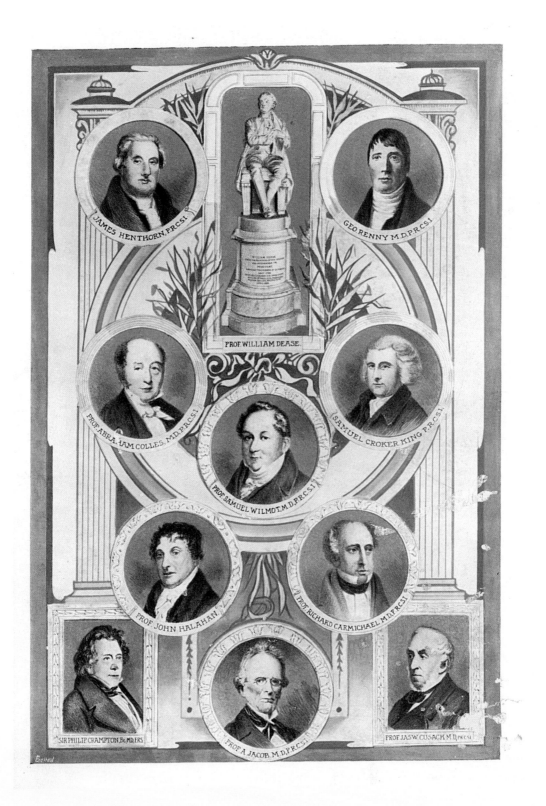

In November, William Dease (c.1752–1798, Prof of Surgery 1785–98, PRCSI 1789) and John Halahan (1753–1813, Prof of Anatomy and Physiology 1785–94 and 1799–1804, Prof of Midwifery 1789–93) were appointed to the first two of these, respectively; the sole applicant for the third chair was rejected, so Halahan double-jobbed until the appointment of RCSI's first knight, Sir Henry Jebb (d. 1811, Prof of Midwifery 1793–94, PRCSI 1800).[10] This marks the start of RCSI as a teaching establishment.

At the time, one spoke of 'the Schools of the College' – that is, 'the School of Surgery' or 'the School of Anatomy' – a locution derived from the Collège de St Cosme. Also borrowed from the same source was RCSI's motto: Consilio Manuque, variously translated as 'by wisdom and dexterity', or 'by scholarship and skill', or 'by the head and the hand'. To readers of Latin, both words also have a collective, rather than individual, inference.[11] The motto appears in both the College Seal, used from 1784 to 1907, and the Coat of Arms, which replaced it.

These new professorships were unsalaried positions, on the basis that a regular salary would only reward the work-shy. Instead, payment was a percentage of student fees, so the ability to attract and keep students was vital. In the continued absence of a College 'Hall', tuition took place in private residences or rented rooms. Halahan fitted up a dissection room at his own expense (he was later reimbursed), while Dease made available his private collection of 'anatomical preparations' – that is, preserved human parts.

From the students' point of view – or 'pupils', as they were called – there was nothing cheap about a surgical education. They paid per course: two guineas for 'registered pupils' – that is, apprentices to Members of the College, who passed a preliminary exam in Greek and Latin and also paid a registration fee of five guineas – or three guineas for 'strangers'. On top of that was the great bane of student life, accommodation: residency in a master's house cost at least 200 guineas, half that if one lived elsewhere. Members of the College were restricted to two apprentices at a time, except by special dispensation.

Facing pages: RCSI's first Presidents and Professors: Dease, Halahan and others. Illustration from Cameron's *History of RCSI* (1886).

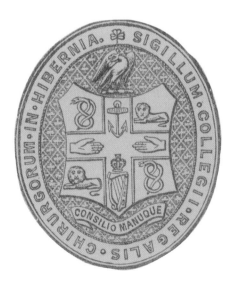

The College Seal, with old Arms.

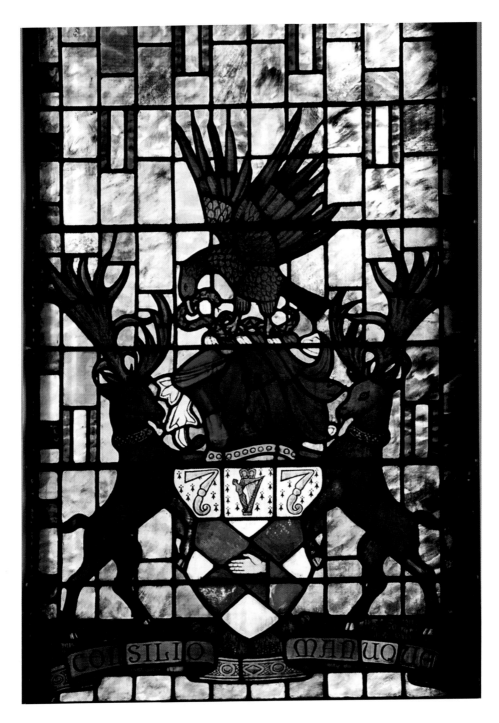

The College Coat of Arms, in use since 1907. Its official description runs: 'Argent on a Saltire gules, a dexter hand apaumée fessewise, couped at the wrist proper; on a Chief ermine a harp crowned between two fleams or; for CREST on a wreath of the Colours an Eagle preying on a serpent proper; for SUPPORTERS two Irish Elks each gorged with a Chaplet of Shamrock all proper; and for MOTTO "Consilio Manuque".'

A HOUSE ON MERCER STREET

The absence of premises is a running theme in the College minutes of the period, and piecemeal measures such as levies on Members or student fees were not about to supply the lack. In January 1785 the RCSI drafted an eloquent petition to Parliament on the subject. What they needed, they said, was a permanent home 'where the various branches of the profession might be regularly and scientifically taught by Practitioners in Surgery, and where they might be able to co-operate with the other physic schools in this city so as to be able to establish a complete system of surgical education in this Kingdom'. Ireland, they pointed out, 'was the only nation in Europe destitute of such an establishment'.[12] In a show of collegiality, the petition was presented by the Provost of Trinity (he was also, usefully, Secretary of State). Parliament, however, declined.

After about a year, RCSI left the Rotunda. (On the way out, they made a thank-you contribution of ten guineas to the hospital's building fund, and tipped the servants two guineas.) Thereafter, a peripatetic period began, with RCSI drifting from one rented room to another. At one point, the idea of settling in a former opera house in Capel Street was considered; at another, an attempt was made to lease a substantial property in Golden Lane. For a time, they met at the City Assembly House on South William Street (currently home to the Irish Georgian Society). Later again, they met at Secretary Henthorn's house on Andrew Street.

All the while, petitions to Parliament continued to be made – three in 1787 – all to no avail, bar the tantalising (not to say maddening) hint that 'it was probable they would succeed eventually'. A year later, even that vague hope suffered a blow:

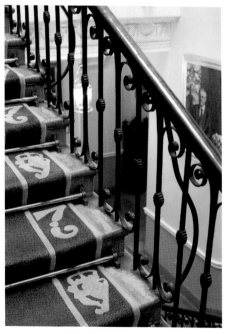

Elements from the Arms, the crowned harp and the fleam (an early lancet), provide motifs on the main staircase.

> ... though the Government highly approved of their institution, and of the measures the College had pursued since their incorporation, it was highly impossible in the present state of the countries [*sic*]

finance to allow any aid in money towards the erection of a hall for the purposes they have lately stated.[13]

In late 1788, RCSI found itself engaged in a little brinksmanship on the subject. At this time, an Act of Parliament permitted the supply of a small number of bodies of executed criminals for dissection at educational institutions. When a city high sheriff contacted RCSI with one such offer, Secretary Henthorn pointedly replied by return of post:

> I am to acquaint you that the College regret it is not in their power to comply with the Act by receiving the body, as Government has not yet enabled them to procure a hall for public dissection.[14]

Unsurprisingly, this did not suddenly alter the government's position; nor did it later, when subsequent RCSI petitions attempted to leverage the incident. What happened to the malefactor's corpse is unclear, though popular tradition says it inspired a famous Dublin ballad, 'The Night Before Larry was Stretched'.

In any event, RCSI found – not for the last time – that it was better off steering an independent course. In August 1789, then – some five and a half years since obtaining its Charter – the College finally took on a property of its own. This was a house in Mercer Street, discovered for them by their appointed bookseller

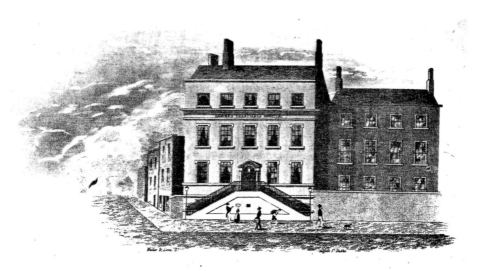

Mercer's Hospital, founded 1734.

MERCER'S HOSPITAL.

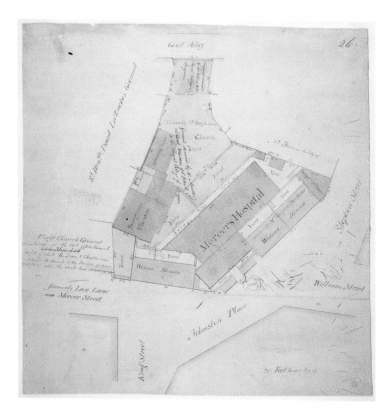

Location of the original College premises at the rear of Mercer's Hospital. Reproduced courtesy of the National Library of Ireland (21 F 89 / 186).

and printer – and, apparently, estate agent – Patrick Byrne. The lease (for 999 years) refers to 'the Premises in Mercer Street lately occupied by the Charity Children of the Parish of St Peter in the City of Dublin'.[15]

This ecclesiastical detail is noteworthy, as the site had medical associations reaching back to the fourteenth century. Originally there was a chapel here, St Stephen's – from whence the nearby eponymous Green – attached to which was a 'lazar house', or leper hospital, medieval healthcare being, as noted earlier, an essentially clerical concern. Some three centuries later, a woman named Mary Mercer opened a stone-built house on the spot as a shelter for impoverished young women, and in 1734 this became Mercer's Hospital. Famously, a fundraiser for the hospital in 1742 featured the world premiere of Handel's *Messiah*.[16]

RCSI's new property was adjacent to the hospital. After all the rootlessness, the College authorities were happy to have it, though it was in fact a dilapidated wreck. Rent was significant – £26 per annum, when the College income that year was £65 8*s* 1½*d* – but the much greater expenditure was on making the premises fit for purpose. Carpenters, plumbers, ironmongers, stone cutters, painters, paperers, upholsterers and glaziers were set to work; teaching supplies were ordered from druggists, glass manufacturers and instrument makers. These bills totalled more than £435 10s 11d – on top of which the architect's fee was £100.

Teaching seems to have begun in October 1789: a few semicircular rows of pinewood seating made a 'theatre', which was also used as a dissection room. The first meeting of the President, censors and assistants in their new home took place on 4 January 1790, at which Dease was commended for 'his very proper conduct in the Chair and for the active part he has taken in establishing a school for the younger part of the profession'. Another resolution thanked Secretary Henthorn for 'his very active and successful cooperation with our late President (Dease) in Establishing an Institution so Essential to the future interests of the Profession'.[17]

A little later that year, the College made another substantial disbursement: 100 guineas to purchase outright an adjoining house. Such an outlay might seem extravagant, but it was in fact vital for the College's operation. The legal provision of cadavers for dissection – noted earlier – was nowhere near adequate, so the College quietly relied on other means. The new house provided convenient access to Goat Alley (now Digges Lane), and it was through this quiet back street that bodies – called 'subjects' – lately and illegally exhumed from graveyards, could be discreetly delivered into the dissection room. There will be more on this activity anon.

WAR — WHAT IS IT GOOD FOR?

How did RCSI pay for all this expansion? For the Goat Alley house, Professor Dease (also President that year) lent the money, as he had done for the earlier Charter expenses. But some of the craftsmen who had toiled on the leased Mercer Street house were left waiting two years for payment. Their ship – and the College's – finally came in when a government grant of £1,000 materialised in April 1791. This was less a change of heart than an expression of hard-headed realpolitik: since the Revolution, thunderclouds had been building over France – and sure enough, following Louis XVI's appointment with Madame La Guillotine, Britain and France went to war in 1793. By then, the army had done much preparation, including the widespread recruitment and training of surgeons. RCSI was happy to play its part: of thirty-five candidates examined by 1790, twenty-four were for the military, while from 1791, fees for lectures in the School were waived for army and navy candidates.

The individual who pushed the College's case hardest with the authorities was a Scot, George Renny (1757–1848, PRCSI 1793). Usefully, he was Surgeon at the Royal Hospital, Kilmainham, and from 1795 until – impressively – 1847, he served on the Irish Army Board. (He also worked hard on behalf of the city's poor, notably at the Foundling Hospital and Cork Street Fever Hospital. One hot day, while making his way from Kilmainham to Cork Street, he was struck by the 'want of water by the poor'; he put together a committee and subsequently had some forty street fountains installed, fed by the Grand Canal.)

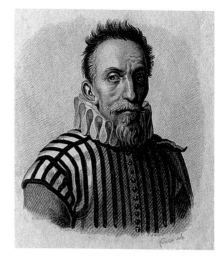

Ambroise Paré. Stipple engraving by C.A. Forestier, c.1823. Wellcome Collection.

Famously, the great barber-surgeon Ambroise Paré (1510–1590) maintained that the only people who benefit from war are young surgeons. Truth be told, it is probably the institutions that train those young surgeons who benefit most of all. For the next quarter of a century, the conflicts that destroyed the lives of millions provided an unrelenting windfall for RCSI, the benefits of which – financial, at least – cannot be overstated.

ABRAHAM COLLES AND HIS PROFESSORS

In 1792 – the oldest date for which detailed student records survive – there were 100 students, many of them military, attending lectures at RCSI. One of this number was Abraham Colles of Kilkenny, who had enrolled as a 17-year-old 'registered pupil' two years earlier. In time – indeed, in a very short time: he was elected President before the age of 30 – Colles would become the single most influential figure in RCSI's early history.

Family lore has it that his interest in surgery began early: as a pupil at Kilkenny College, he is supposed to have found an anatomy textbook floating in the Nore after a local doctor's house had flooded. Seeing the boy entranced, the doctor told him to keep the book. But surgery was also in the family: his great-grandfather William Colles had started life as a ship's surgeon. After some amorous scrapes in the north of England, this Colles settled in Ireland. In the family he was known as 'Brown Billy' on account of the deep sepia

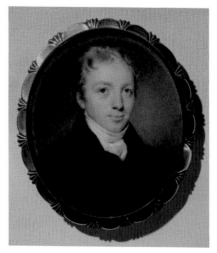

Abraham Colles as a young man. Artist unknown.

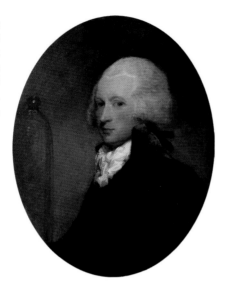

Prof William Hartigan (*c.*1793) by Gilbert Stuart. Oil on canvas. National Gallery of Art, Washington D.C.

portraits he commissioned of himself every seven years.

The story is told that young Aby would stare at one such portrait and plot his own career – much encouraged in this by his doting mother. Right through his life, Colles kept up a constant, affectionate, often comic correspondence with his mother – even when the subject was medical ('As to your question What am I to do for the itch?' he once replied to her, 'I must tell you that the practice here which seems to be most pleasant to the generality of patients is to scratch!'[18]).

Colles' father, who ran a successful marble-works, died when his son was four years old.[19]

Interestingly, Colles also registered at Trinity College five days after he enrolled at RCSI – but in Arts, not Medicine.[20] Although Trinity's 'School of Physic' had been established since 1711, it was by 1790 at perhaps its lowest ebb; in fact, no students at all matriculated that year. That said, Colles took at least two courses therein: Chemistry, under Robert Perceval, author of the first *Dublin Pharmacopoeia* (1805); and Practice of Medicine, under Stephen Dickson, which probably was not too taxing, as Dickson was dismissed later for 'persistent neglect of his duties'.[21]

At least that left time for other pursuits: Colles, along with his brother William, also a Trinity student, joined the Historical Society – the famous 'Hist' – membership of which was, for many, the whole point of a Trinity education. Reputations were made here, and in Colles' lifetime few public figures of Irish life did not pass through its precincts – Burke, Grattan and Wolfe Tone before him, Robert Emmet and Thomas Moore shortly after. Frustratingly, as only surnames were recorded, it is not known which Colles brother was the more active in the Society; either way, within a few years Abraham had developed a reputation as 'an experienced and polished performer'.[22]

Facing page: *A Syllabus of a Course of Lectures on Anatomy and Physiology* (1796) by William Hartigan and William Lawless.

Colles' time at RCSI is better recorded, not least as his admissions cards to lectures and dissections survive. In the house on Mercer Street, Dease taught him Surgery, while Halahan was joined by William Hartigan (*c.*1756–1812, Prof of Anatomy and Physiology 1789–99, Prof of Surgery 1798–99, PRCSI 1797) for Anatomy and Physiology. A former member of the Dublin Society of

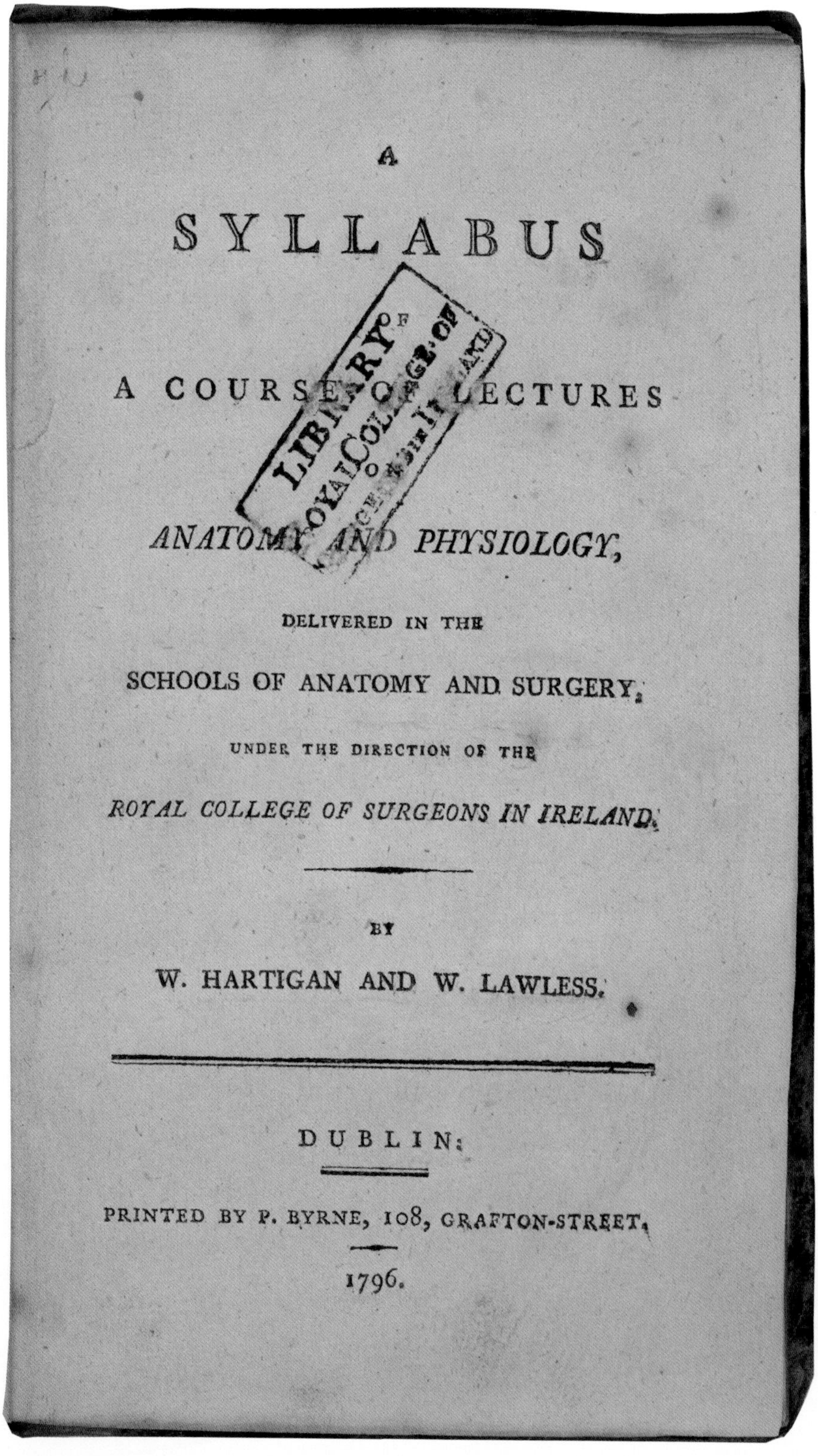

A

SYLLABUS

OF

A COURSE OF LECTURES

ON

ANATOMY AND PHYSIOLOGY,

DELIVERED IN THE

SCHOOLS OF ANATOMY AND SURGERY,

UNDER THE DIRECTION OF THE

ROYAL COLLEGE OF SURGEONS IN IRELAND,

BY

W. HARTIGAN AND W. LAWLESS.

DUBLIN:

PRINTED BY P. BYRNE, 108, GRAFTON-STREET,

1796.

Surgeons, Hartigan had impeccable credentials and was immensely popular with his students. He was also famous for his inordinate affection for cats, and while making his rounds would often carry a pair of kittens around with him in the deep pockets of his greatcoat (pet therapy *avant la lettre*?).

Hartigan collected his teaching in a book, co-authored with William Lawless, initially a Demonstrator in the dissecting room, then Halahan's successor, and published by Patrick Byrne. Called *A Syllabus of Lectures on Anatomy and Physiology, Delivered in the Schools of Anatomy and Surgery, Under the Direction of the Royal College of Surgeons in Ireland* (1796), this was more or less the curriculum that Colles followed as a student. Later, it would be the exact terrain he revolutionised.

Colles' lectures on Midwifery were delivered by Halahan, Jebb and John Creighton (1768–1827, Lic. 1792, MRCSI 1792, Prof of Midwifery 1794–1819, PRCSI 1812, 1824). This was the first such chair in the country, not least as midwifery was considered *infra dig* by most physicians; indeed, taking the College of Physicians' diploma in the subject automatically forbade its holders from later taking a degree in medicine. As a result, it was often a surgeon – or, in the parlance, a 'surgeon and man-midwife' – who assisted at births. Creighton's great claim to fame was ahead of him: in 1800, at the Cow-Pock Institution in

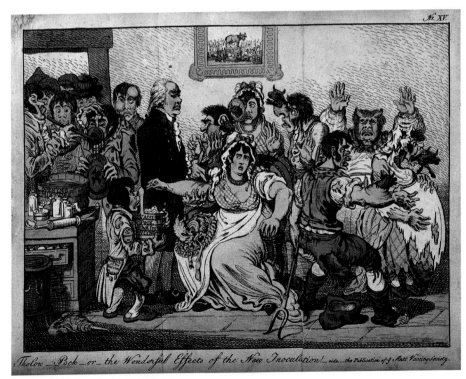

Edward Jenner vaccinating patients in the Smallpox and Inoculation Hospital at St Pancras: the patients develop features of cows. Coloured etching, 1803, after J. Gillray, 1802. Wellcome Collection.

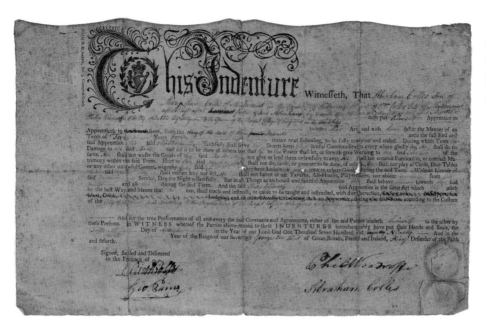

Abraham Colles' Certificate of Indenture to Philip Woodroffe (1790).

nearby Exchequer Street, he introduced Jennerian vaccination to Ireland.[23]

In addition, Clement Archer (1748–1803, Prof of Surgical Pharmacy (aka Materia Medica, aka Clinical Pharmacology) 1789–1803, PRCSI June–December 1795) lectured on Surgical Pharmacy (and much else: he received an official reprimand for consistently wandering off topic). Botany was also introduced in Colles' time, taught by Walter Wade (d. 1825, Prof of Botany 1792–1825), an early advocate of what would become the National Botanic Gardens.

COLLES THE APPRENTICE

Also surviving is Colles' 'Indenture Certificate', dated 15 September 1790, which gives a vivid glimpse of the apprentice–master relationship. Colles signed up for a term of five years' duration – in accordance with the College bye-laws – thereby binding himself to a sweeping range of commitments, some of which are ordinary enough:

> … the said Apprentice his said Master faithfully shall serve, his Secrets keep, & his lawful Commandments everywhere gladly do… He shall do no Damage to his said Master nor see it to be done of others… He shall not waste the Goods of his said Master, nor give or lend them unlawfully to any…

Other, more niche prohibitions suggest the life an average apprentice might prefer to live:

> He shall not commit Fornication, or contract Matrimony... He shall not play at Cards, or Dice-Tables or any other unlawful games... He shall not haunt or use Taverns, Ale-Houses, Play-Houses, nor absent himself from his said Master's Service, Day nor Night unlawfully...[24]

It is hardly surprising that apprentices might like to blow off some steam: theirs was a generally arduous and expensive existence. Day and night they were at their master's beck and call, oftentimes poorly fed, spartanly housed in 'any old corner of the hospital', and expected to jump to any and all duties, whether menial or medical. Apprentices as young as 14 or 15 were in the thick of things, helping to tie or hold down the patient, or wipe a blade on their sleeve before they passed it to their master.

The wards they worked in were often overcrowded nests of infection; in those pre-Listerian days, all wounds went septic and indeed the flow of so-called 'laudable' pus was welcomed as a necessary step towards recovery. As Lombe Atthill (1827–1910, Lic. RCSI 1847, PRCPI 1888–90), later Master of the Rotunda, recalled:

> When anaesthetics were unknown, patients had always to be held, often strapped down to the table while operations proceeded, and the groans and screams, especially in the case of women and children, were most distressing to hear. Instead of the deliberate care with which operations are now performed, surgeons vied with each other as to which would perform an operation in the shortest time. Much blood was lost. A tourniquet would be applied were a limb to be amputated, but beyond this no attempt would be made to temporarily arrest haemorrhage; the bone being sawn through, then the arteries would be ligatured with silk and the stump dressed. But the mortality, even after the simplest operations, was great, and sloughing of the integuments quite common; even simple incisions seldom healed by 'first intention.' I have a vivid recollection of having seen two operations for strangulated hernia performed, I think, on the same day, both patients being healthy men; both were dead a few days later. Cutting for stone too, was a not uncommon operation, and very frequently fatal.[25]

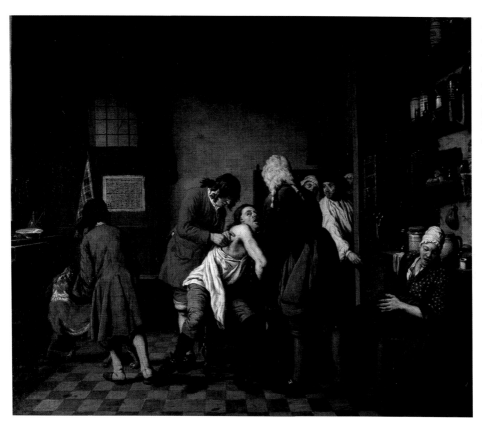

Interior with a surgeon and his apprentice attending to a patient. Oil painting by Jan Josef Horemans, 1722. Wellcome Collection.

For his apprenticeship, Colles fared better than many. His Master was the forward-thinking Philip Woodroffe (d. 1799, PRCSI 1788), Resident Surgeon at Dr Steevens' Hospital. Woodroffe had been a member of the Dublin Society of Surgeons; he is one of those named in RCSI's Charter, and was present at the first meeting in the Rotunda. In addition to his large private practice, he was also civic-minded: he was Surgeon to the Foundling Hospital, the Hospital for Incurables, and Consulting Surgeon to the House of Industry (later the Richmond Hospital). Under Woodroffe's guidance, Colles had little difficulty obtaining his Licence on 24 September 1795. He had already collected his BA degree from Trinity in April.

COLLES THE 'POSTGRAD': EDINBURGH AND LONDON

He left Dublin within days of his qualification, traveling north to Donaghadee, Co. Down, where he boarded a packet boat for Scotland. The sea turned rough and it took three days to reach Portpatrick. 'Such a tossing and such an escape no set of devils ever had,' he wrote home. 'You shall have a journal when I get

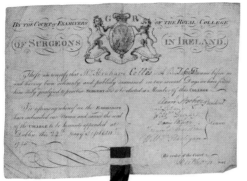

Abraham Colles' 'Letters Testimonial', or Licence, from RCSI (1795).

to Edinburgh.'[26] 'Auld Reekie' was the logical destination for an ambitious young medic. It was not just the capital of Scotland, but the capital of medicine in the English-speaking world. Much of this was owed to Alexander Monro *primus* (1697–1767) and Alexander Monro *secundus* (1733–1817), the former having introduced Boerhaavian clinical teaching at the purpose-built Royal Infirmary.[27]

Students came to the University of Edinburgh from all over Europe, but in Colles' time the Irish were the largest contingent (of the 800 graduates in the last quarter of the eighteenth century, 237 were Irish, 217 English, 179 Scottish and 167 'colonists and foreigners'[28]). This Hibernian brain-drain – or at least, *fee*-drain – was not lost on the newcomer; he noted that Irish students were collectively shelling out £20,000 per annum in Scotland. In time, he would do much to stanch this flow.

In contemporary terms, Colles had landed himself a place on the best possible postgraduate course available. His teachers were eminent: as well as Monro *secundus*, there was Benjamin Bell (1749–1806), author of the landmark six-volume *System of Surgery* (1783–88), and an Honorary Member of RCSI since 1784. Colles was especially fond of Bell, and would later make many references to him in his writings. Another important influence was John Bell (1763–1820; no relation to Benjamin – in fact the namesakes could not stand each other). This Bell was a pioneer of surgical anatomy, and in Colles' *Lectures on Surgery* (1811) the influence resonates loud and clear. (Incidentally, John Bell died in Rome, where he is buried in the Protestant Cemetery next to a young Englishman, a licenced apothecary who had trained as a surgeon – and who also wrote poems – John Keats.[29]) Colles' clinical lectures were in the Royal Infirmary and he also took a three-month course at the Edinburgh General Lying-In Hospital. He worked diligently – his landlady in Nicolson Street worried he was 'reading himself into a coffin' – and he steered clear of his compatriots' excesses ('all people make it a rule to fight and quarrel with their own countrymen rather than with any other'[30]).

In June 1797, Colles was awarded his doctorate. Both his thesis, entitled *De Venaesectione* ('On Bloodletting'), and his *viva voce* defence of it were in Latin (in later life Colles would recommend to his students that they 'refresh and extend your knowledge of the classics at your leisure hours'[31]). Phlebotomy might be prescribed today for conditions such as haemochromatosis, but even in Colles' time bloodletting was part of an old-guard orthodoxy – essentially, it was ancient humeral doctrine in action. Its efficacy – or, more to the point, its lack thereof – was hard to prove: if a patient recovered, it was interpreted as thanks to the treatment; if they unfortunately died, well, that was simply because they were beyond salvation already. Two years after Colles submitted his thesis, US President George Washington developed a sore throat after horse-riding in the rain. He might have gone to bed with a hot whiskey and lived to tell the tale;

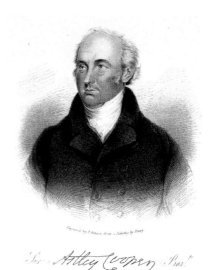

Portrait of Sir Astley Cooper. Wellcome Collection.

instead, his doctors bled him over two days and he died.

Colles next headed south, to London. Little is known of the six months he spent in the city, except that he 'walked the hospitals' and that he made the acquaintance of Astley Cooper (1768–1841), then on the cusp of becoming one of Britain's most celebrated anatomists. Five years Colles' senior, Cooper had married into money and so had little interest in tending to a practice; instead, having already studied with the great John Hunter, Cooper devoted himself to research, in particular a monumental two-volume study on hernias. It is likely that Colles assisted with dissections for that work, though he is not credited. Colles and Cooper corresponded frequently for the rest of their lives, and in 1820 Cooper was made an Honorary Member of RCSI.

RCSI AND THE 1798 REBELLION

The Ireland that Colles returned to in November 1797 was simmering towards insurrection, stirred by a group called the United Irishmen, who took their cues from American and French revolutionary ideals. There had already been a near-miss – from the authorities' point of view – the previous December, when a fleet of French warships slipped past the Royal Navy blockade and made for south-western Ireland. They came 'near enough to toss a biscuit ashore' at Bantry, but atrocious weather prevented them from landing and they sailed away again.[32] Counter-revolutionary measures swiftly followed, and as the noose tightened, RCSI's radical connections began to come to light.

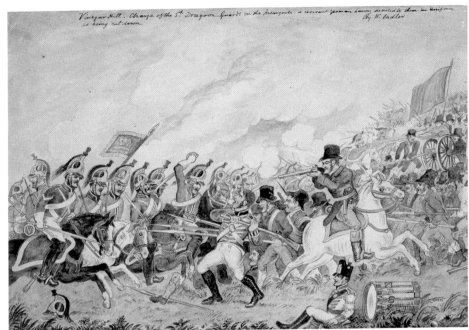

Insurrection in the summer of 1798. The text reads: 'Vinegar Hill, charge of the 5th Dragoon Guards on the insurgents - a recreant yeoman having deserted to them in uniform is being cut down. By W. Sadler.' Reproduced courtesy of the National Library of Ireland (PD 3176 TX 4).

In some respects, these were natural affinities: as the surgeons had liberated themselves from their former guild-mates, the United Irish Society looked to liberate Ireland from colonial rule. Moreover, the United Irishmen were avowedly non-sectarian, and so too was RCSI. In a country divided along confessional lines, RCSI's liberal stance was not just anomalous, but something of a wonder. As one early commentator put it:

> Their projects for the public good and for the advancement of the profession were not circumscribed by narrow tenets nor actuated by those selfish monopolising motives which so frequently influence the acts and proceedings of incorporated societies. Men of all persuasions were permitted, and the most lucrative and honourable situations were as open to the licentiates of every sect as to those of the Established Church.[33]

True, Protestants dominated the surgical field: according to *Wilson's Dublin Directory* (1780), there were sixty-six surgeons in the city of Dublin, of whom perhaps ten were Catholic (including PRCSI Dease).[34] Change came slowly, of course, and subtler social and financial barriers endured, but from the outset RCSI willingly embraced a policy that many other institutions would accept grudgingly only when it was thrust upon them.

In May 1798, two days before rebellion finally exploded, the bookseller Patrick Byrne – who had been instrumental in securing the Mercer Street lease, and who had published Hartigan and Lawless' *Syllabus* – was

Historic salute to Napoleon's famous Irish surgeon

* Lt. Gen. G. McMahon, Chief of Staff, Irish Defence Forces, Prof. T.P. Hennessy, President RSCI, General Amgrall, Director, Medical Corps, French Army

Lawless tomb is restored in Paris

Restoration of William Lawless' resting-place and reputation, *Surgeons' Fleam* (1996).

arrested and his Grafton Street shop ransacked (an eyewitness recalled: 'it was a pitiful sight to behold the amount of property in beautifully bound books ruthlessly torn to pieces and tossed out of the windows into the street'[35]). Byrne was imprisoned for two years without trial, fleeing to Philadelphia upon his release.

The summer's violence resulted in some 30,000 deaths, making it probably the most concentrated period of bloodshed in Irish history. In June, the rebel aristocrat Lord Edward Fitzgerald was captured; in his final illness he was attended to by John Armstrong Garnett (1767–1831, Lic. 1798, MRCSI 1800, Prof of Surgical Pharmacy 1803–13, PRCSI 1810). Garnett left a long memoir of his treatment of Fitzgerald that ends: 'Two o'clock. – After a violent struggle, that commenced at a little after twelve o'clock, this ill-fated young man has just drawn his last breath.'[36]

In the rebellion's aftermath, the authorities rooted out surviving rebels and sympathisers. As ever, there were tip-offs, and one of those who fled was RCSI's Professor of Anatomy and Physiology (1794–98), William Lawless (*c.*1764–1824, Lic. 1788, MRCSI 1790). This was a major embarrassment to the College: intellectual affinity was one thing, but supporting armed insurrection against the very forces who provided your bread and butter was quite another. The College Minutes record the moves against Lawless:

> November 4, 1798. Whereas it appears by an Act of the last Session of Parliament that William Lawless, Esq., one of the Members of this College, has been notoriously engaged in the late Rebellion, and hath fled from Justice, and that unless he shall surrender himself to one of the Judges of His Majesty's Court of King's Bench, or to some Justice of the Peace within this Kingdom on or before the first day of December

next in order to abide such Charges as shall be made against him he shall stand attainted of High Treason. Resolved – that the name of the said William Lawless be omitted in the printed lists of the College.

The December deadline came and went:

January 7, 1799. Resolved that notice be given in the Summons that the College will on their next Quarterly Meeting take into consideration the conduct of William Lawless Esquire one of the Members.

Such 'consideration' ultimately meant the following:

February 4, 1799. Whereas William Lawless, Esq., one of the Members of this College, hath not surrendered himself to take his Trial for such Charges as should be made against him pursuant to the Act of the last Session of Parliament – Resolved that the said William Lawless be, and he is hereby expelled.[37]

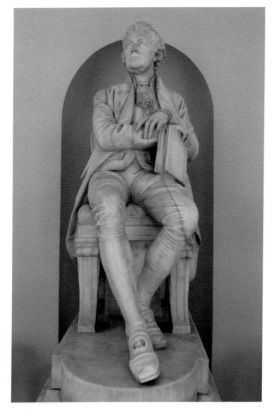

William Dease by Thomas Farrell (1886) in the Entrance Hall.

In fact, Lawless escaped to Paris, where he was appointed captain of Napoleon's Irish Legion. He served at Vlissingen and Dresden (where he lost a leg) and was decorated with the Legion of Honour, France's highest order of merit. He died in 1824 and is buried in Père Lachaise Cemetery, where, over the next 172 years, his gravestone fell into disrepair. The time elapsed gave RCSI a new perspective on its rebellious professor, and on 16 February 1996, a delegation led by PRCSI Tom Hennessy re-dedicated Lawless' restored tomb. In addition, Lawless was re-instated as a Fellow – *antea* Member – of RCSI.[38]

Lastly, Dease was also implicated, not least by the mystery that surrounds his sudden death on 21 January 1798. The nineteenth-century historian (and doctor) R.R. Madden suggested that Dease received advance word of his imminent arrest as a suspected United Irishman from the Surgeon-General to the forces, George Stewart (1752–1813, PRCSI 1792, 1799). 'He went home from the College, where the intelligence was given to him,' Madden wrote, 'opened his femoral artery and died of haemorrhage.' An entirely different story has it that a colleague misdiagnosed a suppurated aneurysm as an abscess, which Dease subsequently opened, causing the patient's death; in a fit of remorse, he supposedly took his own life.

In either case, there was never any inquest, suggesting that Dease's death was owed to natural causes.[39] The truth may never be known, but it certainly spared the College's blushes not to have to expel one of its leading lights. Rather, as the years rolled by, they were able to celebrate the man. In 1812, they commissioned a bust of Dease, sculpted by Edward Smyth, and in 1886 a full-size seated statue by Thomas Farrell was unveiled in the College Entrance Hall. For whatever reason, this statue subsequently developed a crack along the subject's left thigh – exactly, it turns out, along the line of the femoral artery.

TOOLS OF THE TRADE

Westminster's reaction to the insurrection was the Act of Union (1800), which at a stroke converted Dublin into the ghost of a capital. Most narrative histories of Ireland posit the half century that followed as a time of terminal decline, reaching a nadir with the horror of the Great Famine.

But there is another story, too. The same period was a golden age in Irish medicine, later characterised as 'the Dublin School'. The leading lights of the movement were the physicians Robert Graves (1796–1853) and William Stokes (1804–1878). As Stokes put it, looking back:

> It is admitted on all hands that during the last half century a great School of Practical Medicine, Surgery, and Midwifery, has in Dublin grown to such dimensions, and established such a character, as to constitute at least one source of legitimate national pride, so much wanting in Ireland; a possession which to any country is more to be valued than wealth or power, or the barbarous triumphs of war.[40]

The Irish 'bedside' ethos was followed both in Britain and in the US: indeed, William Osler's overhaul of twentieth-century medicinal teaching at the Johns

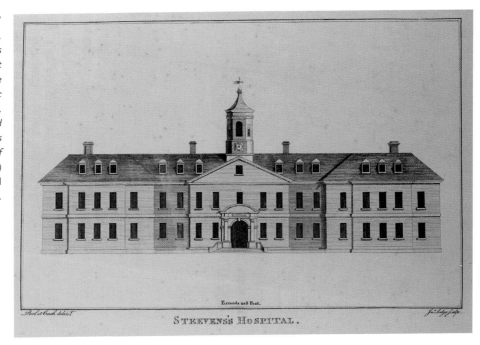

STEEVENS'S HOSPITAL.

Hopkins Hospital in Baltimore arguably has its roots in the 'Dublin School'.

Colles was the surgical counterpart of Graves and Stokes, completing a sort of triumvirate. The eldest of the three, his career took off following the death of his former master, Woodroffe. Within a month, Colles was appointed resident surgeon at Dr Steevens' Hospital, for which he earned £55 a year, plus '£5 per annum in lieu of furniture'. In November he was elected a Member of RCSI, meaning he could now take on apprentices. These represented sea changes in his fortunes; previously he had eked out a precarious living ('feeless' ran one plaintive entry in his monthly records).

One of Colles' first tasks in his new post was to compile a list of all the surgical instruments belonging to the hospital. This *armamentarium chirurgicum* includes cases of amputating instruments, sets of dissecting knives, sets of 'scarifying and cupping instruments', the paraphernalia of lithotomy — staffs, sounds, gorgets, double-edged scalpels, forceps, scoops — male and female catheters, harelip pins and tobacco bellows with tubes attached. This last item was used to treat dislocations and hernias: a rectal injection of tobacco smoke caused the patient to faint, thereby allowing the affected muscles to relax. Alas, this caused 'many uncalled-for and even disastrous result', so Colles abandoned its use, favouring instead a tobacco enema.[41]

As noted earlier, such instruments set surgeons apart from their physician colleagues. In many cases, pioneers were obliged to commission cutlers to make up their bespoke instruments. Croker-King, for example, experimented with a blended form of the trepan (which bored a hole in the cranium) and the trephine (which cut a small disc of bone). In his accompanying *Description of an Instrument for Performing the Operation of Trepanning the Skull, with More Ease, Safety and Expedition, than those in General Use* (1794), he observed that while the trepan was fast, it was prone to slippage ('the

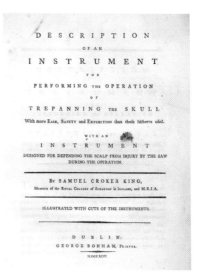

Title-page and illustration (below) from Croker-King's guide to trepanning and trephining.

difficulty of keeping a patient quiet... is known to every operator'). The trephine, on the other hand, required less pressure but was slower ('not only fatiguing to the operator, but tiresome to the patient').

Dease, likewise, attempted to improve on the lithotome and became an expert in its use. 'Even at the dinner table,' Colles recalled, 'while speaking to someone, he might often be detected moving his knife and fork as if pushing the scalpel and staff on together without thinking of what he was doing...'[42] Whether bespoke or not, such instruments were costly and one did not want to lose them – a point illustrated by a story concerning Ralph Smith Obré (d. 1820, PRCSI 1790) and Solomon Richards.

One night, these two close friends were in a carriage together when they were held up by a highwayman. Richards, a famously corpulent gourmand, duly handed over his money, his watch and his case of surgical instruments, but Obré – 'of very small stature'[43] – remained hidden behind his friend. The robber was set to ride away until Richards drew attention to the oversight. Obré was then obliged to hand over his valuables, at which point Richards asked if he might get his watch and surgical instruments back, seeing as he had been so helpful. The thief, apparently, agreed.[44]

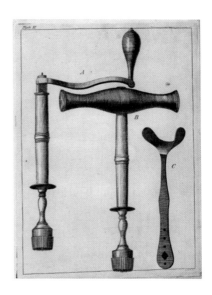

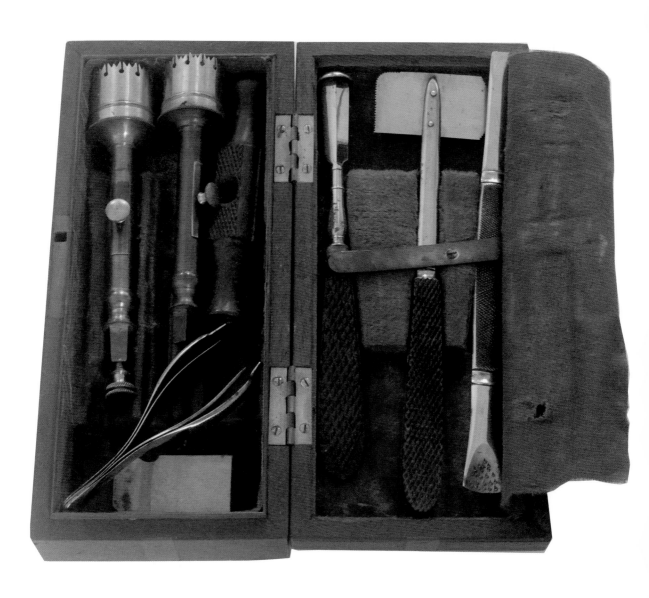

COLLES' APPOINTMENTS

After his election to Membership, Colles rocketed through the ranks at RCSI: he was elected an assistant in 1800, a censor in 1801, and then, in January 1802, in recognition of his evidently outstanding abilities, President of the College. He was just 29 years old.

Curiously, being elected President did not prevent Colles from the temptation to jump ship to his other alma mater. When the Chair of Anatomy opened up in Trinity, Colles competed for the post against his cat-loving former teacher, William Hartigan. The elder man won, whereupon Colles lodged a legal challenge on the grounds that Hartigan was unqualified (his MD had been granted *honoris causa*, as opposed to Colles' shiny Edinburgh imprimatur).

Happily for RCSI, the challenge failed, and it has been suggested that this disappointment led Colles to redouble his energies where he was. In 1804 he was appointed to two chairs at once: Anatomy and Physiology, which he held for the next quarter of a century; and Surgery, which he occupied even longer, until his retirement in 1836.[45] (Meanwhile, at Trinity, Hartigan steered the sleepy School of Physic further into the doldrums; after his death, his widow pointed to RCSI's success as the source of her straitened finances: 'The exertions of the College of Surgeons to draw all the pupils they could to their school... reduce our income very much.'[46])

Under Colles' stewardship, student numbers at RCSI begin to speak for themselves: in 1804 there were about 100; soon after, as his reputation as a teacher spread, that figure rose steadily. *The Lancet*'s scabrous Dublin correspondent, the pseudonymous 'Erinensis', painted this pen-portrait of Colles in full flight:

> ... the bell rings – Mr. C's carriage is at the gate – the benches fill – confusion in all its fantastic forms of juvenile levity prevails throughout the scene. The whole artillery of confectionery, from *canister* lozenges to the heavy grape-shot of spice nuts, is flying on all sides... the folding doors open – and in hurries Mr. C – with a slip of paper, twisted round his index finger – a simultaneous burst of applause greets his welcome entry, but modestly declining the honour intended him, he instantly proceeds, without even returning the salute, 'Gentlemen, at our last meeting'. &c. &c. (...) Short as our digression has been, Mr. Colles has already described the symptoms, and detailed the treatment of, perhaps, five or six different forms of disease, and having unloaded his memory of a variety of information,

Facing page: Boxed trepanation kit.

he has laconically consigned the hopeless cases to the grave. In his dogmatic effusion, books, authors and authorities are all run over, to arrive at one arbitrary and everlasting conclusion, 'the truth is, gentlemen, those men knew nothing of the matter!' (...) he is still the laborious, shrewd, observing, matter-of-fact and practical surgeon... in advice, from long experience and a peculiar tact of discovering the hidden causes of disease, he has scarcely a rival.[47]

A ROMAN TEMPLE ON THE GREEN

If Colles was responsible for attracting students to RCSI, some credit must also go to Napoleon Bonaparte, whose accession to power stirred his enemies into a fever of military spending. In the year in which Colles was appointed to his teaching chairs, there was widespread speculation that French troops would once again attempt to land in Ireland. Within weeks of Napoleon's coronation as Emperor of the French (2 December 1804), RCSI found itself in receipt of a government grant of £6,000 — a vast sum compared to that year's ordinary annual revenue of £251 6s.

Having outgrown the Mercer Street premises, RCSI was now in the financial position to establish for itself a new, permanent home. It was George Renny who

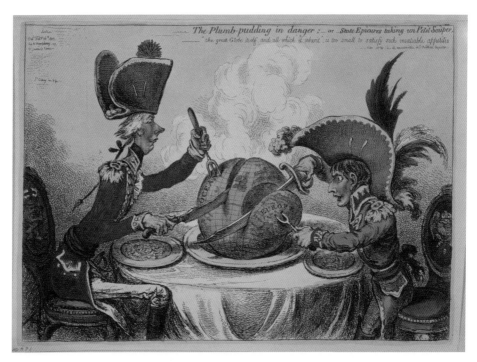

The Plumb-pudding in danger (1805) by James Gillray, depicting William Pitt the Younger and Napoleon Bonaparte carving up the globe. © Creative Commons.

ascertained that further funds for building would follow, and so in July 1805, RCSI entered into an agreement with the Society of Friends – also known as the Quakers – to purchase a plot of land on the corner of York Street and St Stephen's Green West. This was a desirable location: York Street was well-to-do, with many medical connections,[48] while this side of the Green was originally known as Frenchman's Walk, owing to the number of Huguenot refugees who settled in the vicinity in the seventeenth century. They gave Gallic names to some of the surrounding streets (such as the aforementioned Digges – or *Digue*'s – Lane), and they also left a small graveyard – still extant – off the Green's north-east corner.

The Quakers, too, had a graveyard on their York Street plot, which gave rise to a proviso in the RCSI purchase. The deed of conveyance included the restriction that the purchaser, 'under the penalty of Two thousand pounds Sterling... shall not nor will not at any time during the space of one hundred years from the date hereof raise or dig up for any purpose whatsoever' a part of the site fifty-six feet wide and one hundred feet long, situated eighty-three feet back from the St Stephen's Green end.[49] RCSI accepted these terms, and by 12 December 1805, the sum of 4,000 guineas was paid to the Quakers.[50]

RCSI had its architect working even before the plot of land was secured. This was a man called Edward Parke, who some have described as a 'puzzling' choice: he was considered competent rather than 'of the first rank', and one detects again the hand of Renny and his connections.[51] Based on Parke's plans, RCSI petitioned the government for £15,467 10*s* 7*d* for 'a Hall, Theatre and Dissecting rooms for the use of this College'. The foundation stone of the new building was laid 'with great ceremony' by the Lord Lieutenant on St Patrick's Day, 1806.[52] Such official endorsement was vital, and no doubt carefully shepherded at every stage by Renny. Construction commenced about June 1806, continuing until March 1810, during which time no one thanked Napoleon for his 'Continental Blockade' that drove up the cost of materials. Within these four years, RCSI would receive close to £30,000 directly from the Exchequer.[53]

What Parke produced was an unqualified success, a rendering in stone of his client's loftiest

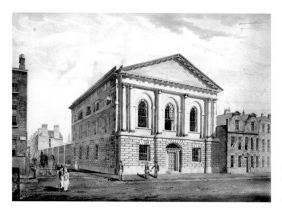

RCSI in 1810. Watercolour. Artist unknown.

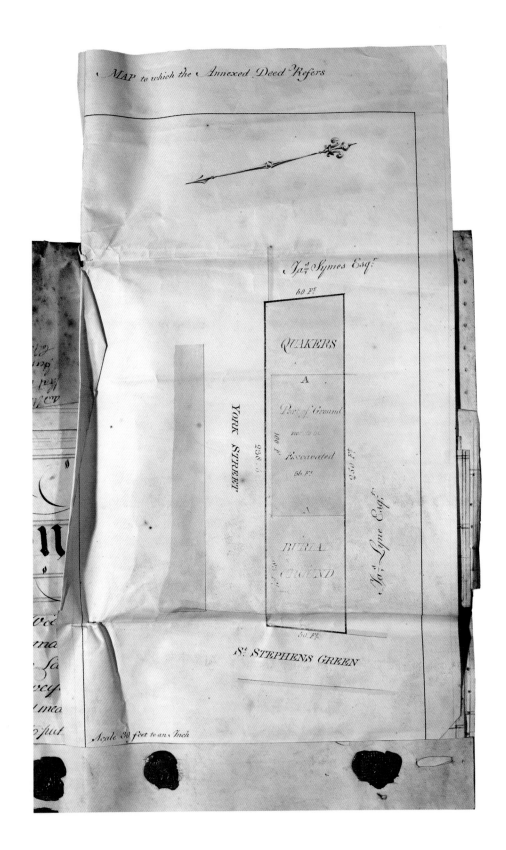

MAP to which the Annexed Deed Refers

Jas. Symes Esqr.
60 Ft.

QUAKERS

A

Port of Ground
now to be
Excavated
56 Ft.

A

BURIAL
GROUND

60 Ft.

YORK STREET

230 6

25d Ft.

Jas. Lyne Esqr.

St. STEPHENS GREEN

Scale 30 feet to an Inch

professional aspirations, obliterating from memory the days of playing second fiddle to barbers. In architectural terms, Parke's design is firmly Neoclassical — essentially, a Roman temple atop a Wicklow granite podium. As the sun rises over the canopy of the Green, light streams into the double-height, barrel-vaulted Board Room via a trio of tall round-headed windows. Remarkably, this elegant and airy room remains essentially unchanged to this day. Also largely unchanged from Parke's design is the cantilevered main staircase and the floral and ox-skull frieze in the former Entrance Hall (now the Robert Smith Room). Even *The Lancet*'s 'Erinensis' — who liked to find fault with everyone and everything — was unexpectedly impressed: 'Solid and substantial... it stands, the pride of Irish surgery and the terror of many a candidate whose fate depends on its decrees.'[54] Inside, he admired the giraffe skeleton (as he put it, 'of gigantic dimensions, a cameleopard'[55]) rising up in the main stairwell.

In contrast to the façade, the York Street elevation was conspicuously plain, albeit relieved somewhat by the upper lunette windows that alternate between semi-circular architraves and rectangular recessions. The windows below this line are blocked to protect the College 'museum' — that is, a collection of animal and human anatomical specimens for teaching and research (and very much not, as the name might imply, a cabinet of curios). An expanding library was located directly underneath the museum.

Facing page: Site-plan showing Quaker burial-ground, from a deed of conveyance to RCSI (1805).

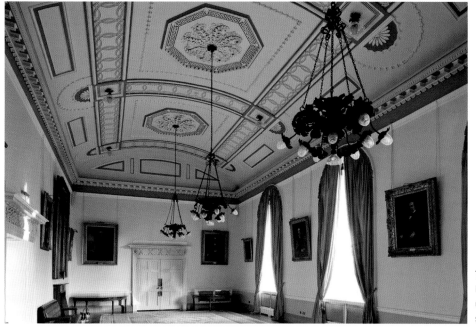

The Board Room, largely unchanged since 1810.

A watercolour (see p. 47) from 1810 shows a brick wall extending along York Street. Missing from this image is a break in the wall: the entrance to the School, whose various buildings (a theatre, a dissecting room, another small museum, possibly a stable and coach-house too) were scattered over this area. But what of the terms of the contract with the Quakers? It is perhaps a matter of interpretation, but it seems that RCSI violated this agreement almost immediately.[56] In any case, the magnanimous Quakers never demanded their £2,000. In addition, in 1809, RCSI purchased more ground to the north, pushing their boundary wall as far as Glover's Alley (the specific reason for this will be discussed in the next chapter).

Soon after the new building opened, the College Minutes record the resolution that:

> the grateful thanks of the College be given to our worthy member, George Renny, Esq., for his uniform and zealous exertions for the honour and advancement of Surgery, and for his able and successful applications to Government, by which our applications to Parliament always met with the desired success whereby we have been able to erect our new hall, etc.[57]

In addition, by way of a 'Testimony of the High Respect we entertain for him', Renny was invited to sit – or rather, to stand – for a full-length portrait that hangs to this day in the Board Room. Under his right hand is an architectural drawing of the three-bay building he had done so much to bring into being. (For a time, this portrait was known to staff and students as being of 'George Penny', as some practical joker had scraped off the leg of the 'R'. Wrong as this was, the fiscal implications were not entirely inappropriate.) From 1812, RCSI was financially self-sufficient, thanks to the steady stream of students and candidates for the Licence. This was just as well: once Napoleon met his Waterloo in 1815, RCSI's golden age of government hand-outs was gone for good.

SHOOTING DEAD MEN

While war with France allowed RCSI to flourish, it did the same for RCSI's competitors. Going back to the barber-surgeon days, there had always been professional anatomists who gave instruction to pupils other than their own apprentices. These small-time operators now set themselves up as 'schools', preparing their pupils to sit for the RCSI licence. In some instances, these competing schools were run by RCSI personnel. For example, Sir Philip Crampton

Facing page:
Portrait of
George Renny
by William
Cuming (1810).
Oil on canvas.

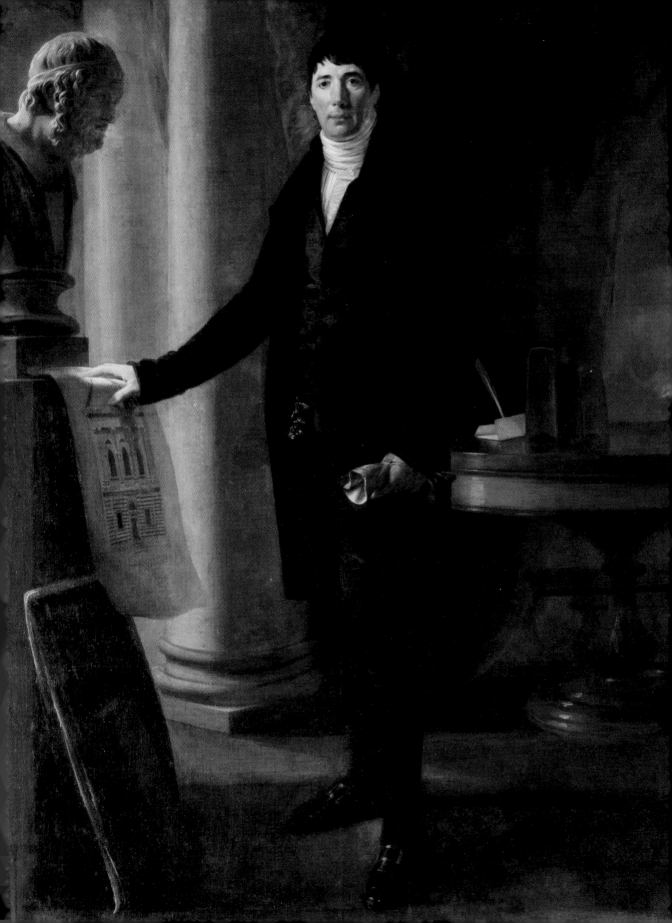

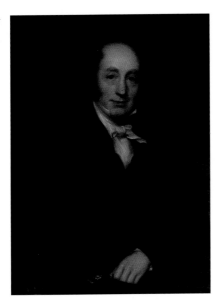

Portrait of
Abraham Colles
by Martin
Cregan (1838).
Oil on canvas.

(1777–1858, Lic. 1798, MRCSI 1801, PRCSI 1811, 1820, 1844–45, 1855–56) continued to run his private school in Dawson Street during his first tenure as RCSI President. Samuel Wilmot (1772–1848, Lic. 1801, MRCSI 1804, Prof of Surgery 1826–36, Prof of Anatomy and Physiology 1826–27, PRCSI 1815, 1832) and Richard Dease (*c.*1774–1819, Lic. 1795, MRCSI 1795, Prof of Anatomy and Physiology 1798–1819, Prof of Surgery 1799–1819, PRCSI 1809; son of the late William) both taught at the Jervis Street Hospital School.

Some of these schools came and went quickly; others lasted many decades, establishing themselves as serious rivals. In the latter category was John Timothy Kirby's School, first located at the rear of a laundry in Stephen Street (Kirby's many foes rejoiced in the sign out front saying, 'Mangling Done Here'); later he moved to Peter Street, where he flourished ('This aroused envy,' he wrote[58]) until RCSI decided that if they couldn't beat him, then he could join them: he was appointed to a professorship in 1832 and Peter Street closed. Many colourful traits attach to Kirby (1781–1853, Lic. 1805, MRCSI 1808, Prof of Medicine 1832–36, PRCSI 1823) – he was dandyish in his attire and drove a flashy carriage – but one in particular stands out, as recollected by 'Erinensis':

> For the purpose of demonstrating the destructive effects of fire-arms upon the human frame, Bully's Acre [a graveyard] gave up its cleverest treasures for the performance of the experiment. The subjects being placed with military precision along the wall, the Lecturer [i.e. Kirby] entered with his pistol in his hand, and levelling the mortiferous weapon at the enemy, magnanimously discharged several rounds, each followed by repeated bursts of applause. As soon as the smoke and approbation subsided, then came the tug of war. The wounded were examined, arteries were taken up, bullets extracted, bones were set, and every spectator fancied himself on the field of battle, and looked upon Mr. Kirby as a prodigy of genius and valour for shooting dead men.[59]

A TREATISE ON SURGICAL ANATOMY (1811)

In spite of all such rivals, RCSI saw its student numbers nearly quadruple inside a decade, from 55 at the turn of the century, to 162, 185 and 204 in the years 1809, 1810 and 1811, respectively.[60] 'Erinensis' again cast his jaundiced eye over such hopefuls:

> … when we had the honour of addressing you last, we supposed you were seated beside us on one of the benches of the great theatre of Anatomy at the Royal College of Surgeons in Ireland, surrounded by one of the largest classes that has been at this Institution since the peace, in all perhaps about two hundred, a hundred and fifty of whom have dissected, or intend to dissect, this season. We also told you, that they were very noisy and ill-behaved. More than three parts of them are apprenticed to surgeons, and being neglected by their masters, and suffered to do as they please by the College, many of them must, of course, be guiltless of any knowledge of the profession! The conduct of youth thus left to themselves, without any restraint to check their levity, cannot be expected to be decorous or attentive. Their mere appearance is our present concern, and as they sit in the panorama before us, they do not much accord with the notions which might be formed of a body of medical students. The same number of young men taken from the various counting-houses or haberdashers' shops through town, would present as much of the elements of genius, as much of the deep traces of thought, and as much of everything else which gives a studious character to the countenance, as this blue-frocked, black-stocked, Wellington-booted assemblage of medical dandies. Gold-rings, broad and bright, glitter here and there among the artful labours of the friseur, as the hand supports the head, thrown into the attitude of mental abstraction; steel-guard chains, often without watches

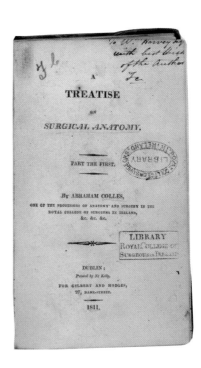

A Treatise on Surgical Anatomy (1811).

View of the Principal Arteries & Veins.

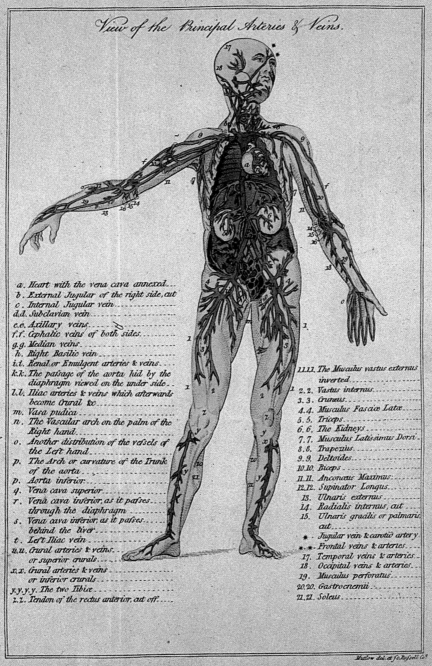

a. Heart with the vena cava annexed.
b. External Jugular of the right side, cut
c. Internal Jugular vein
d.d. Subclavian vein
e.e. Axillary veins
f.f. Cephalic veins of both sides.
g.g. Median veins
h. Right Basilic vein
i.i. Renal or Emulgent arteries & veins.
k.k. The passage of the aorta hid by the diaphragm viewed on the under side.
l.l. Iliac arteries & veins which afterwards become Crural &c
m. Vasa pudica
n. The Vascular arch on the palm of the Right hand.
o. Another distribution of the vessels of the Left hand.
p. The Arch or curvature of the Trunk of the aorta.
p. Aorta inferior.
q. Vena cava superior.
r. Vena cava inferior, as it passes through the diaphragm
s. Vena cava inferior, as it passes behind the liver
t. Left Iliac vein
u.u. Crural arteries & veins. or superior crurals.
x.x. Crural arteries & veins or inferior crurals.
y.y.y.y. The two Tibiæ
z.z. Tendon of the rectus anterior, cut off

11.11. The Musculus vastus externus inverted
2.2. Vastus internus.
3.3. Gruneus.
4.4. Musculus Fasciæ Latæ.
5.5. Triceps.
6.6. The Kidneys.
7.7. Musculus Latissimus Dorsi.
8.8. Trapezius.
9.9. Deltoides.
10.10. Biceps.
11.11. Anconeus Maximus.
12.12. Supinator Longus.
13. Ulnaris externus.
14. Radialis internus, cut
15. Ulnaris gracilis or palmaris, cut.
*. Jugular vein & carotid artery
. Frontal veins & arteries.
17. Temporal veins & arteries.
18. Occipital veins & arteries.
19. Musculus perforatus.
20.20. Gastrocnemii.
21.21. Soleus.

Mutlow del. et sc. Russell Co.

Published by G. Kearsley, Fleet Street, May 1st 1809.

to protect, sparkle almost in every breast, and quizzing-glasses hang gracefully pendant from every neck; in short, the whole paraphernalia of puppyism are displayed here in the greatest possible profusion.[61]

Colles himself was more sympathetic; indeed, much of his success as a teacher was owed to his ability to imagine – or remember – his subject from the far side of the lectern. In 1811 he published a short volume entitled *A Treatise on Surgical Anatomy*, which opens with these words: 'The author of the following work had observed with regret, the slow progress, which, even the most assiduous of the Pupils of the College of Surgeons, generally made in the acquirement of anatomical knowledge.' Whereas any number of professors would assume the students simply needed to apply themselves harder, Colles had a different interpretation: 'A close consideration of the matter led him to apprehend, that this originated from some material defects in the established mode of teaching this science.'[62] Or, to give this statement its full impact, Colles was suggesting that the teaching of anatomy had been fundamentally misconceived since the time of Vesalius.

It is never easy to innovate, especially when others are invested in an earlier way of thinking. When Vesalius pointed out errors in Galen, his teachers told him that the human body must have changed since Galen's time.[63] Undeterred, Vesalius pioneered what became known as *systemic* anatomy: in one limb the entire musculature would be dissected and displayed, in another it would be the nerves or blood vessels, and so on. The result could seem quite perfect and complete, and Renaissance textbooks often feature astonishingly beautiful plates illustrating the entire muscular, vascular or nervous systems, all neatly separated. For several hundred years, anatomy students followed suit; as a student himself, Colles would have dissected one system at a time: the arteries this week, the veins the next... But as a working surgeon – and now teacher – Colles found the method manifestly deficient:

Thus the student who has been shown the distribution of the venous, arterial, and nervous systems of the arm, does not know how each of them lies with respect to the other, at the bend of the elbow, and therefore he knows not how he should attempt, in cases of aneurism, to pass a ligature round the artery, without at the same time including its accompanying nerve, which communicates sensation to the principal part of the limb. Nor can he, in the common operation of bloodletting, account for that sharp pain of which the patient

Facing page: An écorché: seen from the front, with left arm extending to the side, showing the principal veins and arteries. Coloured line engraving by H. Mutlow, 1808. Wellcome Collection.

particularly complains, when the basilic vein is opened, because these detached descriptions of the different systems did not lead him to observe, that some considerable branches of the nerves run down along the face of the vein...[64]

One might as well, he says, take apart a watch and describe each cog and spring in detail, but never say a word about how they work together. Little wonder, then, that the poor student should find the study of anatomy 'so difficult to acquire, and almost as difficult to retain'.[65] What Colles advocates instead is a *regional* or *topographical* approach – that is, the study of how the various systems function relative to one another in any given part of the body. The *Treatise* is laid out according to this new principle: there are sections on the abdomen, the thorax, the pelvis, the neck and throat, and so on. Page by page, Colles focuses on the practical implications – 'the connexion between the anatomical structure of each part, and the surgical diseases and operations to which it is subject'.[66] Any student who learns in this manner, he predicts, will have 'a lively interest excited in his mind... and must have fixed in his memory an indelible impression of the structure of the parts'.[67]

In passing, Colles makes observations that would become eponyms in themselves – Colles' fascia and Colles' ligament. He also gives the first recorded account of the spread of mammary cancer to adjoining lymph glands. Slim as the volume is – it was meant to be the first instalment of a larger work, though no sequel followed – it had an immense influence, initially as part of the celebrated 'Dublin School', subsequently in the wider medical world. Regional, as opposed to systemic, anatomy became the new orthodoxy. Along the way, however, Colles' pioneering role was often forgotten. In some respects, he was a victim of his own success: so completely had he transformed his subject, the world came to believe it was always ever thus.[68] In any case, Colles did not need posterity to confirm the superiority of his method. In the *Treatise*, he

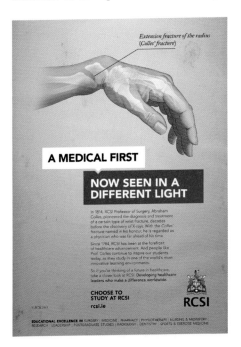

Illustration of a Colles fracture from a student recruitment campaign, 2015.

Extension fracture of the radius (Colles' fracture)

A MEDICAL FIRST

NOW SEEN IN A DIFFERENT LIGHT

In 1814, RCSI Professor of Surgery, Abraham Colles, pioneered the diagnosis and treatment of a certain type of wrist fracture, decades before the discovery of X-rays. With the Colles' fracture named in his honour, he is regarded as a physician who was far ahead of his time.

Since 1784, RCSI has been at the forefront of healthcare advancement. And people like Prof. Colles continue to inspire our students today, as they study in one of the world's most innovative learning environments.

So if you're thinking of a future in healthcare, take a closer look at RCSI. Developing healthcare leaders who make a difference worldwide.

CHOOSE TO STUDY AT RCSI
rcsi.ie

RCSI

EDUCATIONAL EXCELLENCE IN SURGERY · MEDICINE · PHARMACY · PHYSIOTHERAPY · NURSING & MIDWIFERY · RESEARCH · LEADERSHIP · POSTGRADUATE STUDIES · RADIOLOGY · DENTISTRY · SPORTS & EXERCISE MEDICINE proudly notes the 'rapid advances in useful knowledge, made by the Pupils, since the adoption of such a plan'.[69]

THE COLLES FRACTURE

In 1814, Colles published an article in the *Edinburgh Medical and Surgical Journal* entitled 'On the fracture of the carpal extremity of the radius'. Accident and emergency departments the world over know the description therein as a Colles fracture. The cause is a fall on an out-stretched hand, and its fame is owed to its prevalence, affecting both young adult and

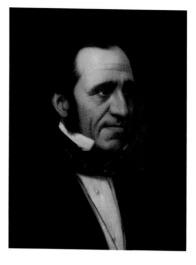

Portrait of Robert W. Smith by John Chancellor. Photograph finished in oils, 1874.

older populations (thanks, respectively, to high- and low-energy falls, or ski-slopes and slips). Nowadays, diagnosis is by X-ray; in Colles' time it depended on external observation of the characteristic 'dinner-fork' deformity.

Colles' classic description might have been lost to posterity had it not been for Trinity College's first Professor of Surgery, Robert William Smith (1807–1873, Lic. 1832, FRCSI 1844, Vice PRCSI 1873), who drew attention to his predecessor's work in 1847: 'It is certainly very extraordinary that... not a single British or foreign author who has written since has made the slightest reference to Mr. Colles' name in connection with the subject, even when almost quoting his words.'[70] Ever since, the names of Colles and Smith have been handed down together: a 'reversed' Colles fracture – the result of force applied to the back of the wrist – is known as Smith's fracture.

JOHN CHEYNE, RCSI'S FIRST PROFESSOR OF MEDICINE

Born in Leith, Scotland, John Cheyne (1777–1836, first Prof of Medicine 1813–19) – or 'big John Cheyne' as he was known, owing to his height – first came to Ireland as a 21-year-old surgeon attached to the army tasked with suppressing the 1798 rebellion. After seeing action at Vinegar Hill, military life bored him ('my time was spent in shooting, playing billiards, reading such books as the circulating library supplied, and in complete dissipation'[71]). He returned to Scotland to help with his father's medical practice – he had earned his own medical degree in 1795 – and there he developed the ambition to 'establish myself as a physician in a large city'.[72] He worked diligently and published three books in quick succession, but medicine in Scotland was full of internecine rifts and biases, and Cheyne could not make progress.

Robert Smith manipulating a dislocated shoulder. Artist unknown.

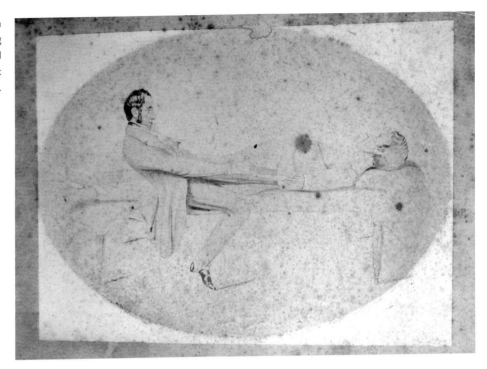

Recalibrating, he applied to the Army Medical School at Woolwich, but did not even receive an answer. Then, while on an information-gathering visit to Dublin in 1809, he found that he liked what he saw: 'the field was extensive,' he wrote, 'and the labourers liberally rewarded'.[73] After a slow start, in 1811 Cheyne was appointed physician to the Meath Hospital, then located in the Coombe. The place was, he said, 'small, mean, and gloomy',[74] but at least in this smaller pond, he was at last the big physician.

Meanwhile, over on St Stephen's Green, RCSI received a very important letter from the Army Medical Board on 23 April 1813. Thus far, RCSI diplomas provided proof of *surgical* ability, but now the Board wanted to raise the bar: henceforth, they would require evidence of *medical* education too. RCSI's response was immediate: on 3 May the College authorities met to consider the idea of 'a professorship of the practice of physic', and on 27 May it was resolved that:

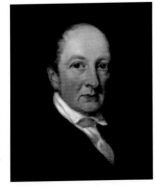

Portrait of John Cheyne. Artist unknown. Courtesy of RCPI.

… in order to facilitate the Education of Surgeons and Assistt. Surgeons for the Army and Navy, it is highly expedient that a professorship of the practice of physick be annexed to the School of Surgery in the College, and that no person shall be deemed eligible to such professorship who is not a regularly educated and practising physician.[75]

Days later, advertisements for the position were placed in Dublin newspapers. For whatever reason, there was only one applicant, and so the College minutes for 15 June 1813 record:

That Doctor Cheyne… is hereby appointed Professor of the Theory and practice of Physic, in the School of Surgery under the direction of the Royal College of Surgeons in Ireland for one year from the 14th day of September next.[76]

The importance of this development should not be underestimated. It signifies that, to the Army at least, the centuries-old division between medicine and surgery was outdated, possibly even dangerous; anyone they were sending to battle needed to be competent in both fields. For RCSI, it represents a giant leap from O'Halloran's purely surgical vision. By name it remained a 'College of Surgeons', and its regulatory role was unaffected, but as a teaching institution its remit had suddenly widened: henceforth, RCSI was home to surgery *and* medicine.

THE HOUSE OF INDUSTRY HOSPITALS AND THE *DUBLIN HOSPITAL REPORTS*

Towards the end of his tenure at RCSI, Cheyne was appointed physician to the House of Industry Hospitals. (This was the collective name for the Hardwicke, Richmond and Whitworth Hospitals; later it would become St Laurence's Hospital, and when it closed in 1987, its staff, along with the staff of the Charitable Infirmary, Jervis Street, transferred *en masse* to Beaumont Hospital.) At the Hardwicke Fever Hospital, Cheyne set about re-organising the nursing service (his instructions have been described as 'of prime importance in the history of nursing'[77]). He also noted that, in the miserable summer of 1817, when a typhus epidemic gripped Dublin, nurses were amongst the first healthcare workers to get sick, particularly

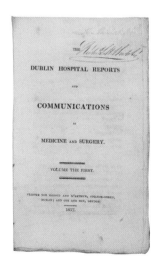

Dublin Hospital Reports, Vol. 1.

'unseasoned nurses', who undressed patients as they were admitted. It was not known at the time that typhus was louse-borne. Over a two-year period, perhaps one and a half million people were infected nationwide, while some 65,000 people are thought to have died.

Cheyne left a vivid account of the epidemic in a new publication he started with Colles and others, the *Dublin Hospital Reports* (1817–30). He noted symptoms as they developed: first a period of dejection, followed by headache, loss of appetite and constipation, then severe muscular pains and delirium as the fever presented: 'We had many patients who created a great disturbance by wandering about the wards all night, prying into closets, and looking under the beds... One man, by trade a cooper, endeavoured to pull his bed to pieces, in order to make a tub of the spars...'

The *Dublin Hospital Reports* filled a gap in medical publishing in Ireland; previously, Irish authors were obliged to send their work to Edinburgh. As well as being the most energetic of editors, Cheyne was also a prolific author, contributing ten articles to the first five volumes. In 1820 Cheyne was appointed Physician-General to the Army, which, he proudly noted, was 'the highest medical rank in Ireland'.[78] In general, however, he was not happy; increasingly prone to bouts of 'nervous fever', he retired to England in 1831 and five years later he breathed his last.

'CHEYNE-STOKES BREATHING'

For the second volume of the *Dublin Hospital Reports* (1818), Cheyne wrote an article entitled 'A Case of Apoplexy in which the Fleshy Part of the Heart was Converted into Fat'. In it he described the phenomenon of rising and falling respiration in a dying man: 'For several days his breathing was irregular; it would utterly cease for a quarter of a minute, then it would become perceptible, though very low, then by degrees it became heavy and quick, and then it would cease again.'

Cheyne's paper was later recalled by the aforementioned William Stokes, when he wrote about one of his own patients: 'so long would the periods of suspension be, that his attendants were frequently in doubt whether he was not actually dead. Then a feeble, indeed barely perceptible inspiration would take place, followed by another somewhat stronger, until at length high heaving, and even violent breathing was established, which would then subside till the next period of suspension.'

For the nineteenth-century medical community, Ludwig Traube (1818–1876) named this pattern 'the Cheyne-Stokes phenomenon'. It entered the mid-twentieth-century common consciousness in 1953, when the Soviet press

announced that Joseph Stalin was ill and had
'Cheyne-Stokes respiration' (he died the next
day).[79] All else being peaceful, it is the last
thing anyone does in their life.

STANDARDS AND SMITHEREENS

Through these early years in its stately new
home, RCSI carefully protected its hard-won
reputation. Even before students were allowed
to register, the bar was high: there were
entrance exams in Greek and Latin (minutes
from 1814 refer to Sallust, Lucien, Virgil's
Aeneid and five books of Homer's *Iliad*). Those
who could not make the grade often went

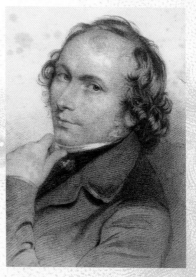

William Stokes.
Engraving after
a portrait by
Frederic Burton.

to the Royal Colleges in London or Edinburgh, where no such classical barrier
obtained. Moreover, the student in Dublin had to serve an apprenticeship of five
years before facing the strenuous two-day Licence exam, but in London one could
earn a diploma in less than half that time: all that was required was a year's worth
of certificates of attendance at a hospital and proof of having followed two courses
of anatomy and surgery. (The remarkable story of Dr James Barry (*c.*1789–1865)
deserves recording here. Born Margaret Anne Bulkley in Cork, Barry lived all of
his adult life as a man, earning his MD at Edinburgh (1812), his surgical diploma
in London (1813) and rising to the rank of Inspector General of Hospitals.)

Fairly or otherwise, Irish students in London gained a reputation for being the
worst students of all. Sir Astley Cooper told the story of how he examined one
such Irish student by asking him the difference between a simple and a compound
fracture. 'A simple fracture is where the bone is broke,' answered the student, 'and
a compound fracture is when it is all broke.' What, Cooper asked, was meant by
'all broke'? 'I mean,' said the student, 'broken into smithereens to be sure.' When
Cooper inquired what were 'smithereens', the student apparently offered him an
intense expression of sympathy, and said: 'You don't know what is smithereens?
Then I give you up!'[80]

This sort of paddywhackery was harmless enough – until, that is, legislation
threatened to punish RCSI for holding elevated standards. Twice, in 1816 and
1818, bills were introduced at Westminster that would allow any diplomate
of each of the three Royal Colleges to practise anywhere in Britain or Ireland.
In other words, poorly trained surgeons could flood the Irish market. On both
occasions RCSI successfully protested against this legislation, forcefully making

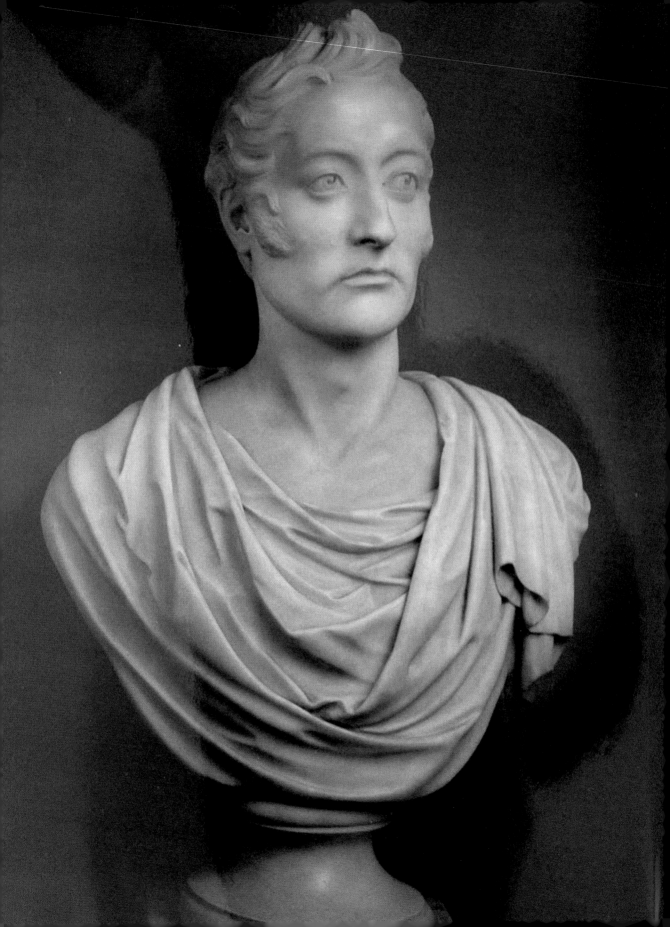

the point that, where standards were concerned, RCSI did not wish to engage in a race to the bottom. Any action that would 'materially tend to lower the profession of surgery in the confidence and estimation of the public' was to be strenuously resisted.[81] In 1817, too, RCSI wrote directly to the sister Colleges about unifying standards in surgical education, but to no avail. In general, this sort of atomised, ad hoc approach to standards would endure until the clean sweep of the Medical Act of 1858.

Facing page: Bust of John Shekleton by John Smyth, c.1824.

THE CONSEQUENCES OF A SCRATCH

In little more than three decades, RCSI had gone from being an idea in a tavern, then a set of ideals without a roof over its head, to where it was now: firmly established in impressive premises, energetic as an advocate and authority in its field, with its destiny and day-to-day affairs steered by celebrated practitioners. And yet, for all this achievement, life at the forefront of surgical and medical endeavour often meant a dive into the unknown, and the unknown could be dangerous.

On Saturday, 13 February 1819, Richard Dease was lecturing to his students on the subject of cervical nerves and the brachial plexus. The subject he used for demonstration was a woman who had died of a pulmonary infection less than forty-eight hours earlier. Dease was known as 'an accomplished anatomist', and yet at some point during the class, without noticing it, he very slightly abraded his skin.[82] The next morning he awoke feeling very ill and sent for Colles, who suspected Dease had cut himself while dissecting. Dease denied this until they discovered the tiny scratch on his hand, where a vesicle had appeared. For the next week the inflammation progressed, and on the following Sunday, the 45-year-old Dease died.

This was not an isolated incident. A few years later, a very talented demonstrator in anatomy, John Shekleton (c.1795–1824, Lic. 1816, MRCSI 1819), pricked himself in a similar manner; ten days later he was dead. In 1834 an unnamed student met a similar fate. Why did this happen? 'Does the infection enter by the wound and cause all the mischief?' Colles asked in the pages of the *Dublin Hospital Reports*. 'Or are the symptoms to be accounted for by some peculiarity in the constitution of the individual?'[83] In the absence of knowledge about micro-organisms, all he could do was guess – and grieve. As an institution, RCSI, too, reacted in its own way: Dease's son, a student of the College, had his fees reimbursed, and in 1958 a Research Fellowship in Microbiology was named in honour of Shekleton. Out of delicacy, the unfortunate student's name was not recorded, but his case at least led to a research paper by his professor.[84] Progress, invariably, comes at a price. ∎

Chapter 3:
Expanding Ambition, 1821–43

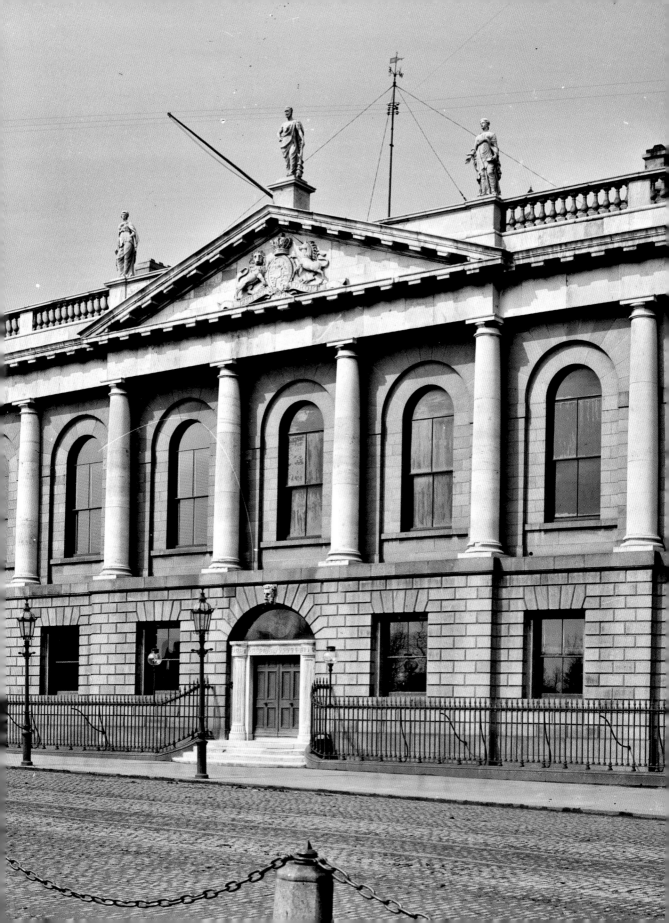

Chapter 3:
Expanding Ambition, 1821-43

AT THE DRAWING BOARD

The fact that RCSI was flourishing brought with it what was, in the scheme of things, a good problem to have: no sooner had the new home on the Green been completed than there was a need to expand it. Overseen by Parke, piecemeal alterations took place, notably including the addition of a 'theatre for anatomical demonstrations'.[1] A publication from 1818 describes a room capable of accommodating

> between 300 and 400 students, besides what the gallery may contain, which is opened for the public during the dissection of malefactors. Adjoining the theatre are the professors' dissecting room, and two museums... the dissecting rooms are very commodious, and were added but lately to the building.

These 'commodious' rooms seem to refer to the octagonal structure, dating from about 1812, that appears on later architectural plans. Elements of these early buildings survive in the southern wall of the current Anatomy Room, where the two tall round-headed windows once looked onto an open passage. The public dissecting room was furnished with twenty tables, none of which came cheap: account books record that £28 8*s* 9*d* was paid for a single dissecting table 'made on a particular construction for demonstrations and lectures'. In addition, there were 'suitable apartments and lofts' for making and drying anatomical preparations.[2]

Elsewhere, in the original 1810 building, poor air circulation in the museum next to the Board Room (in part, today, the Sir Thomas Myles Room) was proving inhospitable to its collection of valuable preparations. In 1819, a new architect, Francis Johnston, was commissioned to produce an inspection report. Johnston had excellent credentials, having recently completed the General Post Office on Sackville (later O'Connell) Street – nor would it have hurt that his brother Andrew (1770–1833, Lic. 1794, MRCSI 1805) was a past-President of RCSI (1817), treasurer (1820) and, successively, Professor of Surgical Pharmacy (1813–19) and Midwifery (1819–23).

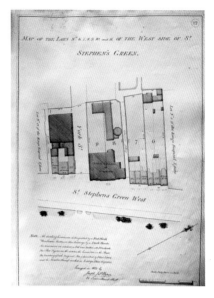

Map showing RCSI property on Lots 8 and 9, St Stephen's Green (1832). Courtesy of the King's Hospital.

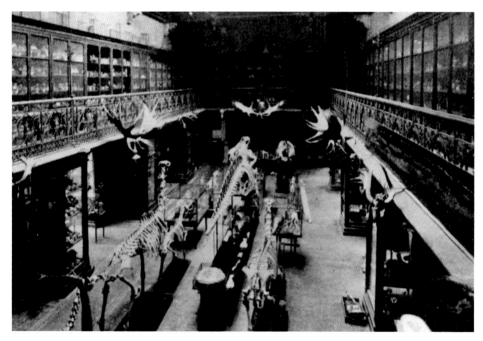

The College Museum, adjacent to York Street. This photograph taken after its c.1880 refurbishment.

67

As it happens, that initial inspection report came to naught — until the matter was revisited some years later, in 1824, by which time the scope of RCSI's ambition had literally and figuratively widened significantly. An airier new room was no longer enough; now RCSI wanted an entirely new building. Johnston was not in a position to take on the project, but he passed it to his assistant (and cousin), William Murray.

GREEK GODS ON THE GREEN: ATHENA, ASCLEPIUS AND HYGEIA

Murray's draft plans show him grappling with the 'aesthetic problem' of how to enlarge a building that was never intended to be enlarged.[3] His first proposal was relatively simple: a four-bay extension to the north, set back slightly from Parke's temple. However, this cost-effective proposal was rejected in favour of

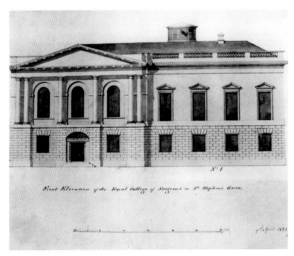

Unexecuted proposal for front elevaation by William Murray, April 1825.

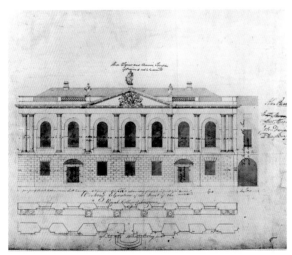

Unexecuted proposal by Murray, dated July 1825, for front elevation (extending over Glover's Alley) with false door on the right-hand-side for symmetry. The plan for the executed façade appears at the bottom of the drawing.

something much more daring and complex. The new version consisted of a symmetrical façade with a false hall door balancing the original; this would have the benefit of preserving the old Entrance Hall.

In an extraordinary architectural coup de grâce, the entire pediment would be lifted and moved several metres to the right, giving the whole a more Palladian than Neoclassical accent. The project moved fast: tendering began on 1 July 1825, and less than eight weeks later, on Thursday, 25 August, at three o'clock in the afternoon, the Lord Lieutenant laid the first stone.[4]

At some point during construction, the two-door option was superseded by the decision to create a sin-

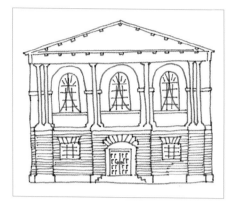

RCSI's original
and expanded
façades. Sketch
by the author.

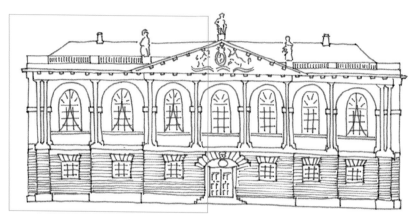

gle central main entrance, replacing the original door with a window – thereby creating the façade as it is today.[5] On the first floor, the Board Room was untouched, but space for a vast new museum was created next to it. To protect the specimens within, this was a windowless room: the façade's fourth, fifth and sixth bays are in fact cleverly disguised 'dummy' windows (a detail which would prove very important some eighty-nine years later, in 1916). The northernmost window lights up what an early plan designates a 'Small Museum'; it is now the Council Room.

Whereas Parke's building was largely austere, Murray's featured a variety of new flourishes. Either side of the new entrance stand two rounded and panelled pilasters (derived in part from Francis Johnston's gate piers at Áras an Uachtaráin, and in part from James Gandon's support piers for Carlisle (later O'Connell) Bridge[6]). Above, and curving into the rounded capitals, is an unusual Greek-key frieze.[7] Asclepius, the Greek god of medicine, keeps watch from the keystone over who comes and goes.[8] (The pale-blue-banded clock by J. Booth & Sons was a Victorian addition, immortalised in James Joyce's *Dublin-*

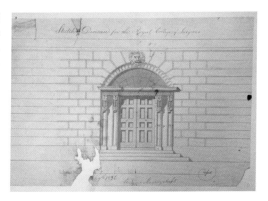

Proposed entrance doorway, February 1826.

ers: 'He went as far as the clock of the College of Surgeons: it was on the stroke of ten.'[9])

At roof level, the northwards transport of the great pediment must have been an extraordinary sight to behold. Into its previously bare tympanum was now placed a bas-relief Royal Arms, with – in heraldic parlance – the lion dexter, the unicorn sinister.[10] Higher again stand three stone newcomers to the city skyline: at the apex, Asclepius again, seven foot tall (2.13m), with his serpent-entwined staff; to his left, his daughter Hygeia, goddess of health and cleanliness; on his right, the goddess of wisdom and war, Athena. All three, and the keystone image, were the work of sculptor John Smyth (he was also responsible for Mercury, Hibernia and Fidelity atop the GPO).[11] Along York Street, a balustrade was added, for the sake of 'the uniformity and general appearance of the Building'.[12]

Inside, the new doorway led to a new Entrance Hall. Originally this was to be 'fitted up plain',[13] but Murray revisited this, adding four free-standing col-

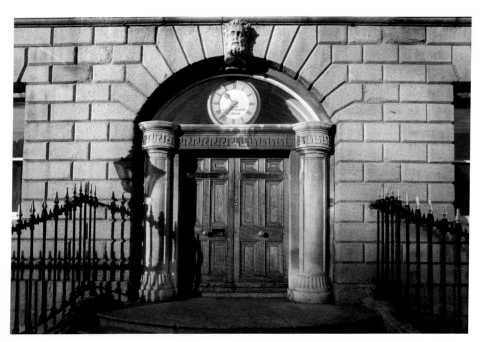

The finished doorway, with its keystone of Asclepius by John Smyth.

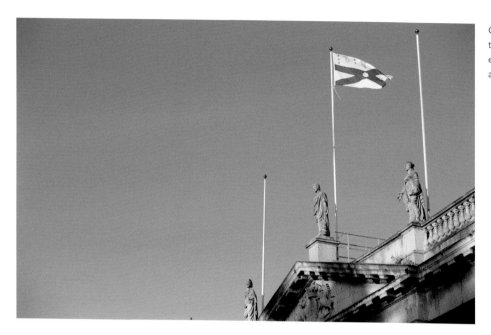

Greek gods on the Green: Athena, Asclepius and Hygeia.

umns and a segmented ceiling to create an impression of height in an otherwise constrained space. The walls feature simple square or rectangular panels, and the Greek-key motif continues on the undersides of the ceiling beams. The recession in the back wall – from which, since 1886, the fissured William Dease has been emerging – was for a stove. The floor is of Yorkshire flagging, famous for its durability.

Even so, the polish shows up shallow concavities here and there: two hundred years' worth of footsteps coming and going have made their mark. The new room to the right – now the President's suite, called the Abraham Colles Room – belonged to the housekeeper, with a narrow vestibule for the porters. Upstairs, the great innovation was the new museum, naturally lit by four large circular roof-lights, or 'lanterns', embedded in a false-vault ceiling. The contents of this space will be discussed below, as will its central place in the story of Irish independence. For now it is enough to note the fluted Ionic columns that supported the ceiling, and the existence of a railed gallery that ran around three sides of the room – so that visitors had the opportunity to stand at orbit level with the skeletons of massive animals.

The entire renovation project ended in December 1827.[14] It is not a straightforward task to discover all the costs accrued, but £7,500 seems a conservative estimate.[15] Fortunately, the RCSI's income had been rising annually: £2,906 1*s* 4½*d* in 1825, £3,912 2*s* 7*d* in 1826, and £4,779 7*s* 0*d* in the year the extension

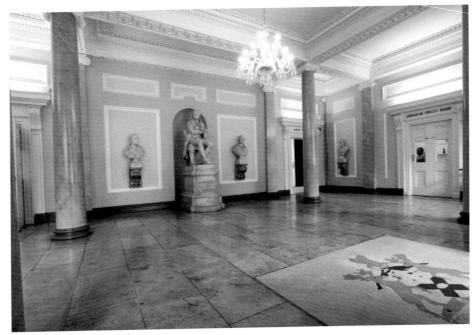

The new Entrance Hall, with the seated William Dease.

was completed.[16] In 1832, candles were quenched as the Dublin Oil Gas Company installed the latest bright idea: gas lighting.

THE SECOND CHARTER (1828) AND THE FIRST REGISTRAR

RCSI's physical changes were matched by revisions in governance and housekeeping. Monday, 2 June 1828 saw the granting of a second Charter, this time

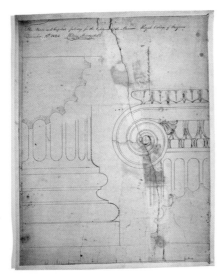

Murray's drawings for base and capitals of columns in the new museum, December 1826.

under the auspices of George IV. As lengthy a document as its predecessor, written in rolling legalese, its most significant change to the College's constitution was to admit for examination those candidates who were not indentured apprentices but had instead been educated via lectures and hospital attendance. There had been some internal resistance to this — certain surgeons valued the apprenticeship system as a lucrative earner — but after 1828 apprenticeship was rendered optional. Additionally, the Vice-President, heretofore appointed by the President, was now elected by the College at large. The cost of procuring the new Charter was an eye-watering £728 8*s* 4¾*d* (as Cameron commented, 'Note the farthings!'[17]).

The day-to-day running of the expanding institution also came under scrutiny. Initially this fell to the 'Clerk and House-keeper', a role that came with in-house accommodation. A man named Joseph Humphreys was the first incumbent (1816); alas, the only other mark Humphreys made in the annals was when he was arrested owing to 'pecuniary difficulties' and escorted to the Debtors' Prison on Green Street.[18] At first, his employers looked sympathetically upon his travails, giving him three months' leave

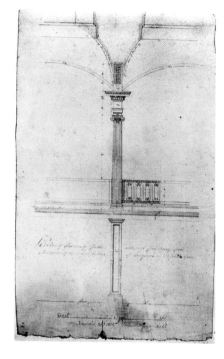

Working drawing by Murray of a detail for the new museum's gallery.

of absence to compose his affairs and take advantage of the Insolvents' Act. But a year later, in 1819, when Humphreys' wife was discovered pawning College property, the couple was invited to exit for good. His successor's successor, one Cornelius O'Keefe, was appointed under the new title of 'Registrar' in 1832.

THE BUSINESS OF BODYSNATCHING - OR, AN OPEN SECRET

The year 1832 saw the end of one of the odder, grislier chapters in the medical history of Ireland and Britain — one in which RCSI, from its inception, played its part in full.

RCSI Library is in possession of a very early edition of the single most famous anatomical atlas of all time, *De Humani Corporis Fabrica* by Andreas Vesalius. The frontispiece depicts Vesalius dissecting in the presence of a large number of his students at Padua. The central subject — the figure undergoing dissection — would have been an executed criminal, probably a murderer, and

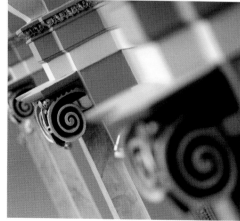

Scrollwork in the College Hall.

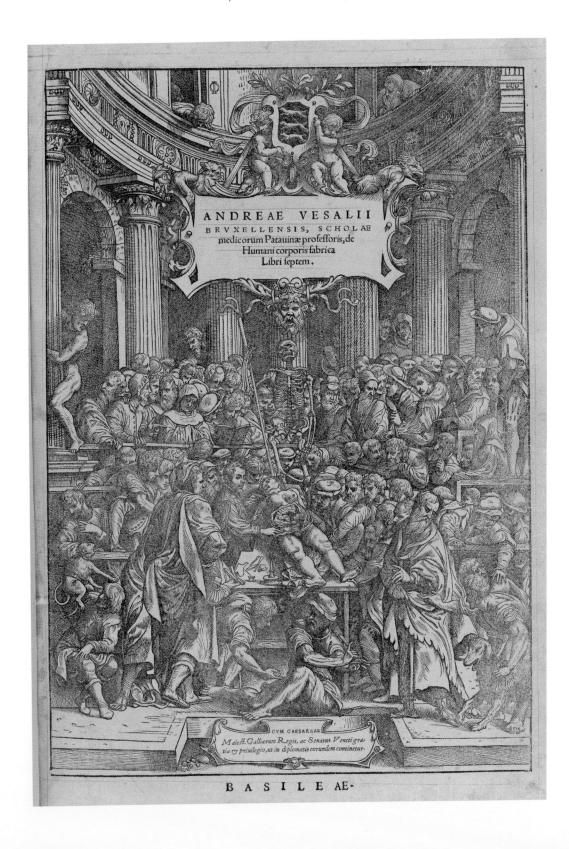

the fact that his cadaver was being dissected was intended to add a metaphysical element to his punishment. The logic was that the greater good was doubly served: justice was done and, at the same time, medical knowledge was expanded.

Indeed, Vesalius is known to have pleaded with judges not to sentence criminals to quartering as this would damage their value as teaching tools.[19] This symbiotic relationship of the law and medicine was found all over continental Europe. Meanwhile, closer to home, in their Seal of Cause (1505), the barber-surgeons of Edinburgh were granted the body of one executed murderer to dissect per annum;

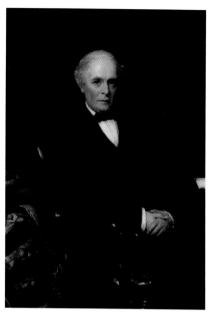

Sir Dominic Corrigan by Stephen Catterson Smith. Courtesy of RCPI.

in 1541, Henry VIII gave London's barber-surgeons the right to four bodies a year; and, as noted earlier, the first recorded dissection of a criminal in Dublin took place in 1676. 'For better preventing the horrid act of murder,' ran the legislation of 25 George 2 c. 37 – aka the Murder Act of 1752 – 'in order that some terror and peculiar mark of infamy be added to the punishment of death, it was laid down that the bodies of all executed murderers were to be handed over to the appropriate surgeon to be dissected and anatomized.'[20] This act was in operation when the College received its Charter – in fact, the act was not repealed until 1973 – hence, Secretary Henthorn's 1788 invocation of the law as a bargaining chip in RCSI's early quest for a home.

When the law was upheld, not everyone, of course, was happy. Records of that 1676 Dublin dissection include the expense of £13 6s for soldiers to 'protect' the cadaver from being seized by distraught relatives. Not long afterwards, another cadaver was successfully rescued 'contrary to a warrant'.[21] 'I well remember,' wrote Sir Dominic Corrigan, who was a medical student in Dublin in the 1820s, 'the bodies of two young men executed for a trades' union murder, carried in an open cart from the prison, Newgate, where they were hanged, to the College of Surgeons, followed by a crowd of howling and yelling relatives and friends.'[22] In Glasgow, a medical school was set on fire.[23] In contrast, others were fascinated by the promised spectacle – note the reference above to a gallery in RCSI's new dissecting room 'which is opened for the public during the dissection of malefactors'.

Facing page: *De Humani Corporis Fabrica* by Andreas Vesalius. Wellcome Collection.

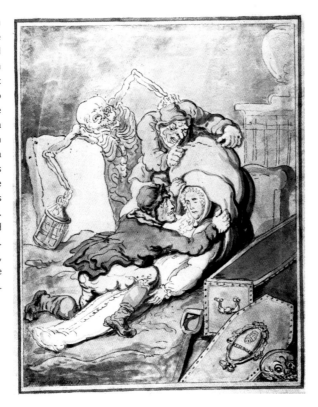

Two men placing the shrouded corpse which they have just disinterred into a sack while Death, as a nightwatchman holding a lantern, grabs one of the grave-robbers from behind. Coloured drawing by T. Rowlandson, 1775. Wellcome Collection.

In theory, then, there was legal provision for anatomical dissection. But in practice the supply of executed criminals never came close to meeting demand (in the 1600s, William Harvey was so short of subjects that he dissected his own father and sister). And so committed anatomists obtained their subjects the only other way they could: they stole them from graveyards. From the time of Vesalius — who himself admitted he engaged in the practice — 'bodysnatching', or 'resurrectionism' as it was sometimes called, was treated as something of an open secret.

From the 1750s, as anatomy was increasingly established as a field of study by the Hunters in London and the Monros in Edinburgh, formal demonstration by the lecturer at the top of the room no longer sufficed; students were expected to dissect for themselves. And in the absence of a suitable fast-acting preservation technique — formaldehyde was not discovered until 1869[24] — a steady supply was required, at least in winter months (in summer, when olfactory issues would be more pronounced, school was fortunately in recess).

Discretion was the order of the day — or, more accurately, the night. Hence the importance of Digges Lane when RCSI was in its Mercer Street location. Hence, too, after the move to St Stephen's Green, the decision to acquire land reaching as far as Glover's Alley. A petition to government for the necessary funds more or less alludes to the open secret involved. RCSI proposed to buy a plot 'sixty feet in breadth and two hundred and fifty in depth... [and to] enclose [it] by a high wall with back entrance from Glover's Alley... [so that] every business connected with the school of Surgery can... be conducted with that Secrecy and Decorum which the nature of an Institution indispensably requires'.[25] Once the subjects had fulfilled their pedagogic function, they were buried within the

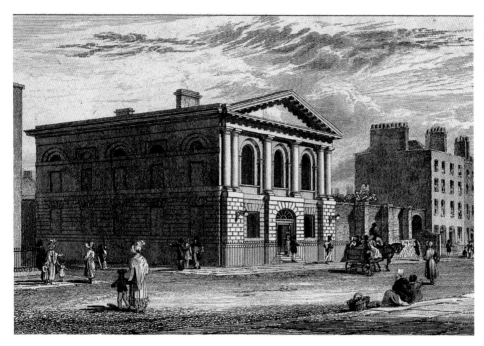

The tell-tale tree behind the wall. Illustration after a drawing by George Petrie, 1821.

expanded grounds. A drawing that pre-dates William Murray's expansion of the façade shows a tree sprouting in this soft earth, where formerly two solid 'Dutch Billy' houses had stood.

In his recollections of the period, Dominic Corrigan put his finger on the pulse of the 'absurd' state of affairs: 'while the law punished anyone found procuring a dead body for dissection, the educational laws required that every candidate should possess a practical knowledge of it'.[26]

Another oddity of the situation was that it was technically not a crime to steal a body from a graveyard. A legal textbook of 1812 noted that 'stealing a corpse itself (though a matter of great indecency and indictable) is no felony unless some of the grave-cloths be stolen with it'.[27] This meant that corpses were either manhandled into 'fresh' rags, heaved into a sack or carted off naked. In general, it was the city's poorest inhabitants who suffered these indignities: a paupers' graveyard at Kilmainham, the Dublin Hospital Fields Burying Ground — known as 'Bully's Acre' — was a favoured spot for resurrectionist activity.

Burial was free here, the graves unguarded and, owing to lamentable living conditions and a concomitant high mortality rate, new arrivals were frequent.[28] There was no such thing as regularly lined and spaced plots; relatives would simply turn up, borrow picks and shovels from a local pub, and begin the dig. Meanwhile, a paid informer — sometimes a dissecting-room porter — would circulate amongst the mourners to glean details as to whether the deceased would be a suitable candidate to revisit once the grieving relatives had gone home.

Corrigan – by this time a knight of the realm and a pillar of the medical establishment – gives a vivid depiction of what happened next:

> Night fell, and our operations commenced. We removed with our hands the recently deposited clay and stones which covered the head and shoulders of the coffin – no more was uncovered; then a rope about three or four feet long was let down, and the grapple, an iron hook with the end flattened out attached to the rope, was inserted under the edge of the coffin-lid. The student then pulled on the rope until the lid of the coffin cracked across. The other end of the rope was now inserted round the neck of the dead, and the whole body was then drawn upwards and carried across the churchyard to some convenient situation, until four or six were gathered together awaiting the arrival of the car that was to convey them to some dissecting theatre... We travelled on our way home safely, sometimes with as many as six subjects in an inside car, until we neared our journey's end, which was either at the College of Surgeons, the dissecting room of Trinity College, or Mr. Kirby's Lecture Rooms in Peter Street; and then occasionally some meddlesome young watchman, not fairly bribed, or busy passer-by, raised a warning shout, and we had to fight our way for half the length of the street. We generally, indeed I may say always, succeeded, for we were young, active and armed with stout sticks, and the gate was ready open for us, and closed on our entrance.[29]

AN INQUIRY INTO COMINGS AND GOINGS IN GLOVER'S ALLEY

It was part of the Professor of Anatomy's remit to take care of RCSI's share of these nocturnal deliveries.[30] If the likes of Dease, Halahan and Colles did not themselves do as Corrigan had done, they certainly employed others to do it for them. The first 'Porter and Messenger' in the Anatomy School was Anthony McMahon: his official income was £20 per annum, but the department accounts show he regularly earned twice that for supplying subjects; he was also given the occasional mysterious 'present' of a guinea or two.[31] The reward, of course, was to compensate for the attendant risk.

Consider the case of Dr Peter Harkan (Lic. 1806), who was employed as a demonstrator in Philip Crampton's private school on Dawson Street. Harkan was 'supervising' students in Bully's Acre when they were surprised by watchmen. Harkan shepherded his charges over the wall first, but when he tried to clamber out, the watchmen grabbed his legs. At the same time the loyal students on the other side grabbed his arms, with the result that Harkan was painfully flossed across the rough wall for several minutes. He escaped, but the internal damage was done and he died afterwards.[32] Then there was Christopher ('Kit') Dixon, a porter in RCSI – and also a known resurrectionist. He was seized by an outraged crowd at Islandbridge, a rope was put around his waist and he was repeatedly immersed in the Liffey until he almost drowned.[33] Another RCSI porter, Luke Redmond, was not so lucky. Caught in possession of a body in 1828, he was killed by an angry crowd. This prompted an internal inquiry at RCSI.

Curiously, this was not the first time a searching light was shined on such night-time activities. In 1805, a city alderman cautioned RCSI over 'the remains of some Human Bodies, taken out of the River Liffey, which were supposed to have undergone surgical dissection'. RCSI thanked the alderman for his 'polite and able communication' and promised they would 'take the same into their most serious consideration'.[34] Colles, Crampton and several others formed a committee to look into the matter. They recommended 'the upmost caution in the disposal of subjects'[35] – which, following the move to St Stephen's Green, seems to have meant that remains were simply buried on-site.

The alderman's light-touch warning was typical of the hands-off attitude of the authorities. Essentially, resurrectionism was accepted as a necessary evil, and as long as the medical establishment kept it under wraps then this was a hypocrisy that everyone could live with. But what happened – and what changed attitudes entirely – was the explosive growth of medical schools in the 1810s and 1820s, not just in Ireland but in Britain, too. (In London, the number of anatomy students in 1798 was 300; in 1820 it was over 1,000.[36])

The corresponding demand for subjects led to a surge in resurrectionism: what might once have been characterised as a distasteful side-line rapidly developed into a large and lucrative profession. In a single year, some 1,500 bodies may have been disinterred at Bully's Acre alone.[37] Prices soared, from a half- or one guinea at the turn of the century to perhaps twenty times that in the new goldrush moment. Graveyard shoot-outs between rival factions were not uncommon (one source claims that a son of Prof Kirby was killed in such a battle[38]).

To satisfy British demand, an export trade boomed. Even with post and packaging (subjects were parcelled into boxes sometimes labelled 'Irish cheddar' or 'salted herring', or for weightier consignments, 'pianos' or 'limestone'[39]), the return was enormous; delivery of a single subject might pay more than most people would earn in a year. London, Glasgow and Edinburgh were the chief destinations; in 1826 the celebrated surgeon – and future RCSI Honorary Fellow (1867) – James Syme even travelled from Edinburgh with a view to setting up a regular supply.[40] To protect their loved ones' remains, some people began installing railed cages, or mortsafes, over graves; those who could afford it invested in heavyweight lead slabs to cover the coffins (ironically, some graves were later raided specifically for the lead). Bloodhounds were used to patrol the newly opened city cemeteries at Goldenbridge (1829), Glasnevin (1832) and Mount Jerome (1836).

In 1826 – even as Syme was sounding out suppliers – RCSI's Prof of Anatomy, Arthur Jacob (of whom there will be more below), proposed a motion that a committee be appointed to prevent such export activity and to examine all other 'irregularities' related to the matter. Nothing happened, however, until the fatal Redmond incident, when, to no one's surprise, the inquiry turned out to be extremely difficult to conduct: 'owing to the evident unwillingness of the resurrection men to disclose the entire truth, and by the contradictory accounts received from them'. But there was no hiding the truth that RCSI had unofficially sponsored bodysnatching, leading the resurrectionists to 'believe that there was no harm in pursuing the trade'.

After all, the professors only objected when the export trade 'increased to such an extent as (according to the acknowledgement of one of the demonstrators) materially to impede the business of the School'. What this meant, in practice, was that there were bizarre occasions when bodies were snatched, delivered, paid for, and snatched back again: 'Bodies have been removed and sold after having been placed on the table of the dissecting room and even partially dissected.' Moreover, RCSI's premises had been used 'as a kind of warehouse' during the bodies' journey to Britain.[41] Controlling the market in this way kept prices inflated (though what it did to the bodies is another matter: as John Cheyne once drily noted, 'the capillary system cannot be well learnt from an examination of the bodies which are usually brought into a public dissecting room'[42]).

The inquiring committee further learned that:

> the exportation of subjects is now principally carried on by a man named Collins, resident in Peter Street, and a man named Wray, resident in D'Olier Street, persons entirely beyond the influence of the College... it is a most unhappy feature in the matter, that this person Wray has often, nay very often, been openly in the College trucking and bargaining for subjects at the time when they were plenty, and

this was the system nurtured and fostered within our walls, which may now tend if not controlled to sap their very foundations.[43]

This admission of corporate culpability notwithstanding, there was insufficient evidence to prove that anyone employed by the professors was implicated in the 'irregularities' (that said, it was noted that 'Kit' Dixon 'scandalously violated the truth in every particular';[44] he remained in the employ of RCSI until 1849, but his responsibilities were much curtailed). Amongst the new recommendations was the appointment of a resident officer ('paid well enough to be incorrupt-ible'[45]); and henceforth, too, the cart for collecting subjects should be controlled only by professors (Dixon and Wray had been in the habit of 'borrowing' it), and no stranger should be allowed to bring in subjects.

As part of the proceedings, Redmond's widow petitioned for £10 in com-pensation ('some small relief'), as her husband had 'died in the service of the College'.[46] The authorities did not share Mrs Redmond's interpretation and the claim was dismissed. Wray (sometimes Ray or Rae), an English navy surgeon on half-pay, was later arrested along with his co-complicit wife.

It is very easy to take the high moral ground when it comes to this chapter in the history of medicine – especially easy, perhaps, for those outside the medical community. Even at the time, Trinity's reforming Professor of Anatomy, James Macartney (1770–1843), decried the inherent hypocrisy of the situation:

> I do not think that the upper and middle classes have understood the effects of their own conduct when they take part in impeding the progress of dissection, nor does it seem wise to discountenance the practice by which many of them are supplied with artificial teeth and hair. Very many of the upper ranks carry in their mouths teeth which have been buried in the Hospital Fields.[47]

Taking the long view of the resurrectionists, the gerontologist and historian Dr John Fleetwood (1917–2007) observed,

> Ruffians, scoundrels, sordid opportunists they may have been, but they played their part in keeping the anatomy schools alive, and with-out the basic knowledge of anatomy there can be no medicine and no surgery, so that without them there would have been no Corrigan, no Graves, no Colles, no Stokes, to bring the fame of Irish medicine to every corner of the then known globe.[48]

The history of resurrectionism reached its grotesque peak – or nadir – in 1828. In Edinburgh, two Irish labourers named Burke and Hare gave up their day jobs to become night-time suppliers of subjects. But their innovation in the practice was to skip the graveyard altogether; instead, they preyed on the living, murdering sixteen men and women, and delivering the bodies to Dr Robert Knox's dissection room in Surgeons' Square ('Burke's the butcher, Hare's the thief,' ran a contemporary street ballad, 'Knox the man that buys the beef'[49]).

Burke and Hare were both arrested in November; the former was duly hanged, dissected and had his skeletal remains publicly displayed; the latter, having shopped his erstwhile partner, was released from prison a week later, never to be heard of again. Dr Knox, meanwhile, left Edinburgh, his career in tatters. (It is salutary to consider that many other eminent anatomists – Colles, say, or Macartney in Trinity – could quite easily have met something like Knox's fate.) The Burke and Hare murders led directly, in 1832, to the passage of the Anatomy Act, which gave surgeons, anatomists and medical students the right to access any unclaimed corpses, in particular those in workhouses, prisons and hospitals. Voluntary donation was also legislated for (needless to say, the only method by which RCSI today obtains bodies for teaching anatomy).

At a stroke, the resurrectionist trade was wiped out. Even so, many graveyards continued to be patrolled; the bloodhounds were only retired from Glasnevin when they attacked the employees' medical attendant, one Dr Kirwan – evidently he still gave off the distinctive scent of a resurrectionist.[50]

BURNS, BLOWPIPES AND SPONTANEOUS HUMAN COMBUSTION – OR, TWO NEW CHAIRS

Also in the year of the second Charter – and, indeed, of RCSI's bodysnatching inquiry, and Burke and Hare's arrests – Colles proposed two new subjects (in the non-anatomical sense): Medical Jurisprudence and Chemistry. The former had the particular advantage of being a low-cost innovation ('the College will have to provide very few materials'), and the first Professor – John Thomas Adrien (1798–1830, Lic. 1821, MRCSI 1824) – was duly appointed in July 1829.

Adrien had an unfortunately short tenure: while experimenting with blowpipes in the School, he suffered a burn to his tongue, which became infected; he died shortly thereafter, in October 1830. He was succeeded by the obstetrician Thomas Edward Beatty (c.1800–1872, Lic. 1821, MRCSI 1824, Prof of Medical Jurisprudence 1830–35, Prof of Midwifery 1842–57). Beatty was elected PRCSI in 1850, but in 1862 resigned his RCSI Fellowship (antea Membership) in order to qualify for Fellowship of the College of Physicians — by the rules of the latter, one could not hold both.

Two years later, Beatty was elected President of RCPI, the first incumbent in their new Kildare Street hall. He remains the sole individual to have been elected President of both institutions. A socialite and *bon viveur*, he died in 1872, having developed septicaemia and cellulitis following a tooth extraction. The Chair of Medical Jurisprudence lasted until 1954, when it became the Chair of Social, Preventive and Forensic Medicine; in turn, this was separated into two Chairs, in 1972, Forensic Medicine and Toxicology, and Social and Preventive Medicine.

Colles' other new subject was Chemistry. On 16 June 1828, James Apjohn (1796–1886; Prof of Chemistry 1828–50) was appointed to the Chair, the first such appointment in any non-university medical school.[51] Colles' application to establish the post outlined some of Apjohn's responsibilities:

> It should be his duty not only to detail and illustrate the principles of this Science, but to enter very fully into the subject of Animal Chemistry — it should also be part of his duty to analyse for any Members of the College such morbid animal products as may be submitted to him, and to deliver in writing the result of his enquiries.[52]

Apjohn proved an inspired hire. His lectures were so well attended — by students from all of the Dublin medical schools — that by 1832 a new 'Chemical Lecture Theatre' and adjoining 'Chemical Laboratory' were built (these were located directly behind Murray's extension, a much-refurbished and -modernised area now known as the Apjohn Laboratory). His interest in humidity led to 'Apjohn's formula' ('It occurred to me that the relation between the Dew-point and the temperature of a thermometer with a moistened bulb might be calculated...'[53]); for his contribution to mineralogy, a manganese alum from South Africa was named *Apjohnite* in his honour; and he was awarded

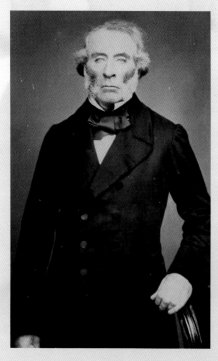

James Apjohn.

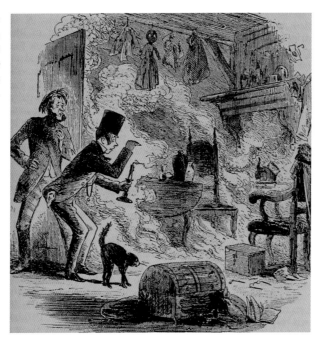

Illustration by Hablot Knight Browne ('Phiz') for *Bleak House* by Charles Dickens.

the Royal Irish Academy's prestigious Cunningham Medal (1837), and elected a Fellow of the Royal Society (1853).

In addition, one of his less scientifically sound contributions had a curious afterlife: between 1833 and 1835, Apjohn contributed articles to the *Cyclopedia of Practical Medicine* on subjects such as electricity, galvanism, toxicology and... spontaneous human combustion.[54] Curiously, this seems to have inspired Charles Dickens in *Bleak House*, when he dispatched Mr Krook in a ball of flame: 'I softly opened the door and looked in. And the burning smell is there – and the soot is there, and the oil is there – and he is not there!'[55]

THE PARK STREET CONNECTION, 1824-49

Before he came to RCSI, Apjohn co-founded and taught at Park Street School, in what is now Lincoln Place. Indeed, five of this rival school's seven founders went on to significant RCSI careers (Cameron called it a 'nursery for College Professors'[56]). They were Apjohn, Samuel Wilmot, Arthur Jacob, James William Cusack (1788–1861, Lic. 1812, MRCSI 1814, PRCSI 1827, 1847, 1858) and Sir Henry Marsh. The founders hedged their bets on the school's viability, commissioning their building to look like a religious meeting house in case they had to offload it in a hurry.

In fact, Park Street operated for twenty-five years, until 1849, when its then-proprietor, Hugh Carlisle, was approached (or poached) for the position of Professor of Anatomy at the newly opened Queen's College, Belfast. Park Street's valuable museum – chiefly the handiwork of a man called John Houston – went north with Carlisle, while the premises were converted into not a prayer house but a site for sore eyes, St Mark's Hospital. This was founded and run by the polymath oto-ophthalmologist Sir William Wilde (1815–1876, Lic. 1837, FRCSI 1844), father of the more famous Oscar.

SIR HENRY MARSH AND THE INSTITUTE FOR SICK CHILDREN

St Mark's was typical of the new nineteenth-century hospital – that is, one founded by a medical practitioner as opposed to a religious order, in the process elevating the hospital setting into the predominant site of modern medical endeavour. In addition, the era's new hospitals established themselves as 'the place par excellence where disease could be displayed to students on what became standard ward rounds'.[57] Four other new Dublin hospitals from the period were also deeply imprinted with RCSI credentials.

The first of these was the Institute for Sick Children, established by one of those who

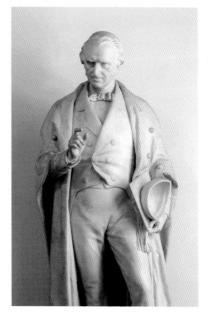

Sir Henry Marsh by John Henry Foley. Courtesy of RCPI.

moved from Park Street to RCSI, Sir Henry Marsh (1790–1860, Prof of Medicine 1828–32). Initially, in 1821, this was located at the rear of Marsh's home in Molesworth Street; subsequently it moved to Pitt (now Balfe) Street, off Grafton Street.[58] This was the first hospital of its kind in Ireland or Britain, treating some 7,000 sick children free of charge in 1826, tripling to 21,000 by 1831. Medical students also gained clinical instruction – including one of its earliest trainees, Charles West (1816–98), in town to imbibe from the 'Dublin School'; returning to London, he established Great Ormond Street Hospital (1852) – while on the wards both nurses and new mothers were educated in paediatric best practice.

In 1884, the Institute would amalgamate with the National Orthopaedic and Children's Hospital – founded by Auckland-born Lambert Ormsby (1849–1923, FRCSI 1875, PRCSI 1902–03); three years later, it relocated to Harcourt Street as the National Children's Hospital, which, in turn, in 1998, would be absorbed into Tallaght Hospital's Children's Services Department. (At the time of writing, the latest iteration of Marsh's idea is under construction at St James's Hospital.)

As a young man Marsh had been indentured to his cousin, Sir Philip Crampton, and had studied at RCSI – but a dissecting-room wound led to the amputation of his right index finger, cutting short at the same time any hope of a surgical career. He turned to medicine, becoming first a Licentiate, then three-time President, of RCPI. A statue of Marsh – Sir Henry from 1839 – stands in the RCPI's Entrance Hall. Restoring in death what was lost in life, Marsh is depicted with his right index finger querulously upraised.

ARTHUR JACOB: 'AN UNCOMPROMISING CHAMPION'

Marsh's neighbour in Pitt Street was the Ophthalmic Hospital, opened in 1829 by one of the outstanding figures of RCSI's second half-century, Arthur Jacob (1790–1874, Lic. 1813, MRCSI 1816, Prof of Anatomy and Physiology 1826–67, PRCSI 1837, 1864).[59] Having earned his Licence, Jacob travelled to Edinburgh for his MD (1814), then walked the length of England, visiting medical institutions. He crossed to France and walked to Paris, where he planned to study, but a political storm blew up – Napoleon had just escaped from Elba – so Jacob erred on the side of caution and returned to London, where he worked with Astley Cooper, Benjamin Brodie (Hon. MRCSI 1838) and, notably, Sir William Lawrence at the Moorfields Dispensary for Curing Diseases of the Ear and Eye (later the Royal London Ophthalmic Hospital). When Jacob returned to Dublin he retained a particular 'Moorfields outlook' as well as enduring friendships with these three mentors. In general, however, Jacob's professional relationships were anything but enduring.

In 1819, Jacob published his most famous research article, 'An Account of a Membrane in the Eye, Now First Described'.[60] This anatomised the light-sensitive lamella of the retina which contains the rods and cones – ever since known as the 'membrana Jacobi' or Jacob's membrane. The familiar condition known as 'detachment of the retina' is, strictly speaking, 'detachment of Jacob's membrane'.[61] By this time, Jacob had already founded his first hospital, the Charitable Institute for the Cure of Diseases of the Skin and of the Eye (1817), in Kildare Street. (The 'Skin' side was handled by TCD's Macartney, but only for a few years, after which that organ was dropped from the name.)

In 1829, Jacob founded the Ophthalmic Hospital in Pitt Street. His description of an operation is worth giving in his own words:

> I seat the patient in a chair and make him sit straight up or inclining, according to his height. If very tall, I raise myself by standing on a large book or two, or anything which answers the purpose to be found at hand. In my own place of business, I find old medical folios answer the purpose well; operating chairs, although very imposing and calculated to produce effect, I have not adopted, not finding myself at ease with such things. When he is seated, I lay the patient's head against my chest, and placing the middle finger of my left hand on his lower [eyelid] and the forefinger on his upper eyelid, and gently holding the eye between them, I strike the point of the needle suddenly into the cornea, about a line from its margin, and there hold it until

any struggles of the patient, which
may be made, cease. There must be
no hesitation here, for if the cor-
nea be touched without fixing the
point of the needle in it, the eye will
turn rapidly and the surface will be
scratched. I advise the operator to
pause here for a moment, holding
the eye firmly and steadily, on the
point of his needle, and if necessary
to say a word of encouragement or
remonstrance to the patient.[62]

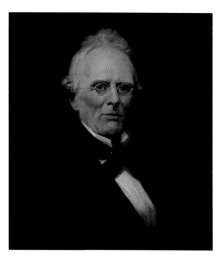

Portrait of
Arthur Jacob,
PRCSI 1837,
by Stephen
Catterson
Smith.

In 1837, Jacob's reforming interests led him to join the editorial board of the
Dublin Journal of Medical Science. However, owing to his vituperative style, he did
not last long, and he was replaced by William Wilde (for which Jacob bore his
rival oculist a lifelong grudge). Two years later, Jacob put his money where his
mouth was and founded, with Henry Maunsell, the weekly *Dublin Medical Press*.
Whereas the older *Journal* concentrated on science and research and tried to
remain above internecine squabbles, the new *Press* revelled in the wider social
and political ramifications of all things medical. For the next twenty-two years
under his editorship, Jacob contributed – often in colourfully scurrilous language – to every single issue (even the work of his celebrated fellow Park Street
founder, Robert Graves, was slated as 'excrementitious discharge'[63]).

In all his (many) arguments, Jacob was fiercely loyal to RCSI, ever ready
to take umbrage at the mere shadow of a slight. Cameron, who knew him
personally, recollected:

He was an uncompromising champion for the College Schools. In the
debates which took place at the meetings of the College he always
took a leading part, and was by no means 'mealy-mouthed' in referring to those from whose opinions he differed... He rarely indulged in
even the mildest festivities, but devoted himself wholly to his professional and editorial work, and to original research. He remained up
till long after midnight as a rule, nevertheless he was always punctu-
ally at work early the next day. He had an intense dislike to charlatan-
ism and humbug of every kind. He took a deep interest in the success
of his pupils, and he labored hard to instruct them.[64]

Arthur Jacob medal. The reverse bears the inscription: 'Arthur Jacob MD FRCS Prof of Anat. & Phys. Roy. Coll. of Surg. in Ireland. In Commemoration of Eminent Services Rendered to Science and the Medical Profession in Ireland. 1860.'

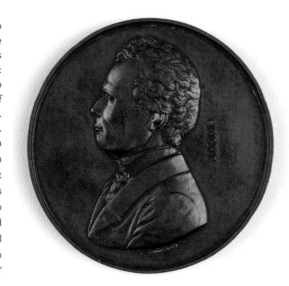

Professionally proud of all that he achieved, Jacob was nonetheless deeply uncomfortable with any celebrations in his name. In 1860, when a testimonial in his honour was proposed, he refused to have anything to do with it. The rebuffed organisers pooled the funds collected and had a medal struck bearing Jacob's profile – but again, Jacob was uninterested. 'I cannot accept this or any other testimonial,' he said: 'but if at death you still think that I deserve it, you may nail it on my coffin.'[65] Jacob died in Barrow-in-Furness in 1874; the medal remains in RCSI Heritage Collections. An open medical scholarship ran in his name from 1961 to 1975 – which begs the question: would he have approved?

THE CITY OF DUBLIN HOSPITAL, BAGGOT STREET

The fourth of these new hospitals with a strong RCSI affiliation had its origins in an argument that pre-dated the enlargement of the St Stephen's Green building. As noted above, John Timothy Kirby, as sometime rival, sometime employee, had a fractious relationship with RCSI – but that did not prevent him from being elected President in 1823. Peace reigned during his year's tenure, at the end of which the minutes record 'the Thanks of the College be Returned to John Kirby late President for the very able and assiduous manner in which he discharged the duties of that Office'.[66] Once out of the presidential chair, however, Kirby stirred up fresh controversy.

Essentially, the debate was between the enlargement project, conceived of primarily to house the museum and Library, and Kirby's proposal for 'the Establishment of a National Surgical Hospital under the management of the Royal College of Surgeons in Ireland'.[67] Noting that London and Paris owed their 'surgical renown' to hospitals, he pointed out the comparative dearth in Dublin:

> Of SEVENTY-ONE Members of the College resident in Dublin, FOR-
> TY-EIGHT are without any Hospital opportunity; and of THIRTY Li-

centiates none are connected with any Institution of the kind. Can it be longer maintained that there is no want of Hospitals, as far as the individuals of the College are concerned? Are those individuals careless on the subject? I say they are not. – Their first ambition is to be connected with an Hospital... They well know [that] without an Hospital, no man in this country has ever taken, or perhaps will ever take, a high station in the profession.

After his presidential stint, Kirby was familiar with RCSI's finances and had the figures to support his arguments: the College had a capital sum of £9,500, of which £6,000 could set up the hospital. Kirby being Kirby, he went public with his argument in a pamphlet (favourably reviewed by *The Lancet*), but to others within RCSI, it surely looked as if the man once famed for his 'mangling' was airing unclean linen again.[68] In any case, it was the extension that won out – while Kirby's hospital was (air)brushed aside. The minutes record:

> First, that the Curators of the Museum be instructed to adopt such measures as they may deem expedient to procure a plan and estimate of a Museum on an extensive scale, to be submitted to the College with as little delay as possible.
>
> Second, that a notice of Motion lately entered on the Minutes of the College, by which it is intended to be proposed that a large sum of money shall be applied, from the funds of the College to the establishment of a National Surgical Hospital be erased from the order of the proceedings...[69]

Later in the year, Kirby resigned from the Building Committee – possibly out of pique, possibly owing to personal tragedy (his wife Lucinda had recently died giving birth to their sixteenth child). Six years on, by which time the extension had proven itself a success, Kirby's ambition for a hospital was reborn.

In 1831, Francis White (1787–1859, Lic. 1813, MRCSI 1815, PRCSI 1836) – himself the proprietor of a small ophthalmic hospital on Ormond Quay – proposed the motion 'that the Establishment of a Clinical Hospital under

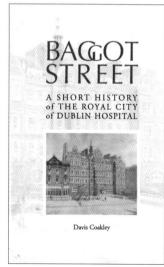

Cover of *Baggot Street: A Short History of the Royal City of Dublin Hospital* (1995) by Davis Coakley.

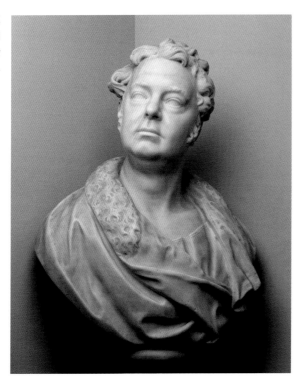

Bust of John T. Kirby, PRCSI 1823, 1834, by Thomas Kirk.

the Superintendence of the College, would greatly contribute to the improvement of surgical education in Ireland'. To no one's surprise, Kirby seconded the motion, but the old objections presented themselves too. Was it a wise use of funds? Colles for one did not think so; he moved an amendment calling for legal advice as to 'the practicability of applying the College Funds to the maintenance of a Clinical Hospital'.

This amendment was defeated, thirty votes to twenty-seven, and so a committee was formed, comprising White, Kirby and others. For whatever reason, no report from this committee reached the minute books — probably the committee was disbanded some time that winter. But from the ashes of that corporate proposal rose a private venture: six RCSI staff members — Jacob, Apjohn, Beatty, and Robert Harrison (1796–1858, Lic. 1816, MRCSI 1818, Prof of Anatomy and Physiology 1827–37, PRCSI 1848–49), Charles Benson (1797–1880, Lic. 1821, MRCSI 1825, Prof of Medicine 1836–72, PRCSI 1854–55) and John Houston — banded together and purchased a three-storey house that opened its doors in 1832 as, officially, the City of Dublin Hospital; though even when a Royal prefix was added in 1900, Dubliners still knew it as Baggot Street Hospital.

Its founders were justifiably pleased with their new premises:

> The situation of the building, and the construction of the wards offers peculiar advantages to the sick. It is on an elevated site, not crowded with surrounding houses. It commands a view of the Dublin and Wicklow mountains, and of the sea. And it possesses a large garden at the rere for convalescents to walk in. The wards have windows at both ends, and thus allow perfect ventilation.[70]

In Baggot Street's first year, nearly 20,000 people were treated as out-patients, 403 as in-patients. The income that year was £766, of which £600 was staff 'donations' – derived, essentially, from RCSI student fees.[71] The fact that this venture was extracurricular to RCSI side-stepped the potentially invidious difficulty of making staff appointments from within the College corps, but in everything but name, Baggot Street Hospital was fundamentally an RCSI-run hospital for the best part of the next fifty years.

Ironically, Kirby ended up unconnected to Baggot Street, having previously committed himself to the Charitable Infirmary, Jervis Street. In June of the year the new hospital opened – 1832 – he was appointed Professor of Medicine, in which capacity one of his first actions, in November, was to resign. This, apparently, was on health grounds ('I was influenced by the severity of my late Attack'[72]), but as he recovered before a replacement was found, he was re-appointed. Thus, despite not actually being retired, he nonetheless made a retirement gift to RCSI:

> SIR
> Having always intended to present my Museum to the College, when-
> ever I retired from the duties of Lecturer on anatomy and surgery, I
> now beg leave to offer it for acceptance, and I trust the Collection will
> be found not unworthy of a place in our National establishment.
> I have the honor to be
> Your faithful Servant
> J. Kirby[73]

RCSI gratefully accepted the offer – after all, they now had ample space for it – and as a mark of gratitude a bust of Kirby was commissioned. At the time of writing, it occupies a prominent place on the return of the Main Staircase in 123 St Stephen's Green – that is, neither up nor down, but fitting for a figure who never quite saw eye to eye with anyone for long.

THE RISE AND FALL OF JOHN HOUSTON'S MUSEUM

Had he not been so generous, Kirby might easily have sold his collection for a tidy sum. A short time after this – in 1836 – Trinity declined to purchase James Macartney's similar collection; it went instead to Cambridge, who offered £100 a year for ten years, and forty years later one TCD professor was still lamenting the loss: 'The board... were unacquainted with the importance of such an adjunct to medical education, and allowed it to pass into the hands of a more enlightened body.'[74]

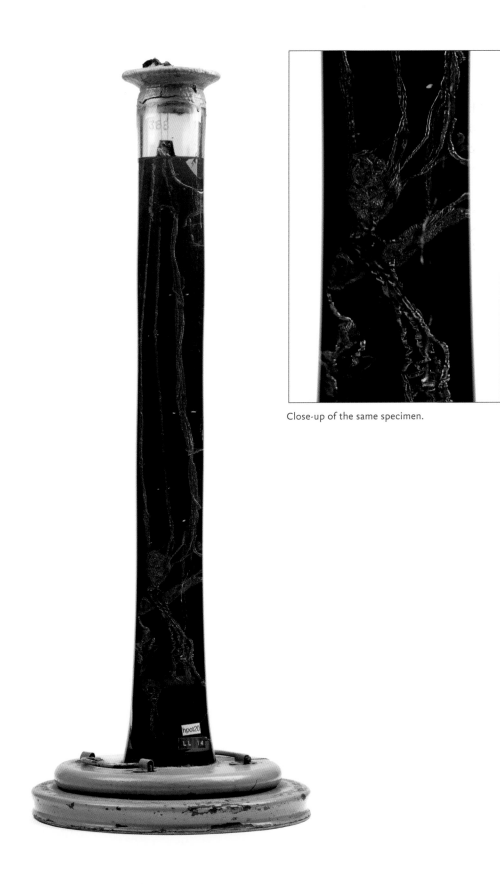

Close-up of the same specimen.

The role of such collections is perhaps obscured by the word 'museum', which has changed its meaning over time. In the medical world at this time, 'museum' denoted a collection of wet and dry specimens and preparations. ('Wet' means preserved in fluid; 'dry' implies desiccated; 'specimens' generally exhibited the exterior, whether in part or whole; 'preparations' were internal parts usually obtained by dissection.) Such a 'museum' was a state-of-the-art *desideratum* for any ambitious medical institution; it was a hands-on teaching resource, a research laboratory and a three-dimensional reference library, all rolled into one. (The more familiar concept of a museum as a silent, spick-and-span domain, where the eye is privileged over all other senses, dates from a later period.)

From the outset, then, the establishment of a museum at RCSI was a priority. Its beginnings were modest, when Professors Dease and Halahan made available their private collections. (By contrast, the London College began life with a 15,000-piece collection, bought for them by the government from John Hunter – hence, the Hunterian Museum.) Once the Mercer Street house was acquired, more contributions and purchases were added. By 1795, a catalogue was required to keep track of everything.

After 1810, the museum was slow to follow to St Stephen's Green; by the end of the decade a stable and coach house in the College's yard were converted into a 'School Museum'. This was unsatisfactory, however, and a committee was formed to establish the museum 'upon a scale commensurate with their other departments'. An annual budget of £200 was devoted to the museum, and in June 1820 the first official Curator (later Conservator), the ill-fated John Shekleton, was appointed. A mercurial injection of the lymphatics of the lower extremity that Shekleton produced as part of his application for the post remains on display in the Anatomy Room.

At the close of 1822 the museum held some 600 preparations; a year later this rose to 1,300, the bulk of which was donated by staff and licentiates (notably Colles, Robert Harrison (1796–1858, Lic. 1816, MRCSI 1818, Prof of Anatomy and Physiology 1827–37, PRCSI 1848) and Rawdon Macnamara (d. 1836, Lic. 1812, MRCSI 1815, Prof of

Facing page: Shekleton's mercurial injection of the lymphatic of the lower extremity.

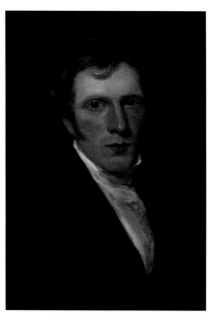

Portrait of John Houston. Artist unknown.

Materia Medica (hitherto Surgical Pharmacy) 1826–36, PRCSI 1831)). Shekleton was succeeded as Conservator by one of his apprentices, the 22-year-old John Houston (1802–1845, Lic. 1824, MRCSI 1826).

In fact, Houston attended his master's funeral in the morning and then in the afternoon sat for his Licence. 'He was a great favourite,' noted a contemporary, 'especially with the students... he possessed that rare faculty in an anatomical teacher, of interesting his audience in the object of his discourse...'[75] Houston wrote many scientific papers over his career, including in 1835 a description of the 'valves' of the rectum – ever since known as the 'valves of Houston'.[76] He was also a pioneer in the use of microscopes in medicine. 'Investigations of this nature,' he told the Surgical Society of Ireland in 1844,

> have opened a new door in the science of pathology, and will lead, it is to be hoped, to an accurate knowledge both of the nature of malignant diseases, and of the diagnostic differences between them and affections of a benign character.

So novel were his points on that occasion that he was obliged to begin with the basics: 'A *cell* is the ultimate limit of organised structure – an atom, beyond which, subdivision is impracticable.'[77] His notebooks, complete with cell drawings, survive in RCSI Heritage Collections.

Culpeper microscope — such as Houston would have used.

Houston's first major responsibility was to supervise the installation of the vast new museum facilitated by RCSI's expansion. Within a decade, when two new Honorary Members visited – Jules-Germain Cloquet (1790–1883, Hon. MRCSI 1836) and Friedrich Tiedemann (1781–1861, Hon. MRCSI 1836) – they both deemed the museum to be 'one of the most valuable in Europe'.[78] Its contents may be imaginatively reconstructed by Houston's 863-page *Descriptive Catalogue of the Preparations in the Museum of the Royal College of Surgeons in Ireland* (vol. 1, 1834, vol. 2, 1840).

The work is evidently a labour of love, with Houston's scientific rigour complemented by his humane sensitivity. The first entry of the first volume, for example, reads:

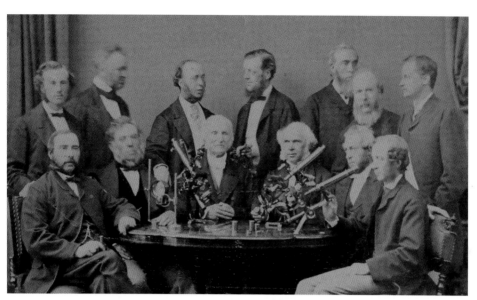

Members of the
Dublin Micro-
scopical Club,
1865.

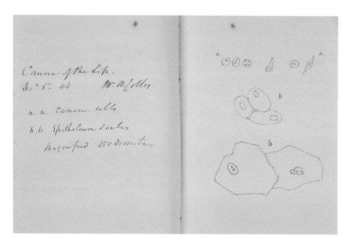

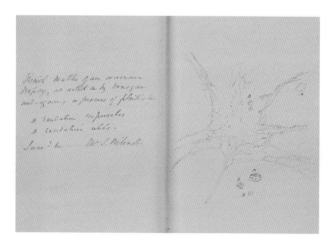

Cancer cells
from Houston's
notebooks.

A finely injected preparation, exhibiting the situation, form, and connections of the pharynx. The subject was that of a female, 13 years old. The posterior part of the head and the vertebral column have been removed, so as to expose the cavity from behind... The injection has nearly restored the natural colour of the lips and tongue, and given prominence to the villi of the mucous membrane. Artificial eyes, which have been substituted for the original, give a striking expression of life to the countenance...[79]

All human – and animal – life is here. Discussion of a human tongue is followed by comparison with the tongues of monkeys, lions or parrots ('no resemblance whatever can be traced... as an organ of speech'). The variety of animals is Noachian: in part or whole, wet or dry, there are swans, seals and scorpions, possums, pikes and panthers, cats, camels and chameleons.[80] There are he bones and innards of buffalo, elk and elephants, often acquired at considerable expense. The eight-foot whale prepuce, 'stuffed and dried',[81] is long gone now, but one of the same creature's vertebrae can still be seen in the Anatomy Room. Houston's second volume, devoted to 'Pathology', features many so-called 'monsters': 'Monsters with excess of parts (human)'; 'Monsters

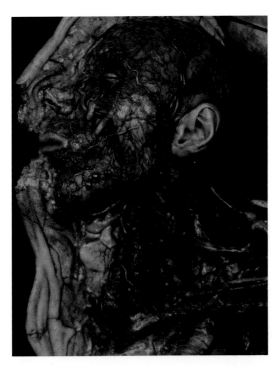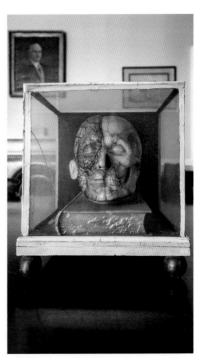

Wax models by Jacques Talrich from RCSI's Northumberland Collection.

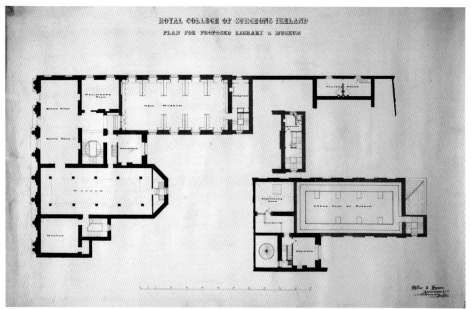

The heyday of the museums. First-floor plan of RCSI by Millar & Symes, c.1875, showing the 'New Museum' adjacent to York Street.

with deficiency of parts (human)'; 'Monsters with irregularity of parts (human)'; 'Specimens of monsters amongst the lower animals'. In addition, Peruvian and Egyptian mummies were displayed – the latter, after Houston's time, was 'unrolled by Professor Jacob at an evening *conversazione*, in the presence of the Lord Lieutenant and many distinguished guests'.[82] The ethics of human exhibition – and the discomfiting language that went with it – were very different in those days.

In an appendix, Houston also discusses one of the great treasures of RCSI: the Northumberland Wax Collection. Such 'ciroplastic' models had been highly valued teaching tools since the 1600s, reaching a sort of zenith in Florence's *Museo della Specola* at the end of the eighteenth century. (In Paris at the same time, Marie Tussaud was learning her trade as an apprentice to a physician, Philippe Curtius; later she moved to London – and Dublin, living in Clarendon Street – before opening her famous 'museum' in 1835.) The pedagogic advantages of wax models were manifold: they were clean, dry, astonishingly detailed, and not about to poison anybody, and before advances were made with preservation they were often more lifelike than the shrunken or discoloured real thing.

In 1829, the Lord Lieutenant, Hugh Percy, Duke of Northumberland, made a gift of £500 to RCSI for the specific purpose of purchasing a 'collection of Anatomical Preparations in Wax',[83] and to this end Houston set off for Paris, commissioning a set of models from the celebrated sculptor Jacques Talrich (1790–1851). The entire Northumberland Collection – which RCSI still holds – comprises forty-four wax models, the majority by Talrich; one is by the multi-talented Houston himself. The duke's gift was generous, but it was not quite on the scale of his uncle John Smithson's gift to the United States, which paid for the entire Smithsonian Museum.[84]

Soon after completing his *Descriptive Catalogue*, Houston resigned his Curatorship. He went on to produce another massive catalogue, this time of the Park Street School's museum (1843). While delivering a lecture in 1845, he was struck with 'violent head symptoms' – the result, claimed Richard Butcher, 'of an overworked brain'.[85] He died a short time later, at the age of 43. For the half-century after his death, the museum collection continued to grow – to the point where an annex was required. By this time the original museum on York Street was gone, converted into the upper floor of an extended library, but in 1875–78 this space reverted to its former purpose to accommodate a 'New Museum', images of which show a bony parade of massive animals surrounded by potted and vitirined specimens and preparations. (Later again, the upper area of this museum was sliced off for an attic laboratory, which in turn became the Nightingale Theatre.)

By the end of the nineteenth century the museum was still valued, but its days were numbered. Ironically, the heyday of medical museums was largely brought to an end by the same microscopes that fascinated Houston: the future of medical research would take place at a cellular level in laboratories. Terminal decline occurred in the early twentieth century, when Houston's museum was cleared out to create College Hall. What remained was housed in the 1870s annex – which itself fell into disrepair: in 1937, the then-Curator, William Boxwell (1875–1943, Prof of Pathology 1918–43), described the space as 'a lumber room and furniture store... what are left of the specimens in separate glass cases are in danger of irretrievable ruin'.[86] A portrait of Houston oversees his successors in the Surgeon Prosectors' Office,[87] while the Houston Lecture Theatre is named in his honour.

MANUSCRIPTS, MAGIC AND A MURDER:
THE BODIES AND BOOKS IN THE LIBRARY

The desire to establish a library dates back to the year of the original Charter. At that time, Members paid one guinea per annum to build up funds, though few books were bought during the peripatetic early years. The first outlay – on 12 January 1787 – was an advance subscription for the 'forthcoming' *Flora Dublinensis* by the Prof of Botany, Walter Wade. This was typical publishing practice

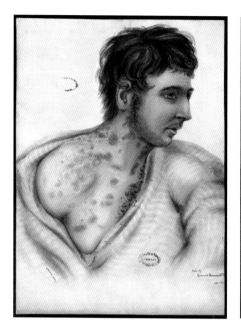 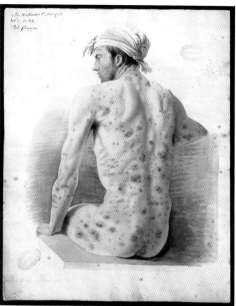

Illustrations from the William Wallace Collection.

in the era, a type of crowdfunding *avant la lettre*. Alas, by the time Wade died, thirty-seven years later, the volume remained unfinished and unpublished.

The collection began in earnest once the Mercer Street house was acquired. Books – and plates and drawings – were both bought and donated (in recognition of his Honorary Membership in 1790, John Hunter sent a gift of his works from London). But facilities were less than ideal: books were kept in an upper room which doubled as an overflow from the dissecting room.

Accommodation was much improved with the move to St Stephen's Green. The Library occupied a generous space on the ground floor with windows on to York Street; expansions and contractions notwithstanding, it stayed in this location until 1991. The first 'librarian' was John Armstrong Garnett (1767–1831, Lic. 1798, MRCSI 1800, Prof of Surgical Pharmacy 1803–13, PRCSI 1810). Garnett answered to a committee comprised of Colles, Richard Dease and Sir Henry Jebb (d. 1811, MRCSI 1784, Prof of Midwifery 1793–94, PRCSI 1800). The lion's share of the work seems to have fallen to the 'assistant librarian', Charles Hawkes Todd (1782–1826, Lic. 1803, MRCSI 1805, Prof of Anatomy and Physiology 1819–26, Prof of Surgery 1819–26, PRCSI 1821), appointed in 1811.

None of these positions attracted any salary, and as Todd's professorial career took off he was glad to give up his library duties. In 1819, James William Cusack was appointed to the 'assistant' role, while the 'Clerk and Housekeeper', Peter

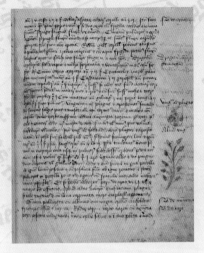

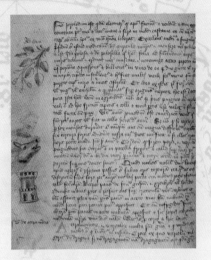

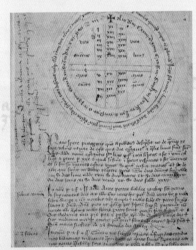

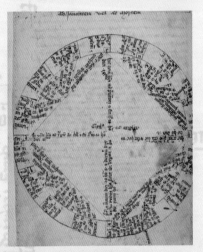

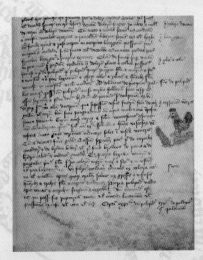

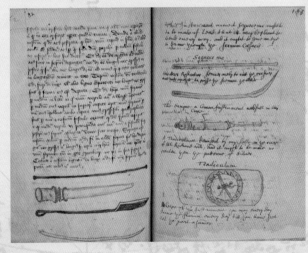

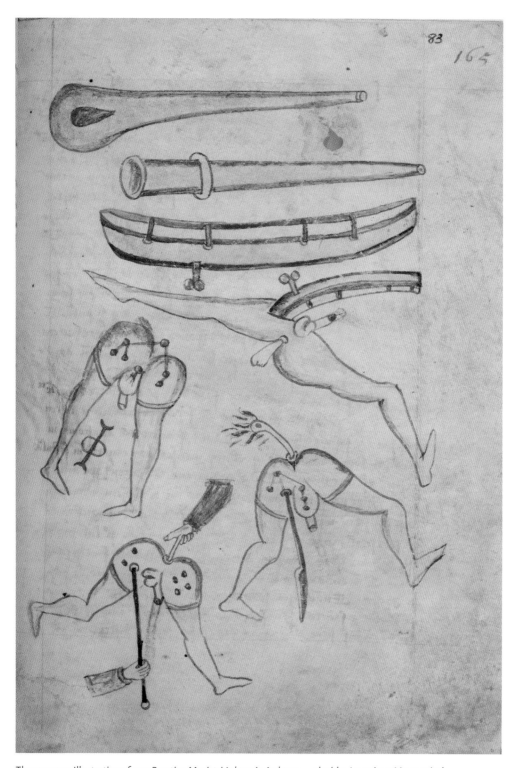

These pages: Illustrations from *Practica Magistri Johannis Arderne* — aka 'the Lentaigne Manuscript'.

Ruttledge (d. 1832), 'took charge of the books'.[88] Other titles and roles would come and go, but for the next century or so a senior member of staff (later a Council-member) served as overseeing 'honorary librarian', while day-to-day tasks fell to the Clerk (later, Registrar). In 1835, when the Library became a 'circulating' one – that is, books could be taken away for reading – Courtney's successor, Cornelius O'Keefe, was obliged to be present between 10 and 11 a.m. on Mondays, Wednesdays and Fridays to issue and collect books, for which he earned an extra £10 per annum.

By this time the collection was 'of respectable dimensions', thanks in part to a number of bulk acquisitions, notably the library of the defunct Physico-Chirurgical Society (1790–1816). Later, Jacob and Sir Philip Crampton both bequeathed significant private collections.[89] To keep track, catalogues were prepared in 1825, 1839 and 1874. From 1830 the Library spread over two floors, one directly above the other. Around the time the Library marked its golden jubilee, the collection numbered more than 14,000 volumes; in the half-century that followed, this figure would double again. Many rare and valuable volumes survive to the present day, including: a 1544 Latin translation of *The Canon of Medicine* (*Canon Medicinae*) by the Persian physician Avicenna, or Ibn Sina in the Islamic tradition; a 1550 copy of Galen's *De usu partium corporis humani* (*On the utility of the parts of the body*); a second edition (1555) of Vesalius' *De Humani Corporis Fabrica* (*On the Fabric of the Human Body*); and a 1660 printing of Harvey's *Exercitatio Anatomica de Motu Cordis et Sanguinis in Animalibus* (*An Anatomical Exercise on the Motion of the Heart and Blood in Living Beings*).

In 1838, the Library purchased for £50 a remarkable cache of clinical notebooks and drawings belonging to William Wallace (1791–1837, Lic. 1813, MRCSI 1815).[90] Arguably the leading figure in the history of dermatology in Ireland, Wallace's interest in skin afflictions began during his apprenticeship (to Charles Hawkes Todd) at the Townsend Street Lock Hospital, after which he studied under the skin specialist Thomas Bateman (1778–1821) in London.

Wallace returned to Dublin to open the Dublin Infirmary for Diseases of the Skin at 20 Moore Street – the first such hospital in Europe (or indeed anywhere in the British Empire). In its first year, Wallace treated some 1,775 cases (scabies was the commonest complaint, followed by measles, scarlet fever, leprosy, lice and smallpox). One of his important innovations was to use potassium iodide in the treatment of venereal disease (as opposed to mercury); this became standard practice until the advent of penicillin. In addition, he proved the contagiousness of secondary syphilitic lesions – unfortunately, he did so by deliberately infecting healthy patients and watching their symptoms develop. His casebooks – which survive in RCSI Heritage Collections – exhibit no scruples whatsoever about this practice.

The accompanying drawings – life-sized and unsparingly detailed – were made by two artists, William Burke Kirwan and James Connolly.[91] (Kirwan later gained notoriety of his own after he was convicted of the murder of his wife on Ireland's Eye off Howth in 1852.) Wallace was by all accounts a difficult colleague, and when he died in 1837 – of typhus, likely contracted from a patient – he had fostered no successor to take over the Infirmary. It closed within months, having treated some 25,000 cases in twenty years. Library ledgers show that Wallace was a voracious reader whose record, as a borrower at least, was unblemished: even the four books he had out at the time of his death were returned on time.

In 1851, the Library acquired its most treasured manuscript, the *Practica Magistri Johannis Arderne*. Its author, John Arderne (1307–*c*.1390) of Newark in Nottinghamshire, was probably the first English surgeon of any repute. The manuscript, which is not in Arderne's hand, dates from the early fifteenth century. Broadly speaking, it has two parts, one astrological, concerned with prognosis; the other, larger, part deals with surgical practice, notably Arderne's treatment of *fistula-in-ano*.

Today, this would likely be diagnosed as pilonidal disease, characterised by a painful cyst at the upper end of the intergluteal cleft, which in Arderne's day was an occupational hazard for knights on horseback (curiously, it made a comeback during World War II as 'Jeep riders' disease'). Before Arderne, the condition was generally considered incurable, and even in the nineteenth century commentators looked on his technique as 'heroic'.[92] The manuscript's many margin illustrations of herbs, flowers, birds and animals are colourful and charming; the sketches of medical instruments and how to apply them offer a vivid glimpse of an era when sharp steel was complemented by magic spells ('write this which I have made known on the handle of a knife and kill therewith a full grown or a young pig, and see that blood has not come forth on it'[93]).

Of the forty-three surviving Arderne manuscripts worldwide, most are damaged or incomplete, whereas RCSI's copy is 'perfect and in an excellent state of preservation'.[94] It was presented to the Library by Sir John Lentaigne (1803–1886, FRCSI 1844) and has been known since as 'the Lentaigne Manuscript'.[95]

RICHARD CARMICHAEL'S *PLAN OF MEDICAL REFORM AND REORGANISATION*

Reform was the watchword of the 1830s. In the political sphere, it was there in the passage of the Catholic Emancipation Act (1829), the Great Reform Act (1832) and the Slavery Abolition Act (1833). In the medical world, it was in

Thomas Wakley's establishment of *The Lancet* (1823) – conceived from the start as the scourge of nepotists, quacks and incompetents – and, closer to home, the *Dublin Medical Press* (1839). But perhaps the most consistent, and most radical, voice for Irish medical reform belonged to Richard Carmichael (1776–1849, Lic. 1803, MRCSI 1804, PRCSI 1813, 1826, 1845).

On 29 May 1839, at a meeting in RCSI, Carmichael founded the Medical Association of Ireland, the purpose of which was 'the protection of its members in their just and legal rights'.[96] In addition, it administered a benevolent fund for doctors and the families who fell into financial distress. One of the most striking proposals made at that first meeting ran as follows:

> It is, therefore, our opinion a legislative measure should be sought for by us, to unite the medical profession in Ireland into a corporation, upon such principles as shall constitute them one National Faculty, and thereby identify, in feelings and interests, the great mass of provincial practitioners with their metropolitan brethren.[97]

Colles, for one, reacted strongly to this suggestion. 'As to the establishment of one school and licensing body,' he wrote, 'that would blast the profession.' As far as he was concerned, RCSI had come too far in its fifty-five years to allow itself to be swallowed whole by some national quango. After all, just recently, in 1837, an editorial in the *Edinburgh Medical Journal* had declared that 'the Royal College of Surgeons in Dublin is, perhaps, the most enlightened surgical incorporation in Europe, and requires from its members a greater range of accurate knowledge than any other body, excepting' – this caveat was no surprise – 'the Medical Faculty of the University of Edinburgh'.[98]

Colles' further comments give a sense of the various pressures then bearing down on Irish medical schools in general, and RCSI in particular. 'Let there be competition,' he argued,

> only for competition with the College of Physicians our scientific meetings would never have been established. Going on with this project is only plunging into a sea of difficulties. It is embroiling us with the other corporations, it will bring down the University upon us... Let us give up parliamentary business and make a new effort in science. Let the hospital surgeons work the hospitals, and let us all show the advantages of Dublin as a medical school, its University, its cheapness. It had been said that steam would take

our pupils and business away from us, but steam went both ways, and the carriages might come here. We ought to bring men here from England to graduate... Let us, instead of quarrelling, put forward our advantages and the steamboats would arrive, loaded with English money. Let us only raise the character of our diploma to its former rank – Let us only be united.[99]

Carmichael and Colles often disagreed – notably in their preferred treatments for venereal disease, their uneasily shared specialty – but in the reformist debate, Carmichael seems to have taken Colles' point. Two years later, in 1841, he published a far-seeing document with a telling subtitle: *Plan of Medical Reform and Reorganization of the Profession, without subverting the existing Colleges of Physic and Surgery.* His comments therein on the 'artificial and unnatural' division of medicine and surgery are worth quoting in full – not least as this would soon become the orthodox view:

PLAN

OF

MEDICAL REFORM

AND

REORGANIZATION OF THE PROFESSION,

WITHOUT SUBVERTING THE

EXISTING COLLEGES OF PHYSIC AND SURGERY,

ADDRESSED TO THE

RIGHT HON. SIR R. PEEL, BART.

BY

RICHARD CARMICHAEL, M.R.I.A.

President of the Medical Association of Ireland; Corresponding Member of the Royal Academy of
Medicine of France, &c.; and Consulting Surgeon of the Richmond, Hardwicke, and
Whitworth Hospitals.

" If the united voice of nearly all the individuals who constitute the
Medical Profession, may be admitted as a just indication of the necessity
for reform, nothing more need be said in proof of the existence of that
necessity ; for that united voice is already raised in favour of the measure."
T. KIDD, M.D.
Regius Professor of Medicine in the
University of Oxford.

DUBLIN

WILLIAM CURRY, JUN. AND CO. SACKVILLE-STREET.
LONGMAN, BROWN, AND CO. LONDON.
FRASER AND CO., EDINBURGH.
1841.

Richard Carmichael's *Plan of Medical Reform (1841).*

Notwithstanding that the Colleges of Physicians of London and Dublin still insist upon a distinct education in physic and surgery, and will not admit a surgeon into either of their respective bodies until he has disenfranchised himself from the College of Surgeons to which he belongs; yet it is now generally admitted that this distinction between physic and surgery is so artificial and unnatural that it is totally impossible to draw any line of demarcation between them, so as to indicate to either physician or surgeon his peculiar province; and it is certain that there cannot be a good physician who has not the knowledge of a surgeon, or a good surgeon who has not the knowledge of a physician; therefore it is obvious that both should be educated alike.[100]

COLLES AND THE QUICKSILVER CURE

By the time of these debates, Colles had relinquished his Chair of Surgery.[101] But if he stepped down from teaching, he was as active as ever in other matters, as a tribute address made clear:

> ... it is the unanimous feeling of the College that the exemplary and efficient manner in which you have filled the chair for thirty two years, has been a principal cause of the success and consequent high character of the School of Surgery in this country. It is gratifying to the Members that although they lose the advantage of your valuable services as Professor in the School of the College, you will still continue to afford your disinterested assistance in promoting the general welfare of the institution, and sustaining the profession of surgery in public estimation.[102]

As tokens of esteem, Colles' likeness was sculpted by Thomas Kirk and painted by Martin Cregan. In his first year of retirement, he finally finished his labour of many years, a 350-page study entitled *Practical Observations on the Venereal Disease and on the Use of Mercury* (1837).

From a modern point of view, Colles and his contemporaries were working in the dark. Syphilis was highly infectious and contagious, but little else could be said with confidence except that it was 'a poison'. Everyone knew how it was transmitted, but conjecture and rumour still abounded ('Erinensis' told the slanderous story that Colles once asked his colleague Ralph Obré if the disease could be contracted from 'sitting on a public privy'; Obré is supposed to have replied that 'it was sometimes the manner in which *married* men contracted it, but *unmarried* men never caught it in this manner'[103]).

Colles' interest in the condition dated back to 1820, when the male patients of Westmoreland Lock Hospital were transferred to Dr Steevens' Hospital (the name 'lock hospital' refers to earlier leprosy hospitals where patients wore rags or 'locks' to cover their lesions). The *Observations* was hailed by many as Colles' 'greatest work', establishing him as 'one of the great authorities' in the field.[104] A good deal of the book charts Colles' favoured mercury treatment – essentially, an early chemotherapy. The element was used externally in the form of ointments, plasters and fumigations, and internally in its crude state and in salts.

The efficacy of treatment was measured by the amount of salivation produced: patients were expected to fill several mugs' worth per day. For 'rubbing', an unction was prepared, often by mixing the mercury with hog lard (profes-

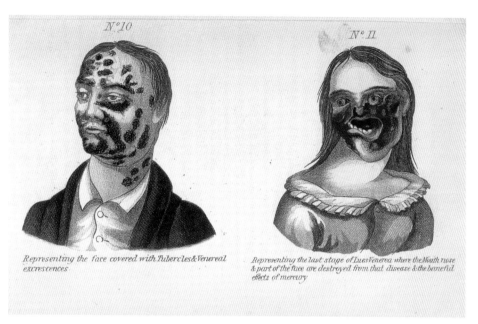

Nº 10

Nº 11

Representing the face covered with Tubercles & Venereal excrescences

Representing the last stage of Lues Venerea where the Mouth nose & part of the face are destroyed from that disease & the baneful effects of mercury

Illustrations of the effects of venereal disease and mercury treatment. Wellcome Collection.

sional rubbers used pig's bladders as gloves to protect their hands). The danger, of course, was from mercury poisoning, and Colles gave a graphic description of how this manifested:

In some case, however, we find that these alarmingly large doses of mercury do excite a ptyalism, not that gentle, manageable kind which is our anxious wish to obtain, but rather a sudden, a violent, and an ungovernable action which overwhelms the system and threatens destruction to life. The day preceding the appearance of this violent salivation the patient announces its approach by informing us that he was feverish and restless the preceding night, and that he has great headaches or tormina, or dysenteric dejections from his bowels. On the following day his cheeks and lips are enormously swollen, there is copious and incessant flow of saliva, the tongue is protruded and swollen, the speech is impaired, and deglutition is so impeded that he cannot even drink without much difficulty. Haemorrhages from the gums to a pretty large amount in many instances occur repeatedly; the tongue continuing swollen and protruded the edges more particularly on their lower surface, become indented and ulcerated from the pressure of the teeth. When awake he hangs his head over some vessel to receive the saliva, which flows copiously and incessantly, and when overcome by fatigue he attempts to sleep, the saliva still flows, and bathes his pillow with a foetid moisture; his sleep is broken and unrefreshing, and is frequently interrupted by a sudden and alarming sense of suffocation... After two or three weeks passed in this way, but with little alteration, the saliva at length becomes more thick and ropy, and the patient feels a strong desire for food, but is totally unable to take any in a solid form, and he suffers exquisitely in attempting to swallow any, even the blandest fluid; and thus he is harassed on the one hand by a craving for food and nourishment, and on the other by the apprehension of acute pain attending every attempt at mastication or deglutition.[105]

The reader is reminded that all of the above is caused by the treatment, not the disease. In subsequent decades, studies established that mercury treatment was iatrogenic – that is, it actively caused harm – but even in Colles' time there was growing 'non-mercurial' school of thought (this was Carmichael's position, but even as he and Colles differed sharply in opinion, the manner of their debate remained 'courteous and friendly'[106]).

After blighting untold numbers of lives for centuries, the end of syphilis came remarkably swiftly. In 1905, its causal microorganism, the single-cell corkscrew-shaped *Treponema pallidum*, was isolated; a year later a blood test was available, and during the next year, at his laboratory in Frankfurt, Paul Ehrlich (1854–1915) synthesized an effective cure, arsphenamine, aka Salvarsan.

A LAST LESSON

In 1839, Colles declined a baronetcy, saying such distinctions held 'no attraction' for him.[107] For some time he had been suffering from gout and bronchitis, and in 1841 he made a tour of Switzerland for his health. He improved temporarily, but in October 1842 he felt the end was approaching; accordingly, he wrote the following letter to his friend (and successor as Chair of Anatomy and Physiology), Prof Robert Harrison:

My Dear Robert,
I think it may be of some benefit, not only to my own family, but to society at large, to ascertain by examination the exact seat and nature of my last disease. I am sure you will grant my request, that you will see this be carefully and early done. The parts to which I would direct particular attention are the heart and lungs, a small hernia immedi-

ately above the umbilicus, and the swelling in the right hypochondrium. From the similarity of the Rev. P. Roe's case with mine, I suppose
there is some connection between the swelling of the hypochondrium
and the diseased state of the heart.
Yours truly, dear Robert,
A. Colles[108]

Colles died a year later, on 1 December 1843, at home in Kingstown (Dún
Laoghaire). When the news reached the city, all of its medical schools closed
immediately as a mark of respect. On the day of the funeral, the north and west
sides of St Stephen's Green were impassable due to the great number of mourners and carriages.

The Fellows of RCPI walked from their President's house in Merrion Square,
joined by members of the Apothecaries Company; members of the judiciary
walked too, headed by the Master of the Rolls. As the hearse passed 123 St Stephen's Green, the doors opened and President James O'Beirne (1787–1862,
Lic. 1810, MRCSI 1820, PRCSI 1843) processed out ahead of the Members
and the Licentiates; remaining on foot, they followed the cortège to Mount
Jerome Cemetery.[109]

Some days earlier, Robert Harrison, Henry Marsh and William Stokes were in
attendance as Robert Smith fulfilled Colles' last request. The findings of their
post-mortem examination were communicated to the Pathological Society of
Dublin. There was evidence of chronic bronchitis, a fibrotic left lung, and a
dilated and fatty heart with no indication of valvular disease. Once a teacher,
always a teacher. William Stokes called this 'the last great act of Mr. Colles's
medical career'. ■

Chapter 4:
Invention and Innovation, 1844–85

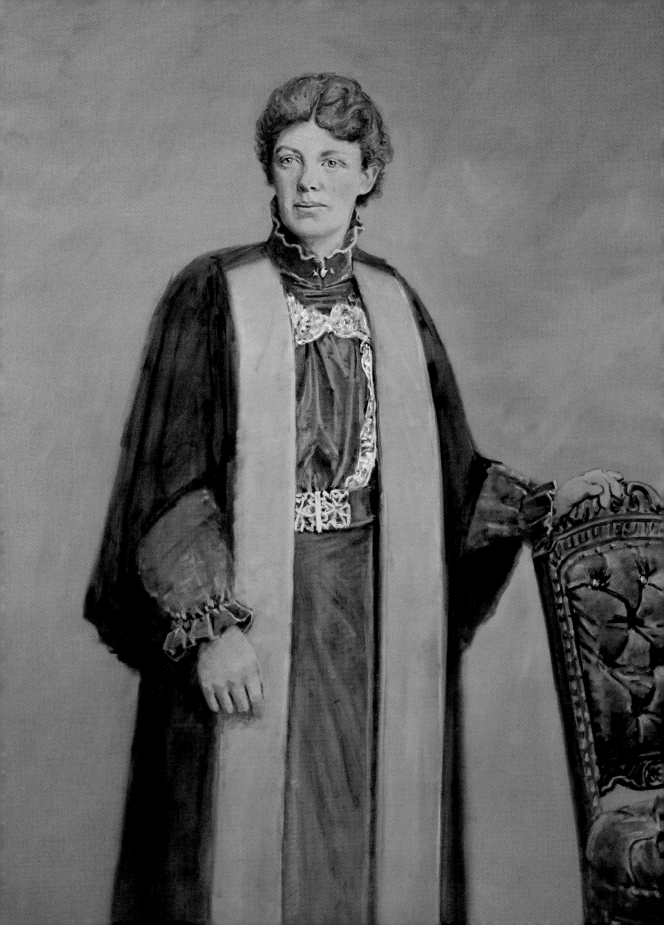

Chapter 4:
Invention and Innovation, 1844–85

EMINENT VICTORIANS

Shortly after the death of Abraham Colles, the grant of a Supplemental Charter (11 January 1844) ushered in a new age at RCSI. For the first time, the royal authority was a woman, Queen Victoria, then in the seventh year of her reign. Five years later, in 1849, her scientifically minded husband, Prince Albert, visited RCSI, afterwards saying he was 'much gratified with the Museum and other parts of the institution'.[1] When he died in 1861, aged 42, RCSI scrambled to memorialise him: a bust was swiftly commissioned and installed, and since renovation work was already underway in a new sunken-floor area off the Entrance Hall, this became the Albert Hall (from 1979, the Albert Theatre).

The Supplemental Charter had three notable innovations. First, it introduced a governing Council, capped at twenty-one persons, consisting of the President and Vice-President, the remainder being elected from a new body – this was the second innovation – the Fellows of the College. Previously – from 1784 – there had only been the Licentiates and, above them, the Members, who had voting rights within the College. A Licentiate could become a Member after they

Previous page: Emily Winifred Dickson by Mick O'Dea (2019).

they had been in practice for three years (four after 1830). However, in London, anyone who passed the Royal College of Surgeons' basic examinations was immediately styled a Member; they had no grade that indicated greater experience or higher achievement.

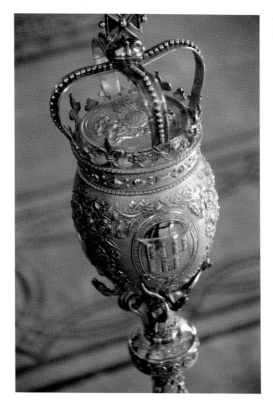

The College Mace.

As part of the general reform and reorganisation of the period, the London College introduced a Fellowship examination to create this tiered distinction. As a result, RCSI was obliged to overhaul its nomenclature too. Henceforth, Members were to be called Fellows. In addition, to level the playing field, for the period of one calendar year, any other working surgeons, whether they were RCSI Licentiates or not, could be granted the new RCSI Fellowship without having to sit an examination; it was in this manner that distinguished surgeons such as William Wilde and Richard Butcher (of whom more later) gained their post-nominal letters FRCSI – and 352 others did the same.

Once the grace year elapsed, prospective Fellows were obliged to sit searching two-day public exams. Day One consisted of a written examination on 'anatomy and physiology, surgery, medicine, midwifery, chemistry, materia medica and medical jurisprudence'; candidates were 'directed to answer as many under each head as time [two hours] would permit'. Day Two required the candidate to 'perform operations on the dead Body' in the anatomical theatre, after which came a final *viva voce* exam.[2] Of the first two candidates who presented themselves, on 27 and 28 May 1845, only one, Joliffe Tufnell (1819–1885, FRCSI 1845, Prof of Military Surgery, 1851–60, PRCSI 1874–75), was deemed to have made the grade.

The third innovation was the establishment of a (paid) Court of Examiners to replace the (unpaid) censors and Court of Assistants. Finally, amongst other lesser developments, there was ordinance 22:

And we do hereby grant and declare that it shall be and may be lawful for the said College, at all times hereafter, and upon all occasions as they shall think proper and expedient, to exercise and enjoy the right and privilege of having a Mace, and causing the same to be borne by such officer as they shall appoint for that purpose.[3]

In 1854, West & Son supplied RCSI with its ornate and weighty ceremonial mace; a similar one is still in use on formal occasions.[4] It cost £110, which perhaps goes some way to explain the decade-long delay. The cost of the Supplemental Charter was to be £220, but on the grounds that it was a 'short period' since the last Charter — fourteen years, in fact — this was reduced by the officers of the Crown to £94 17*s* 3*d*.

THE LIFE AND AFTERLIFE OF 'FLOURISHING PHIL'

The first President under the Supplemental Charter was Sir Philip Crampton (1777–1858, Lic. 1798, MRCSI 1801, PRCSI 1811, 1820, 1844, 1855), the third of his four terms in the chair. While the likes of Colles and Jacob made scientific and pedagogic advances on which their legacies justly rest, Crampton was probably the most famous surgical practitioner in Dublin at this time. And yet, within two

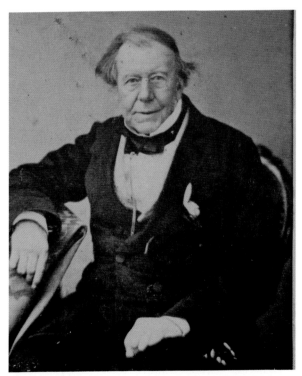

Sir Philip Crampton, PRCSI 1811, 1820, 1844, 1855.

generations, he was all but forgotten: in Joyce's *Ulysses*, Leopold Bloom rides in a carriage past a memorial in Crampton's honour and thinks, 'Who was he?'[5]

Aged 14, Crampton had been indentured to Solomon Richards (the only other four-time PRCSI); he attended RCSI in Mercer Street and took both a surgeon's mate diploma and his Licence in 1798. Three days later, aged 21, he succeeded the unfortunate William Dease as surgeon at the Meath Hospital, a position

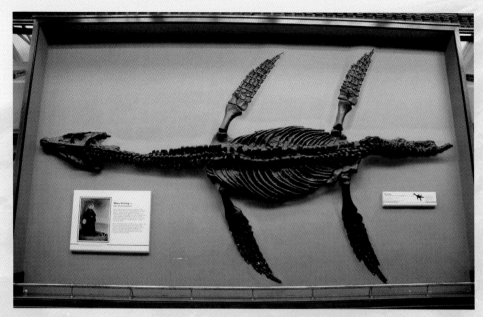

he retained for the next sixty years. A dandiacal dresser and a striking figure ('about six feet in height, slightly formed, elegantly proportioned, and elastic as corkwood'[6]), Crampton revelled in publicity.

Already esteemed by peers, his wider reputation took off following an incident in 1810, when a waiter in a tavern opposite his house in Dawson Street began to choke on a piece of meat. Crampton dashed across the road and performed an emergency tracheostomy; the man recovered and the heroic tale spread like wildfire. In 1813 he was appointed to the important (and lucrative) position of Surgeon-General, at which point he closed the private anatomy school he ran behind his house. Thereafter, 'Flourishing Phil' (as the Dublin wags called him) moved in the most fashionable circles. He bought one house on Merrion Square and another at Lough Bray, County Wicklow. In advanced age he liked to boast that he could still swim across the lough, ride into Dublin and amputate a limb – all before breakfast.

Crampton attained 'every honour which is usually bestowed upon eminent medical men': he was successively Surgeon-in-Ordinary in Ireland to George IV and Queen Victoria; the latter made him a baronet in 1839. A colleague noted that Crampton's great forte lay in acute observation:

> ... a look, a touch, one or two pregnant questions, and the diagnosis was made, and the treatment determined upon. And with this rapidity of judgment – so captivating to the looker-on, and so fatal to those who, with

less accurate eye and feebler powers of deduction, attempt to copy it — he seldom erred. To the last his hand was light and steady, his movements as an operator quietly graceful, devoid of ostentatious show, rapid, but not hurried, cool in every emergency, and prompt in every danger.[7]

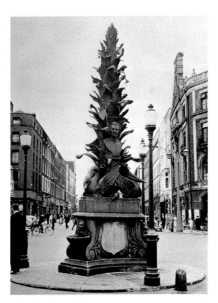

The Crampton Memorial, D'Olier Street. © Creative Commons.

In some respects, Crampton's interests were more zoological than medical (though in the era this was not a distinction that mattered much). He was the first president of the Dublin Zoological Society (established, like RCSI, at the Rotunda) and was instrumental in securing the zoo's home in Phoenix Park. An avian eye muscle, *musculus cramptonius*, and a species of giant, extinct sea reptile, the seven-foot-long plesiosaur, *Rhomaleosaurus cramptoni*, are both named in Crampton's honour.

In contrast to Colles, Crampton did not want anyone learning from his remains, so he ordered that his body should be encased in cement. Four years later, in 1862, the Crampton Memorial that puzzles Leopold Bloom was unveiled at the junction of D'Olier Street, College Street and Brunswick (now Pearse) Street. At the base was a public fountain, reflecting the surgeon's interest in the supply of drinking water to Dublin; this was topped with a bust of Crampton set amid a variety of birdlife; above that towered twenty-five feet of exotic metal fronds.

From the start, opinion seems to have been divided on whether it was offensively hideous or merely laughable. Locals dubbed it 'the Cauliflower' or 'the Artichoke', while Myles na gCopaleen judged it 'an enormous rotting pineapple'.[8] A letter-writer to the *Irish Times* lampooned Crampton's teetotalism by asking if it was erected to frighten passers-by into one of the eleven pubs nearby.[9] Worse was to come: in 1959, part of the sculpture's foliage collapsed on a postal worker who was eating his lunch; he was taken to Mercer's Hospital and made a full recovery. But it was the end of the Crampton Memorial, which was duly dismantled and carted off.[10]

TO THE POINT: FRANCIS RYND AND THE HYPODERMIC SYRINGE

Crampton's cementitious last request was carried out by one of his former apprentices, Francis Rynd (1801–1861, MRCSI 1830). Rynd is widely credited as the inventor of the forerunner of the modern hypodermic syringe. An article in the *Dublin Medical Press* (1845) recorded its first use:

> Margaret Cox, aetat. 59, of spare habit, was admitted into hospital, May 18, 1844, complaining of acute pain over the entire of left side of face, particularly in the supra-orbital region, shooting into the eye, along the branches of the portio dura in the cheek, along the gums of both upper and lower jaw, much increased in this situation by shutting the mouth and pressing her teeth close together, and occasionally darting to the opposite side of the face and to the top and back of her head... On the 3rd of June a solution of fifteen grains of acetate of morphia, dissolved in one drachm of creosote, was introduced to the supra-orbital nerve, and along the course of the temporal, malar, and buccal nerves, by four punctures of an instrument made for the purpose... In the space of a minute, all pain (except that caused by the operation, which was very slight,) had ceased, and she slept better that night than she had done for months.

In November that year, a 28-year-old man who had been bedridden with pain in his right leg for almost three years came under Rynd's care, and a similar injection was performed ('one puncture behind the trochanter, and one half-way down the thigh'): 'He was instantly relieved from pain and walked steadily through the ward'. Rynd administered a follow-up injection some days later, after which the man was 'perfectly well'.[11]

Rynd's purpose-made instrument had a hollow needle but not a plunger, and so relied on gravity to introduce the fluid. In 1853, a French surgeon, Charles Pravaz (1791–1853), adapted Rynd's invention by adding a screw to control the flow. Meanwhile, in Edinburgh and London, respectively, Alexander Wood (1817–1884) and Charles Hunter (1835–1878) both had the idea to add the more familiar plunger – thereby giving rise to a long, fractious public debate about which of them deserved the greater credit.[12]

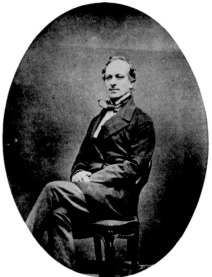

Francis Rynd. Wellcome Collection.

Francis Rynd's
article in the
*Dublin Quar-
terly Journal of
Medical Science*
(1861).

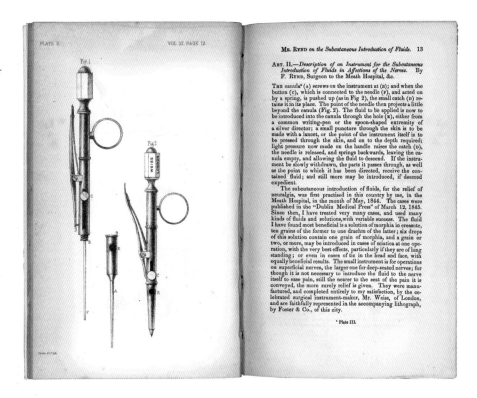

Francis Rynd's article in the *Dublin Quarterly Journal of Medical Science* (1861).

Rynd's contribution looked to be forgotten until he belatedly entered the fray, publishing in 1861 a fuller, illustrated account of his earlier innovation. This secured his reputation – though it came in the nick of time, as he suffered a fatal heart attack that summer following a minor traffic accident in Clontarf. The same issue of the *Dublin Quarterly Journal of Medical Science* in which he published his reputation-saving article also carried his obituary, edged in mourning black.[13]

'IT'S ALL DONE, ALICE': THE AGE OF ANAESTHESIA

Rynd's experiment was part of the great surgical riddle of the ages: how to control pain. To the astonishment of the world, this riddle was solved at Massachusetts General Hospital on 16 October 1846. For the first time publicly, a dentist, William T.G. Morton (1819–1868), administered ether to a patient so that a surgeon, John C. Warren (1778–1856), could painlessly remove a subcutaneous lump from the patient's neck.[14]

Three weeks later, on 7 November, a more testing, 'capital' operation took place. This time the patient was Alice Mohan, a 21-year-old Irish-born servant with a tubercular right leg. As the operating surgeon, George Hayward (1798– 1863), later recalled:

For some months before the operation her constitutional symptoms had become threatening, and the removal of the limb seemed to be the only chance for her life. The ether was administered by Dr. Morton. In a little more than three minutes she was brought under the influence of it; the limb was removed and all the vessels tied but the last, which was the sixth, before she gave any indication of consciousness or suffering. She then groaned and cried out faintly...[15]

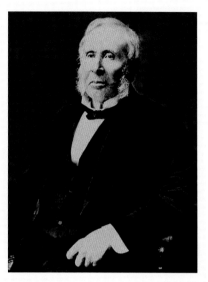

John MacDonnell.

At this point, Hayward indulged in some regrettable theatrics. He bent over her. 'I guess you've been asleep, Alice.' 'I think I have, sir,' she replied. 'Well, you know why we brought you here; are you ready?' 'Yes, sir, I am ready.' Hayward then lifted the amputated limb from the sawdust and showed it to her. 'It's all done, Alice.' Alice's reaction is not recorded, apart from Hayward's comment that 'she seemed much surprised'.[16]

News of the wonder spread fast. On 19 December, having read a letter about events in Boston, an American dentist in London, Francis Boott (1792– 1863), performed a molar extraction on a patient under ether. Two days later, on Monday, 21 December, the Scottish surgeon Robert Liston (1794–1847) performed Europe's first capital operation under ether at University College Hospital, London. The patient was a butler named Frederick Churchill, suffering from chronic osteomyelitis of the tibia. 'Now gentlemen, time me,' Liston told his audience, brandishing his favourite amputation knife (it had notches in the handle to count previous operations). He set to – for twenty-eight seconds, after which the limb lay in the sawdust. As the stump was being dressed, Churchill tried to raise himself. 'When are you going to begin?' he asked; then he said he'd changed his mind, only to have his attention directed to his elevated stump, whereupon he slumped back, wept a little, and was stretchered out.[17]

A little more than a week later – on Wednesday, 30 December – John MacDonnell (1796–1892, Lic. 1821, MRCSI 1827, Prof of Descriptive Anatomy 1847–51) was contemplating a procedure scheduled for the next morning in Dublin's Richmond Hospital, the amputation of a young girl's arm. A colleague drew his attention to an article in an advance copy of January's *British and Foreign*

Early apparatuses for anaesthesia.

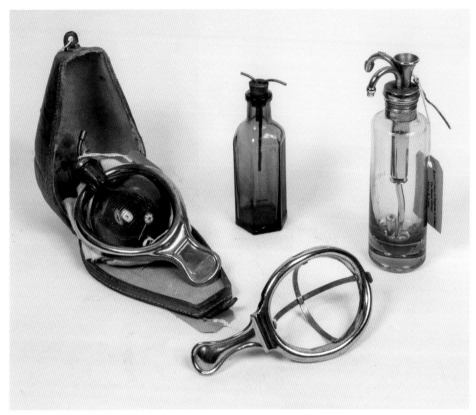

Medical Review, in which Liston's recent amputation under ether was discussed. MacDonnell immediately postponed the girl's operation and set about improvising the necessary apparatus:

> I procured a bottle with two necks, into one of which I introduced the tube of a funnel, made air-tight in the neck of the bottle by adhesive plaster rolled round it, and to the other, I adapted a double tube furnished with Read's ball valve. A sponge being placed in the funnel, and saturated with pure sulphuric ether, the apparatus was now fit for use...

With an assistant present, he tried it out several times, rendering himself satisfactorily unconscious. Then on Friday, New Year's Day, 1847, the patient was brought in. She was Mary Kane, an 18-year-old who had suffered a thorn-prick some six weeks before. Within a fortnight the puncture had turned dangerously ulcerous and she began to lose significant weight. MacDonnell's first attempt to render her insensible failed, but the second was successful. He then amputated her arm.

Twice before the dressing of the wound was completed, the patient gave evidence of suffering, just at the moment of finishing the division of the muscles, and again at the time of tying one of the arteries. Her own testimony is clear and positive, that she had no unpleasant sensation from the inhalation, and that till, as she says, she 'saw me put a thread on her arm,' she felt nothing.

Unlike Liston, who let others tell of his triumph, MacDonnell was taking no chances: he sat down that afternoon and wrote a full account of the operation and fired it off to the *Dublin Medical Press*. His final paragraph reads:

I regard this discovery as one of the most important of this century. It will rank with vaccination, and other of the greatest benefits that medical science has bestowed upon man. It adds to the long list of those benefits, and establishes another claim in favour of that science, upon the respect and gratitude of mankind.[18]

THE BUTCHER'S SAW

At a meeting of the Surgical Society of Ireland – held in RCSI on 9 January – MacDonnell gave a further account of Mary Kane's operation. Joliffe Tufnell also described how he had used MacDonnell's apparatus on four soldiers.[19] Some potential adverse effects were recorded, and it was agreed that patients with cardiac and pulmonary complaints were unsuitable candidates. More tests were planned and (student) volunteers were sought. Thanks to his connections, Sir Philip Crampton exhibited to the Society the very apparatus Liston had used, which was closely compared with MacDonnell's version. The floor was also given to the devil's advocate – in this case, Richard Butcher. If an operation was to take seconds

Butcher's saw.

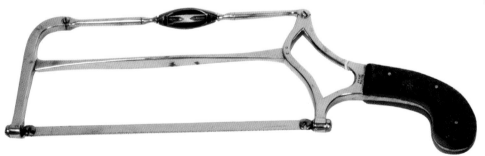

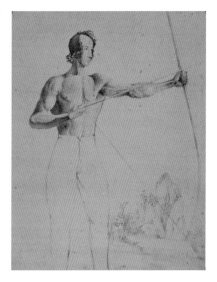

Sketch of Butcher's 'remarkable' appearance. Artist unknown.

only, why run the risks associated with the newfangled gas? 'Severe as the pain of these operations may be,' he reasoned elsewhere, 'it is better endured than the risk of suffocation.'[20]

Butcher (1818–1891, Lic. 1841, MRCSI 1844, PRCSI 1866) was a much-celebrated surgeon at Mercer's Hospital. In an era when speed with the blade was often a surgeon's best quality, Butcher was amongst the fastest. He was fast because he was strong, and he was proud of this fact: 'Early in his career, and for many subsequent years, Mr. Butcher excited the admiration of medical students by exhibitions of his muscular development. He was wont to roll-up his shirt-sleeves before operating, thereby exposing to view biceps of much more than average proportions. His dark complexion, well-oiled, raven-black, long hair and good features rendered his appearance remarkable.'[21]

Butcher's claim to fame was his invention of the somewhat unfortunately named 'Butcher's saw'. He had long noticed that, following amputation, the sharp edges of sawn-off bones were slow to heal and often caused great pain. One day, he observed how cabinet-makers could execute intricate, curving cuts by using a bow-saw whose

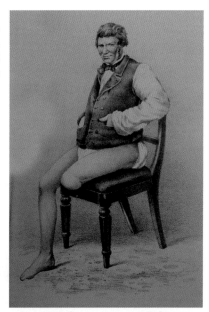

Illustration from Butcher's *Essays and Reports on Operative and Conservative Surgery* (1865).

blade could be rotated to any angle. He adapted his surgical saw accordingly, noting how it 'cuts more evenly than any other saw, and the bones cannot be splintered by it... and lastly it cuts more rapidly than any other saw, owing to the extreme tension of the blade'.[22] Butcher's saws were widely employed on the battlefields of the Crimea and during the American Civil War, where, in the absence of anaesthetics, metal, muscle and speed still had their place.

In fairness to Butcher, he was soon convinced by ether's efficacy after conducting his own experiment in Mercer's (his manuscript casebooks are preserved in RCSI Heritage Collections):

Facing page: Caricature of Richard Butcher, PRCSI 1866. Artist unknown.

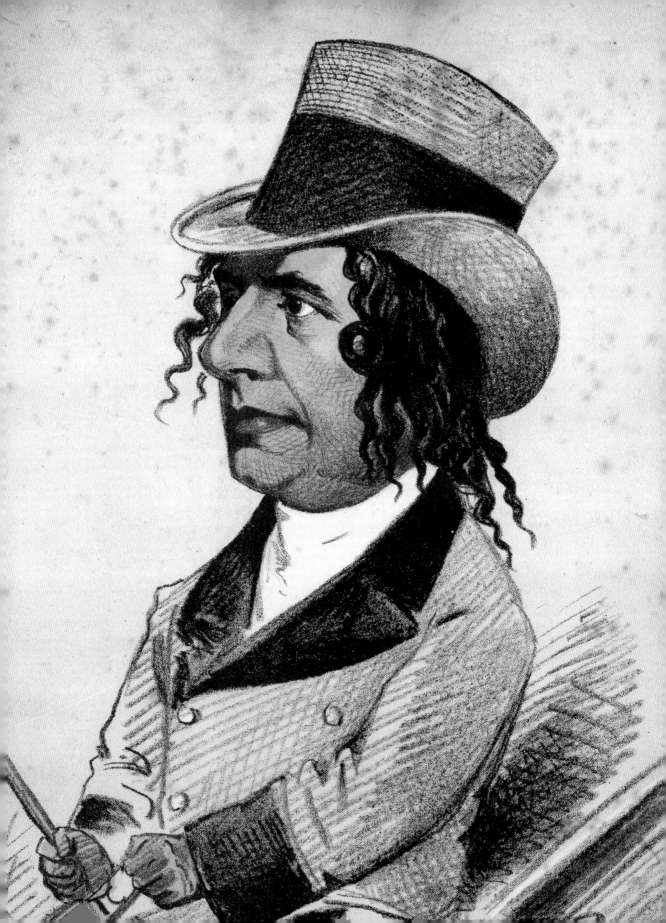

When the patient awoke he was amazed the limb was off; he declared he never felt any part of it, and indeed his statement is beyond dispute, when we recollect the death-like manner in which he lay during all its steps. He laughed after it and was cheerful... From this case and others it is quite clear the powerful agent we have at our command... and it is a truly valuable and splendid invention.[23]

Alas, Butcher also recorded that this cheerful patient subsequently died of post-operative sepsis within a fortnight. This remained an endemic problem whose particular (carbolic) solution was — as yet — just beyond the horizon.

THE BODY'S VOICE AND THE ELEPHANT FOLIO

Another innovation dating from the same year as Butcher's saw is that of the binaural stethoscope — that is, a stethoscope with two earpieces. Its monaural predecessor

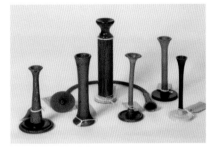

A selection of monaural stethoscopes.

Below: View of the nave, Great Exhibition, 1851. Victoria & Albert Museum, London.

is credited to the French physician, René Laënnec (1781–1826), who in 1816 had been inspired by the sight of two children sending acoustic signals to each other with a length of wood. He found that *mediate* auscultation — that is, using rolled-up sheets of paper to listen to a patient's internal organs — produced louder and

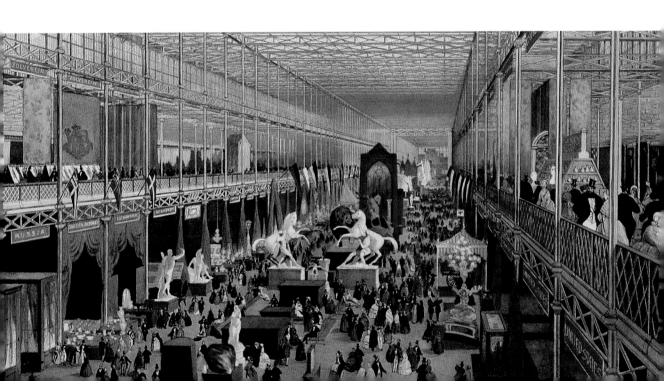

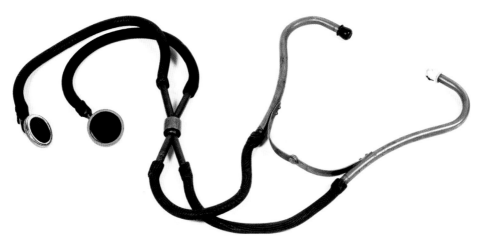

Leared's binaural stethoscope.

clearer sounds than the previous practice of *immediate* auscultation – placing one's ear directly on the patient (which was considered a particularly fraught encounter for women). Laënnec later replaced his rolled-up paper with a simple wooden tube. By the time he died in 1826 (prematurely, of tuberculosis, diagnosed by his nephew using a stethoscope), William Stokes, then still a student, had already published the first book in English on the instrument.[24]

The invention of the more familiar binaural version belongs to Arthur Leared (1822–1879, Lic. RCSI 1846). As with Rynd's needle, the story of Leared's stethoscope is something of a cautionary tale. He exhibited his advance on Laënnec at London's Great Exhibition in 1851 – and then sailed off to serve in the Crimean War (throughout his life he remained an inveterate traveller; he even wrote a book in Icelandic). When Leared returned to London, he found that George Cammann of New York City was manufacturing and selling binaural stethoscopes that were very similar to the one he had exhibited. Leared wrote to *The Lancet* to set the record straight, pointedly noting that 'it is not only possible, but highly probable' that his idea had been pirated.[25]

Medical history, at least in Europe, sides with Leared. Cammann's manufacturer, meanwhile, made a fortune – the company, in fact, is still operating.[26] If, for patients, the stethoscope is perhaps the symbol *par excellence* of the modern physician, for healthcare professionals it might be emblematic of the perils of not publishing – or adequately publicising – one's research.

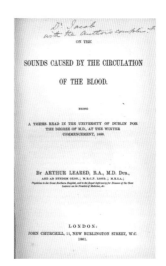

On the Sounds Caused by the Circulation of the Blood (1861).

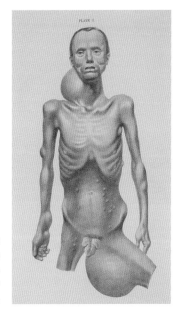

Recklinghausen's syndrome - as illustrated in Smith's 1849 elephant folio.

But publishing on a large scale can have its pitfalls too. In 1849, two years after he secured the legacy of Colles' fracture, Robert Smith published *A Treatise on the Pathology, Diagnosis and Treatment of Neuroma*, in which he gives a full description of neurofibromatosis type 1. To provide life-size illustrations of tumours, Smith's *Treatise* appeared in so-called 'elephant folio' format (about 70 x 48 cm). Being possibly the largest book printed in Ireland up to that time, few benefitted from Smith's labours – so that thirty-three years later, in 1882, when Friedrich von Recklinghausen (1833–1910) published his work on fibromas (including Smith in his literature review), the eponym for NF-1 went to the German.[27]

BLACK '47 - OR, ON THE MORTALITY OF MEDICAL PRACTITIONERS

At the same time as these breakthroughs were occurring, beyond the walls of RCSI the country was experiencing the upheaval and devastation of the Great Famine. Catastrophic crop failures caused widespread hunger, but it was the attendant infections – typhus, dysentery, measles and smallpox – that caused most of the million-plus excess deaths, a fact that neither authorities nor medical experts would understand until the 1880s.

James William Cusack, PRCSI 1827, 1847, 1858. Artist unknown.

Much of the statistical information about the disaster derives from statistics compiled by William Wilde. As both a demographer and medic, he was quick to see – and foresee – the calamitous effects of the 'great social revolution which this country is at present undergoing'.[28] As a million-plus survivors emigrated, the population went into steep decline, from 8.5 million before the Famine to less than half that number in the early twentieth century. It is little wonder that the poet James Clarence Mangan (1803–1848), York Street resident and cholera victim, characterised the country as 'Siberia'.

Little wonder, too, that the artists of the coming Celtic Revival would sense ghosts – absences – all over the west.

Among the dead were many 'frontline' medics. In 1847, the serving RCSI President, James William Cusack (1788–1861, Lic. 1812, MRCSI 1814, PRCSI 1827, 1847, 1858), collaborated with William Stokes on a survey that resulted in an important two-part article entitled, 'On the mortality of medical practitioners from fever in Ireland'. The impetus, as they stated from the outset, was 'to deplore the loss of many of our most meritorious pupils'.[29] (Cusack and Stokes often worked in tandem: previously they had, with others, co-founded the Pathological Society of Dublin, intended to promote cooperation between surgeons and physicians, and in 1843 they delivered a joint report to Westminster on the inadequacies of the medical system.) Their paper presents a number of stark findings, including the statistic that

> during the year 1847 one hundred and seventy-eight Irish medical practitioners, exclusive of pupils and army surgeons, died; being a proportion of 6.74 per cent., or 1 in every 14.83 practitioners in a single year; and of this number, the great majority fell victims to disease contracted in the discharge of public medical duties.[30]

Of those who did not die, very many nonetheless fell ill: 'during the prevalence of the late epidemic, 500 Irish medical men, at the lowest computation, suffered from fever or other epidemic diseases... by which themselves and their families have suffered considerable loss'. Physicians and surgeons, Cusack and Stokes point out, are 'more exposed to the influence of fatal diseases than any other class of the community... from the period of their entering the profession as students to advanced life'.[31] The article closes with a plea for the government to provide for the widows and children of 'those gentlemen whose lives have been sacrificed to the public service'.[32]

DISPUTE WITH TRINITY COLLEGE

Over the course of a long career, Cusack had 'an unusually great number of apprentices',[33] the last being a Dr Tweedy of Rutland (now Parnell) Square, who died in 1911 – that is, an impressive 123 years after his master was born. Cusack also had an unusual pedagogic style, choosing to lecture his students from his bed before he got up each morning. For many years that bed was at 3 Kildare Street, but after being appointed Surgeon-in-Ordinary to Queen Victoria, Cusack grew very wealthy and purchased the Gandon-designed Abbeville in Kinsealy, north

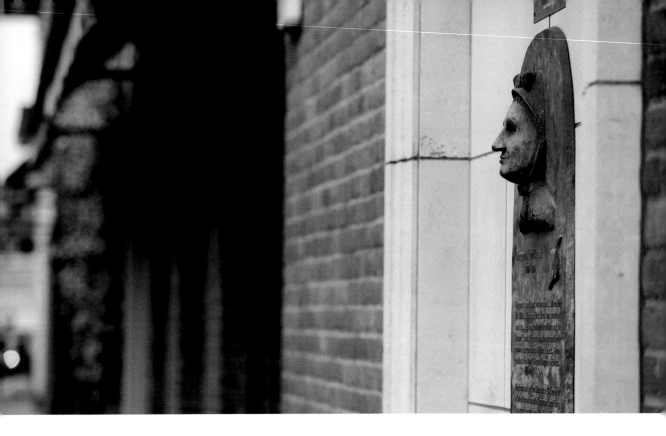

Sculpture of the 'Nun of Kenmare' on Cusack Corner.

Dublin. Cusack Corner – where York Street and Mercer Street meet – was so-named in 1998 for James William's niece, Margaret Anna Cusack (1829–1899), an author and campaigner known as the 'Nun of Kenmare'.[34]

In 1852, Cusack was appointed to the university chair of surgery at Trinity College – the first time a Catholic held a chair wholly under the university's control. The appointment also gave rise to a 'full-scale war' with RCSI.[35] Previously, when Trinity first began surgical instruction in 1849, with Robert Smith as the inaugural professor, there had been tentative negotiations between the two institutions as to the possibility of recognising each other's lectures. At length, RCSI suspected it would be the worse off by the arrangement, but rather than outright refuse, the Council decided to postpone 'further consideration of the subject'.[36]

This led Trinity to proceed with a surgical diploma of their own – to the chagrin of RCSI and, indeed, the Royal College in London: claims were made about 'a violation of the rights of the surgical colleges' and 'a degradation of the profession'[37] – but Trinity held firm, backed up by the attorney general. While the institutions clashed, however, the individuals involved were generally ecumenical in their allegiances. Cusack's successor in the Trinity chair was Robert Adams (1791–1875, Lic. 1816, MRCSI 1818, PRCSI 1840, 1860, 1867), famed for his observation of 'Stokes-Adams syndrome' – fainting spells caused by heart block. This was the first Irish cardiac eponym.

'A GREAT ACT': RCSI AND THE CATHOLIC UNIVERSITY MEDICAL SCHOOL

RCSI and Trinity both felt the pinch in 1845 with the establishment of the Queen's Colleges of Cork, Belfast and Galway, each with their own medical school. These were secular institutions, designed to educate the masses who were effectively disbarred from Trinity. Ironically, the Catholic hierarchy objected to such 'Godless education', choosing instead to form the Catholic University of Ireland (1854); it too opened a medical school, a development that was only made possible by the helping hand of RCSI.

From the start, the Catholic University was obliged to operate with a certain secrecy. Their ambition was to open a medical faculty in Cecilia Street, in a building which previously housed the Apothecaries' Hall medical school – but they did not want to advertise this fact. So a former RCSI President, Andrew Ellis (1792–1867, Lic. 1820, MRCSI 1827, PRCSI 1849), stepped in and made the purchase, then transferred it to the fledgling faculty. As John Henry Newman, first rector of the university, wrote: 'It would never have been sold to us if it had been known that we were trying for it. Dr Ellis told me that for a fortnight he had not been able from nervousness to get a good night. It was a great act.'[38] The Catholic University Medical School thus opened on 1 October 1855 – with Ellis as its first Professor of Surgery.

Even with a home, the new school faced another significant obstacle: in the eyes of the law, it did not exist. It was unlicensed and unchartered, meaning its students would earn essentially worthless qualifications – unless, that is, its teaching was to be recognised by a body that was legally entitled to do so. This was where RCSI stepped in again, committing to that recognition in 1856: graduates of the Catholic University Medical School could thereafter style themselves Licentiates of RCSI.[39] Newman's Catholic University would struggle in general, even as its medical school flourished. In 1909, it was incorporated into University College Dublin (UCD) as a constituent college of the National University of Ireland (NUI). In that guise, some seventy years later, it would return the favour of official recognition at a crucial juncture in RCSI's history – but that is a story for later pages.

OPENING THE MEDICAL REGISTER (1859)

Where reform was the watchword of the previous generation, now the medical world turned its collective attention to regulation. The year 1858 brought the landmark Medical Act – or, to give its full title, *An Act to Regulate the Qualifications of Practitioners in Medicine and Surgery* (21 & 22 Vict c. 90). Its purpose was to allow the public to distinguish between qualified and unqualified practitioners; only the names of the former would appear in the new Medical Register, launched on New Year's Day, 1859. Similarly, those who flouted its standards would find themselves struck off.

In the eyes of the law and the public, surgeons and physicians were now on an equal footing. In theory, the surgeons ought to have been happy about this parity – but in fact both cohorts were miffed to discover that apothecaries, too, were also their legal equals. (Apothecaries' Hall concerned itself with examining and licensing, not teaching, so prospective apothecaries still had to take courses at other recognised bodies. In time, qualified apothecaries generally pursued one of two career paths: either they worked in retail, calling themselves chemists or druggists; or they made a virtue of their broad – that is, general – knowledge to become a new type of doctor, the general practitioner.) One thing the Medical Act did not do was outlaw unqualified practitioners: quacks and amateurs could still operate (literally); they just would not be listed in the Register.[40] The first RCSI entrants on the Register appear as: *Lic.* (or *Fell.*) *R. Coll. Surg. Irel.* followed by the year of qualification.

'EVERY BRANCH OF THE HEALING ART'

In practice, if not hitherto by the letter of the law, RCSI had already placed itself on a par with the best colleges of medicine anywhere. This was a point forcefully made by Arthur Jacob as he welcomed the incoming students of 1844 (in fact, Jacob refused to allow anyone else to deliver this annual address[41]):

> This College, although called a College of Surgeons, is as you all
> know, just as much a College of Physicians. We have the same corps
> of professors, or even a larger one; we require the same course of
> medical studies, or even a more extended one; and we examine as
> carefully on medical subjects as they do in the schools of medicine.
> In fact, this is a College of Medicine and Surgery, and the diploma
> you receive from it is universally accepted as evidence of your fitness
> to practice every branch of the healing art.[42]

As it happened, Jacob was addressing a low ebb of 105 students that year – far off the 1829 peak of 291. Numbers remained close to the 1844 figure through the middle of the century, generally due to competition from the Queen's Colleges, several new English medical schools and Trinity College, especially following their much-resented incursion into surgical teaching.[43]

SALUS POPULI SUPREMA LEX: THE FIRST CHAIR OF POLITICAL MEDICINE

A pioneering expansion of what Jacob called the 'corps of professors' took place in 1841, when RCSI created a Chair of Hygiene, or Political Medicine – meaning, in contemporary terms, public health medicine. Its establishment was spurred by a lecture given in RCSI by Jacob's partner-in-polemic at the *Dublin Medical Press*, Henry Maunsell (1806–1879, Lic. 1827, MRCSI 1832, Prof of Midwifery 1835–41, Prof of Hygiene or Political Medicine 1841–46). For Maunsell, prevention was unquestionably better than cure, from more efficient vaccination to the consistent application of rules on quarantine ('when the country is invaded by an epidemic, all is confusion – no one knows what to do, or where to look for aid'[44]). Medicine, he said, was at its noblest when it 'aims at the higher object of protecting the public health, and providing for the physical well being of the human race'.[45]

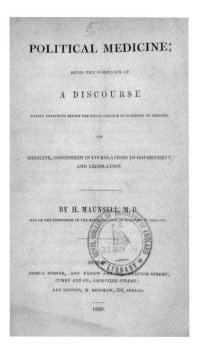

POLITICAL MEDICINE;

BEING THE SUBSTANCE OF

A DISCOURSE

LATELY DELIVERED BEFORE THE ROYAL COLLEGE OF SURGEONS IN IRELAND,

ON

MEDICINE, CONSIDERED IN ITS RELATIONS TO GOVERNMENT AND LEGISLATION.

BY H. MAUNSELL, M.D.

ONE OF THE PROFESSORS IN THE ROYAL COLLEGE OF SURGEONS IN IRELAND.

DUBLIN:
JOSHUA PORTER, AND FANNIN AND CO., GRAFTON-STREET;
CURRY AND CO., SACKVILLE-STREET;
AND LONDON, H. RENSHAW, 356, STRAND.

1839.

The advent of public health medicine: Maunsell's pamphlet on *Political Medicine*.

In an age when healthcare was largely a private, individual concern, Maunsell urged the profession – and the authorities – to look to the bigger picture and to 'promote the common weal'.[46] Radically for his time, he argued that marginalised groups such as prisoners, mariners, asylum-dwellers and 'the poorer classes' deserved the state's intervention and protection – and he excoriated his fellow medics for 'having abandoned the higher and more honorable walks of their profession, to pursue, *exclusively*, the less exalted, though more profitable trade of the empirical curing of diseases'.[47]

The lecture – which Maunsell subsequently distributed as a pamphlet – ends with a quotation from Cicero: *Salus Populi Suprema Lex* (the health of the people should be the supreme law) – which is the same motto that appeared on the masthead of the *Dublin Medical Press*. RCSI's reaction to Maunsell's polemic is recorded in the College Minutes:

> Resolved, that a professor be appointed by the College to deliver lectures on the provisions required for the preservation of the health of the public and the precautions to be adopted for preventing the extension of disease.[48]

This was the first chair of public health medicine in any medical school in Ireland or Britain.

'INTO HER VEINS': IRELAND'S FIRST BLOOD TRANSFUSION, 1865

Eighteen years after John MacDonnell conducted Ireland's first surgical operation using ether, his son Robert McDonnell (1828–1889, Lic. 1851, FRCSI 1853, PRCSI 1877–78) attempted the country's first human-to-human blood transfusion at Jervis Street Hospital. This was fraught with danger, as the concept of compatible and incompatible blood groups would remain unknown until Karl Landsteiner's discoveries at the turn of the century.

Experiments with transfusion go back to William Harvey's discovery of the

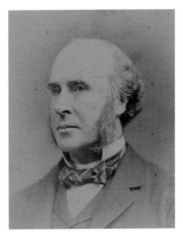

Robert McDonnell, PRCSI 1877.

circulation of blood in 1628. Early animal-to-animal transfusions were successful, but when animal-to-human transfusions proved fatal, all such investigations fell into disrepute. Not until 1818 was the first successful human-to-human transfusion performed, by the obstetrician James Blundell (1790–1878) – but even then, he waited a decade before publishing his research in *The Lancet*. Pre-Landsteiner, transfusion was a form of roulette, and so the procedure was generally reserved as a last resort.

McDonnell was presented with just such a last-resort case in 1865: on 27 March, a paper-mill worker, Mary Ann Dooley, was admitted to Jervis Street Hospital following an accident. Her hand was lacerated and contused, with the little finger entirely destroyed. Within three weeks tetanus had set in, rendering her unable to eat or drink. On 20 April, McDonnell decided to attempt a transfusion. He drew blood from his own arm, which he stirred, strained and syringed into Dooley. 'As the patient was quite conscious during the performance of this operation,' he later wrote, 'she was able to describe accurately her sensations as the blood was thrown into her veins... She expressed herself as feeling an agreeable sensation... of warmth pervading her.'

Unfortunately, Dooley died the next day ('without pain, and quite conscious to the last'), but the experience prompted McDonnell to refine his method. He devised a new instrument to replace the syringe, and this was used successfully five years later, in 1870, following a case of post-partum haemorrhage. On that

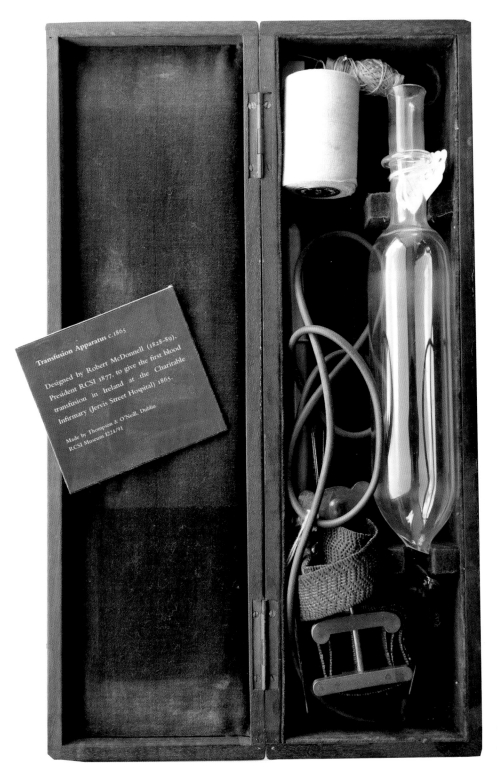

Transfusion Apparatus c.1865

Designed by Robert McDonnell (1828–89), President RCSI 1877, to give the first blood transfusion in Ireland at the Charitable Infirmary (Jervis Street Hospital) 1865.

Made by Thompson & O'Neill, Dublin
RCSI Museum E24/91

Transfusion kit, c.1865.

occasion, the compatible blood came from the woman's husband. Only at this point did McDonnell publish accounts of his research activities.[49]

Amongst those who would have been interested in this work were William Thornley Stoker (1845–1912, Lic. 1867, FRCSI 1873, Prof of Descriptive Anatomy 1876–89, PRCSI 1894–95[50]) and his brothers – two of whom, Richard (Lic. 1873) and George (Lic. 1876), were army surgeons. Another brother, Abraham – better known as Bram – wrote possibly the most famous blood transfusion novel of all time, *Dracula* (1897):

> When I described Lucy's symptoms – the same as before, but infinitely more marked – he looked very grave, but said nothing. He took with him a bag in which were many instruments and drugs, 'the ghastly paraphernalia of our beneficial trade,' as he once called, in one of his lectures, the equipment of a professor of the healing craft. (...) 'My God!' he said; 'this is dreadful. There is no time to be lost. She will die for sheer want of blood to keep the heart's action as it should be. There must be transfusion of blood at once. Is it you or me?' 'I am younger and stronger, Professor. It must be me.' (...) I asked the Professor in a whisper: - 'What do you make of that mark on her throat?' (...) Just over the external jugular vein there were two punctures, not large, but not wholesome-looking...[51]

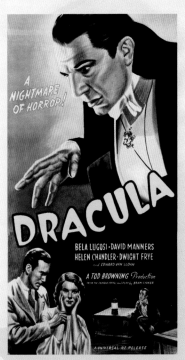

Bram Stoker's endlessly adaptable tale of transfusion — Bela Lugosi in *Dracula* (1931).

Dracula was an aristocrat, albeit a fictional one, but William Thornley Stoker went one better: he received an actual knighthood in 1895, during his RCSI Presidency. Henceforth, with rare exceptions, such automatic ennoblement was one of the perks of the position. The custom ceased with Irish independence.

THE EYE IN RCSI: WILSON, SWANZY AND JACOB *FILS*

The establishment of new subject chairs was a rarity in the period. In fact, the abolition of pre-existing ones was a more regular occurrence, amongst which were Military Surgery (abolished 1860), Logic (a short-lived subject, from 1852 to 1862) and Botany (1889). Thirty-one years passed before a new chair followed Political

Medicine: this was Ophthalmology, in 1872, under the inaugural professorship of Henry Wilson (1838–1877, Lic. 1858, FRCSI 1865, Prof of Ophthalmology 1872–77). It was something of an open secret that Wilson was a 'natural' son of Sir William Wilde, though they conducted themselves publicly as nephew and uncle. Wilson had trained at Bonn, Heidelberg, Berlin, Vienna and Paris, before returning to Dublin and Wilde at St Mark's Hospital.

When Wilde died in 1876, Wilson took over as senior surgeon and trustee. His *Lectures on the theory and practice of the ophthalmoscope* (1868) is considered to be the first text in English on the subject (it is dedicated to Sir William 'by his affectionate pupil').[52] A year after Wilde's death, Wilson himself died suddenly, of pneumonia, aged 39. His half-brother Oscar (who called him 'cousin') travelled from Oxford, where he was a student, to serve as a chief mourner at the funeral – and, it seems, to see what was in his unmarried relative's will. But Wilson left everything to St Mark's.

After Wilson, the Ophthalmology chair passed to Henry Swanzy (1843–1913, Lic. 1866, FRCSI 1873, PRCSI 1906–07). Like Wilson, he had studied at Vienna and Berlin, under Albrecht von Graefe (1828–1870), probably the nineteenth century's leading ophthalmologist. Though respected as a surgeon, it was Swanzy's writings that gave him an international reputation; his *Handbook of Diseases of the Eye and their Treatment* (1884) ran into ten editions over thirty years.

Closer to home, he was central to the establishment of Dublin's Royal Victoria Eye and Ear Hospital on Adelaide Road (1897). His daughter, Mary Swanzy HRHA (1882–1978), was one of Ireland's finest Impressionist artists. Swanzy's successor, in 1881, was Archibald Hamilton Jacob (1837–1901, Lic. 1859, FRCSI 1863, Prof of Ophthalmology 1881–1901), son of the more famous Arthur. From that year on, Ophthalmology became a compulsory subject for the final Licence exam.

How the Licence exam was conducted underwent changes in this era. In 1863, written answers to printed questions were introduced, in addition to the traditional oral grilling. Four years later, graded marks replaced the Examiners' single 'yes' or 'no' votes. Demonstrations of surgical operations on a cadaver were also required. From 1871, clinical examination at a patient's bedside formed part of the final exam (for which the patient was rewarded to the tune of £1 18*s*).

In 1874, histology was an examination subject for the first time. In truth, this was more of a catch-up than the breaking of new ground. As early as 1854, in his *Apology for the Microscope*, Robert Lyons (1826–1886, Lic. 1849) deplored the neglect of microscopy in Irish research in histology and pathology, despite great advances being made on the continent. That same year, as if to illustrate his point, RCSI spent its money on a 'handsome Presidential gown';[53] another eight years would pass before the Council invested in a 'powerful and complete' (and second-hand) microscope, which was entrusted to a 'Microscopic Committee'.[54]

On other occasions, RCSI was at the technological forefront: in 1883, a telephone was installed. There were not many other telephone users to ring, but the Dublin Fire Brigade was one, so the line rental of £12 per annum was a prudent expense.

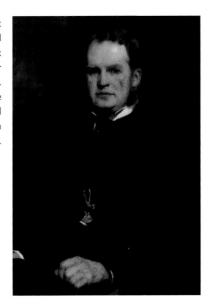

Portrait of Richard Theodore Stack by Walter Osborne. Courtesy of the British Dental Association Museum.

DENTIST STACK AND THE LICENCE IN DENTAL SURGERY

RCSI was responsible for another Irish and British first in 1884, when it created a Professorship in Dental Surgery. The inaugural appointee was Richard Theodore Stack (1848–1909, Lic. 1875, FRCSI 1878, Prof of Dental Surgery 1884–1909), who never intended to be a dentist. He was headed for a glittering medical career when a bout of rheumatic fever left him so deaf, at 26, that he could no longer use a stethoscope.

Three years later, he graduated in dentistry from Harvard. (For the rest of his life, he disliked being called 'Doctor' – his door-plate, visiting cards and book-stamp all read 'Dentist Stack'.) Returning to Dublin, Stack joined the city's sole dental college, the Metropolitan Dental Hospital in Beresford Place. After a time, dissatisfactions with the Metropolitan led Stack and others to found the Dental Hospital of Ireland in 1879, first located at 29 York Street, later moving to Lincoln Place. Until this era, dentistry in Ireland was entirely unregulated.[55]

In some cases, trained surgeons or apothecaries would take care of teeth; elsewhere, barbers, wigmakers or even blacksmiths did their best, or worst, with the tools of their trade. It was a similar situation in Britain, where reformers had unfortunately split into rival factions.[56] Ultimately, this led to parliamentary invention and regulation: the Dental Practitioners' Act (1878). This act, in turn, motivated RCSI to institute a Licence in Dental Surgery, Ireland's first ever dental qualification.

A dental Court of Examiners was set up, consisting of three Fellows and three dentists, including Stack – and two days later the first exams were held. Stack's subsequent professorship underlined the profession's raised status. Undergraduate dental education would continue at RCSI until 1977, during which time some 1,600 students earned their LDSRCSI.[57]

THE COLLEGE AND THE SCHOOL: A FORK IN THE ROAD?

Student numbers fluctuated considerably during these developments, rising steadily through the 1860s and 1870s to a peak of 198 in 1876 – just before a precipitous fall to 111 in 1884. Through the same transformative period, teaching and research facilities required near-constant modernisation. In 1882, a histology lab was built over the School's old dissecting room; the School museum was converted to a 'bone room'; the preparation of subjects now took place in an 'airy, well-lighted apartment'; and the professors were furnished with new rooms.[58] (Up to this point, Anatomy was a co-chair – with the salary split in two. From 1882, this was converted to a single post, in the hope of attracting a 'first-class anatomist' – which is exactly what happened: enticed from Edinburgh, the Scottish anatomist Daniel John Cunningham (1850–1909) took the post. His

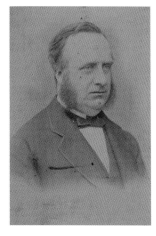

George Hugh Kidd, PRCSI 1876.

Manual of Practical Anatomy, first published in 1896, is now in its third century, in double-digit editions. Alas, Cunningham's tenure at RCSI was short-lived; he left after one year to spend twenty at Trinity before returning to Edinburgh.)

The financial outlay on the School improvements was significant, coming to £3,421 18*s* 10*d*. This displeased some of the Fellows, and at a subsequent meeting on 3 June 1882 the whole policy of the connection between the College and the School was debated at great length. Finally a resolution was passed, seventy-one votes to thirty-nine: 'That the Fellows are of opinion that in the interests of the College and in accordance with the Charter the Council is bound to maintain the School by every means in its power.'[59]

One of the strongest voices in favour of maintaining the School connection was past-President George Hugh Kidd (1824–1895, Lic. 1842, FRCSI 1844, PRCSI 1876). As Master of the Coombe, Kidd had worked with Robert McDonnell to administer last-chance

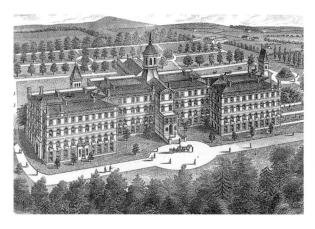

The Stewart Institution, Palmerston, c.1886.

blood transfusions to treat post-partum bleeding (of fifteen cases, nine were successful). Kidd also had an abiding interest in the welfare of children with intellectual disabilities. He visited asylums in England and Scotland, which led to a pamphlet entitled *An Appeal on Behalf of the Idiotic and Imbecile Children of Ireland* (1865); soon after, he co-founded and ran the Stewart Institution, later Stewart's Hospital. This was the first — and for fifty years the only — body providing care of this kind in Ireland.[60]

Agnes Shannon (her name misspelt 'Agnus') enrolled for Chemistry lectures at RCSI, 1885.

'THAT PROGRESS WHICH ACCORDS WITH THE SPIRIT OF THE AGE': THE ADMISSION OF WOMEN AT RCSI

Almost forty years after the last Charter revision, two further 'Supplements' were granted in quick succession in the early 1880s. The first of these, known as the 'Second Supplemental Charter', came in October 1883, and its primary function was to allow all members of Council to vote in the election of the School's professors and examiners. No sooner was this granted than criticisms were aired — specifically, that no provision had been made for Council members to vote *in absentia*. When some grumbled about 'undue haste', a lengthy defensive statement in the end-of-year report closed further comment. The subsequent 'Supplement' — the Third — granted on 23 May 1885 was a good deal more interesting, thanks specifically to amendment number 14:

> And we do hereby, for us, our heirs and successors, grant, declare and appoint, that all provisions of the Charter, Bye-Laws, and Ordinances as to education, examination, and granting diplomas to Fellows or Licentiates shall extend to include women.[61]

At the beginning of the academic year 1885–86, RCSI enrolled the first woman to study at any medical school in Ireland or Britain. Her name was Agnes Shannon.

In taking this pioneering step, Shannon was advancing on the hard-won victories of others. Some twenty-six years earlier, when the Medical Register was published, only one woman was listed therein. This was Bristol-born Elizabeth Blackwell (1821–1910), who had earned her medical degree in the United States – the first woman to do so. In fact, Blackwell had only been admitted to her medical school in upstate New York when the faculty allowed the student body to vote on her application, confident of her rejection. More out of mischief than egalitarianism, the students chose to admit her – then found the joke was on them when she finished top of her class. After a period of further study in Paris, Blackwell began practice at St Bartholomew's Hospital in London. Her appearance on the Register was similarly by dint of a loophole: a clause in the Medical Act recognised doctors with foreign degrees if they were in practice prior to 1858.

In 1865, a mentee of Blackwell's, Elizabeth Garrett Anderson (1836–1917), became the second woman named in the Medical Register – also, more or less, by dint of a loophole. She had earned her qualification at London's Society of Apothecaries (with the highest marks in her class), having enrolled at a time when the society's charter did not expressly exclude women. Immediately after she qualified, the society changed their charter to correct this 'oversight'.

For the next decade, during which time no further women were eligible to appear in the Register, figures such as Sophie Jex-Blake (1840–1912) campaigned tirelessly, and in 1876 the MP Russell Gurney – much influenced by his wife Emelia – succeeded in passing an 'Enabling Act', which meant that British and Irish medical institutions were 'enabled' (but not obliged) to accept candidates with foreign degrees to sit their exams. The first body to act upon this liberalisation was Dublin's RCPI, at that time called the King and Queen's College of Physicians of Ireland (KQCPI).

In January 1877, five years after she earned a medical degree in Zurich, Eliza Louisa Walker Dunbar (1849–1825) became, at once, the first female Licentiate of KQCPI and the first woman to earn a medical qualification in the United Kingdom. Forty-five more women followed this 'Irish route' over the next ten years, including Jex-Blake, who had obtained her degree at Bern. The opening up of the KQCPI Licence was, according to Jex-Blake, 'the turning point in the whole struggle'.[62]

These developments were watched with interest at RCSI. But 'enabled' as it now was, there were no sudden moves to follow Kildare Street. As there were ongoing debates in the period about a Conjoint Licence of both bodes, special efforts by RCSI may have been seen by some as unnecessary. On the other hand, as the KQCPI coffers attested, there was perfect parity between men and women when it came to paying examination fees.

The change finally came at a Council meeting on 23 October 1884, when it was proposed that women might be admitted to the RCSI. The motion passed by nine votes to three. Next, at a meeting in early January 1885, a proposal by the Vice-President, Charles Cameron, went a step further, introducing the language of what would become the fourteenth amendment ('all provisions of the Charters, by-laws, and ordinances as to education, Examination, and granting of diplomas to Fellows or Licentiates shall extend to include women').

It was the word 'Fellows' that caused disquiet for some. Edward Hamilton (1824–1899, Lic. 1846, FRCSI 1852, Professor of Surgery, 1884–98, PRCSI 1875, 1892–93) proposed that the word be omitted, and Joliffe Tufnell seconded this, but they were defeated by eighteen votes to fourteen (for context, KQCPI did not admit women to their Fellowship until 1924). The original wording was then passed by twenty-five votes to eleven. This was potentially far-reaching: it meant that, in theory at least, women were eligible to compete for every office associated with RCSI, including President. In practice, however, RCSI did not elect a female President for another 125 years. This was President Eilis McGovern (FRCSI 1982, PRCSI 2010–12), in 2010.

AGNES SHANNON, RCSI'S FIRST FEMALE STUDENT

Unfortunately, not a great deal is known about the pioneering Agnes Shannon. Before coming to RCSI, she (and her two sisters) attended the Royal College of Science for Ireland, which admitted women from its foundation in 1867; she also sat at least one medical exam at the Royal University of Ireland.[63] She attended three courses of lectures at RCSI, as enthusiastically reported in the *Englishwoman's Review* (1885):

> Neither has she had to wait, as ladies in London were so long compelled to do, for hospital teaching, for instruction is already being afforded her at St Vincent's Hospital. We must heartily congratulate the ladies of Ireland on this important accession to their rights in being able to obtain medical instruction at home, and we no less heartily congratulate the Irish doctors in having had the sense to originate this act of justice and the generosity to carry it out spontaneously.[64]

In the first edition of his *History* of RCSI (1886), Cameron records Shannon's singular presence: 'In the session 1885–86 the School was opened to women

– one only, Miss Agnes Shannon, entered.'[65] Indeed, student records show that Shannon attended Cameron's lectures in Chemistry.[66] After this, however, the trail goes cold. No more is known about Agnes Shannon, except that, for whatever reason, she did not obtain any qualification at RCSI.

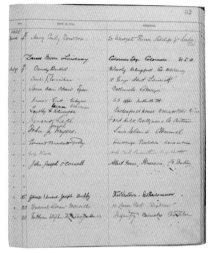

Mary Emily Dowson's signature in the Roll of Licentiates, 1886.

MARY EMILY DOWSON, RCSI'S FIRST FEMALE LICENTIATE

In 1884, a Yorkshire woman named Mary Emily Dowson (1848–1941, Lic. 1886) chose the 'Irish route' to the Medical Register: like Jex-Blake and others before her, she came to Kildare Street and obtained the KQCPI Licence.[67] But Dowson had specifically surgical ambitions: four years earlier, she had passed the Royal College of Surgeons' Preliminary Examination in Arts (coming second in her class), but was not permitted to progress further.

When RCSI opened its doors, she crossed the Irish Sea again, and in June 1886 – aged 38 – she was awarded the RCSI Licence. 'This lady,' the *British Medical Journal* noted at the time, 'has the honour of being the first woman admitted as a surgeon on the roll of the Royal College of Surgeons in Ireland.'[68] In point of fact, this made Dowson the first *qualified* female surgeon in Britain or Ireland. The momentousness of the occasion, both for Dowson and for RCSI, was recorded in the *Medical Press*:

> Although it is not the custom of the Court of Examiners to express any opinion as to the quality of the answering of a candidate, we take the responsibility of breaking the rule, in stating that we have heard that, during the four days' examination to which Mrs. Dowson was subjected, her answering was more than amply sufficient to satisfy the examiners, and would have entitled her to a mark of distinction if such were given by the College. (...) In any case, no one can fail to make obeisance before the persevering energy, steadiness of purpose, calmness under annoyance, and intelligent industry, which a lady must possess who, in the face of the prejudice of centuries, steps across all obstacles to the professional goal. Such qualities are those which make successful practitioners and skilful

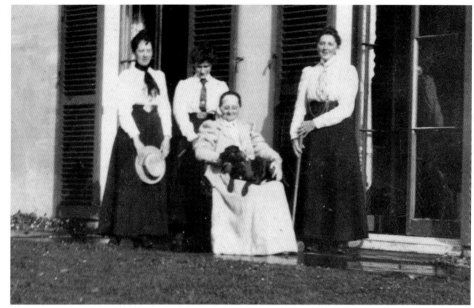

Mary Emily Dowson (standing, right) with her mother and daughters, c.1900. Courtesy of Henfield Museum, West Sussex.

surgeons, and we are, therefore, glad to welcome Mrs Dowson within the 'pale' which has, heretofore, been barred against her sex. We are also, we believe, justified in congratulating the College upon having shown itself superior to the prejudices which might have been expected to influence the acts of an institution of its years. In this, as in other of its proceedings of the last few years, the College has shown that it will not be precluded by an obstructive medical conservatism from pursuing that progress which accords with the spirit of the age, and we are convinced that even those who dislike the invasion of surgical precincts by ladies will consider that the College has acted properly in sacrificing the feeling which many of its Fellows must entertain for the sake of doing what seems right and just.[69]

Subsequent volumes of the Medical Register record aspects of Dowson's career: medical tutor and lecturer in forensic medicine at the London School of Medicine for Women, lecturer on hygiene for Queen's probationer nurses, and assistant physician and pathologist at the New Hospital for Women, Euston Road (from which she stepped down in 1888 owing to concerns about standards). There is also brief mention of further training in Vienna. In 1912, the Register described Dowson as 'retired'; for some time by then, she had been devoting her energies to literary practices, generally in the religious mode. In 2019, a conference room in 123 St Stephen's Green was named in her honour.[70]

Facing page: Portrait of Mary Josephine Hannan by Molly Judd (2019).

Upon retirement, Hannan lived at Hartbeespoort for number of years. She died in Irene, south of Pretoria, on 7 July 1936, aged 78. An obituary notice recorded:

> Mary Hannan in her life played many parts but her most useful and let it be added most characteristic role was that of a medical woman who had a deep interest in her calling, and was ingrained with a passionate devotion to truth. A strong character, her outspokenness and her contempt for everything that savoured of dishonesty created enemies for her. She was not afraid to criticise prominent politicians... In some ways she was leavened with the missionary spirit, though her strong fund of commonsense, and her appreciation of the humorous, made her less aggressive and one sided than she would otherwise have been.[76]

As part of the Women on Walls project (2019), RCSI commissioned a portrait of Hannan by the artist Molly Judd. Prior to this restorative initiative, next to nothing was known about this remarkable woman – not even her birth and death dates.

EMILY WINIFRED DICKSON, RCSI'S FIRST FEMALE FELLOW

While history eclipsed Hannan, the first female Fellow of RCSI, Emily Winifred Dickson (1866–1944, Lic. 1891, FRCSI 1893), left a more indelible mark – at least for a time.

Initially, Dickson attempted to enrol at Trinity, but while the School of Physic itself was amenable, higher powers objected (women were finally admitted to TCD in 1904; Cambridge and Oxford, meanwhile, would resist until 1916 and 1917, respectively). Instead, Dickson enrolled at RCSI in 1887 – the only woman in her class – winning an Anatomy medal in her first year. Having earned her Licence (1891[77]), she gained further wide-ranging clinical experience at Sir Patrick Dun's Hospital, the Rotunda, the Eye and Ear, Donnybrook Dispensary and the Richmond Lunatic Asylum.

In 1890 – that is, just prior to Dickson's RCSI qualification – the Royal University of Ireland decided to allow women to take their medical degree; the first to do so was

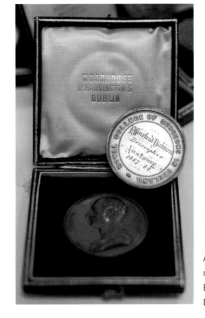

Anatomy medal won by Emily Winifred Dickson, 1888.

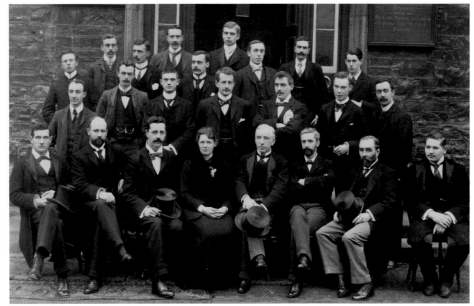

Eleanora Fleury. Dickson duly followed suit, collecting her RUI degree in 1893 – with first-class honours and an exhibition prize. (In later life, Dickson made light of her academic ability, saying: 'exams are merely a "knack" which I possessed. I often beat people who knew more than I because I could put my goods in the shop window and was not nervous.'[78] The evidence suggests this was excessively modest.) The year 1893 was also the one in which Dickson passed the Fellowship exam at RCSI – making her the first female Fellow of any College of Surgeons in Ireland or Britain (for context, the RCS in London did not admit women until 1911, nor female Fellows until 1920). In the period 1893 to 1922, twenty-six women attained the Fellowship of RCSI.

A six-month travelling scholarship from the RUI enabled Dickson to study at Vienna and Berlin. Indicative of the times, an older female relative went with her as chaperone. In the latter, she attended lectures by the celebrated pathologist Rudolf Virchow (1821–1902), but generally the city was 'a waste of time' because she was refused entry to the classes that interested her. Her place had been confirmed by letter, but, as a friend of Dickson recalled, 'when she arrived, [the professor] looked her over, declared she had cheated, that "Winifred" was a man's name, and would have none of her'.[79]

Returning home, Dickson set up a practice in her father's house on St Stephen's Green (during her undergraduate years, Thomas Dickson had been MP for the Dublin St Stephen's Green constituency); later, on her own, she relocated to

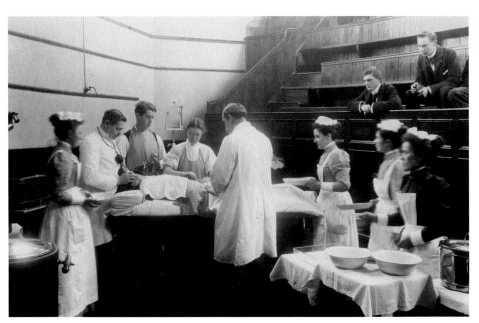

Dickson (centre) in the operating theatre.

Upper Mount Street. In 1894, on the opening of the Extern Department for Diseases of Women at the Richmond Hospital, Dickson was appointed as its first female gynaecologist (for a time, the adjectives 'first female' precede almost all of her appointments).

From 1895, Dickson was assistant master, later supernumerary assistant, at the Coombe Lying-In Hospital. She put her exam 'knack' to use again in 1896, qualifying as MD and MAO (with first-class honours) from the RUI, following which she was appointed Examiner in Midwifery and Gynaecology at RCSI, a first for the RCSI and a first for any woman in Ireland or Britain. This appointment, however, caused a stir: students protested at the idea of being examined by a woman and went so far as to organise a petition – running to fourteen pages of signatures, including those of students at the Catholic University Medical School – for Dickson's removal. The Council received the petition but declined to act on it.[80]

This was a rare display of prejudice – at least in such an overt, formal expression. Generally speaking, the Irish medical establishment was favourably disposed to women doctors – more so, it seems, than their counterparts in Britain. And amongst students, relations between women and men seem to have been essentially egalitarian. Tuition was entirely integrated, with one exception: men and women were separated for anatomical dissection. This was typical in the era: from 1892, RCSI had 'a ladies' dissecting room' and a 'suite of apartments for female students'.[81] In 1896, one RCSI student, Clara Williams, gave a very favourable report to the in-house magazine of the London School of Medicine for Women:

> ... nothing in the slightest degree unpleasant has ever occurred, and the professors are unanimous in stating that far from regretting the admission of women to their classes, they consider it has improved the tone of the College considerably. The students are all friendly, there is a healthy spirit of emulation aroused in working together for the various prizes, and an absence of jealousy which augurs well for the future of medical women in Ireland, and reflects favourably on the men as well; we all help each other, and I, for my own part, owe a great deal of my success to the assistance of a few of the senior men students.[82]

On the other hand, Williams also reported that the absence of segregated student accommodation deterred many would-be female medical students (or, at least, deterred their parents). For this reason a committee of women doctors – including Dickson as honorary secretary – was formed to help those coming behind them; they offered advice on practical issues, such as housing, as well as professional matters.[83]

Through the 1890s, Dickson was a strong advocate for women, both in medicine in particular and in society in general. Her correspondence with the British Medical Association seems to have been instrumental in extending its membership to women; when this happened, in 1892, Dickson was amongst the first women to join. She published in the *BMJ* and the *Irish Times* on the necessity of women

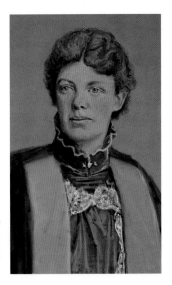

Portrait of Emily Winifred Dickson by Mick O'Dea (2019).

as workhouse doctors, not least as inmates were predominantly women and children. As a member of the Irish Suffrage Association, she urged women of her class to take an interest in 'questions which affected working women', and she decried corsets as unnecessary, unnatural and ungainly. She was also involved in the National Society of Prevention of Cruelty to Children and the Irish Association for the Prevention of Intemperance – both, to some extent, considered women's issues at the time.

And yet in spite of this litany of achievement, Dickson's career did not flourish in the following century. 'After 1900 her name no longer appears in the Medical Directory,' noted the *Journal of the*

RCSI in 1969: 'It might be presumed she died in or about that year...'[84] Not quite: in 1899, Dickson married and ceased to practice. For a time at least, Dickson chose 'the profession of marriage' over the 'profession of medicine' (these were her own terms, from a lecture she delivered at Alexandra College). By 1910, she was the mother of five children; in the 1911 Census, she is listed as 'Medical Doctor Retired'. Dickson's marriage effectively ended at the outbreak of the First World War. Her husband, who was ten years her junior, had been a successful businessman, but from the time he enlisted and was posted overseas, he allocated to his wife sixpence per day from his pay, or £9 per annum.

So Dickson went back to work – now in England, where her children were at boarding schools. She took posts close to these schools, the first of which was at Rainhill Mental Hospital outside Liverpool. From 1917, she worked as a war locum in Ellesmere, Shropshire, and even bought a practice – but she gave this up in 1919 owing to the double blow of bronchial pneumonia brought on by the 'Spanish Flu' and the return of her shell-shocked husband. The couple officially separated soon after, and for the rest of her life Dickson was the sole breadwinner for her family. She moved often, taking short medical postings, and suffered general ill health.

In 1940, she returned to Rainhill Hospital, by then struggling with its status as one of the largest mental hospitals in the world. Dickson worked until two months before her death, aged 77, in 1944. Two years previously she had written:

> I don't regret anything, even the foolish things, but I see in countless ways that I missed many priceless chances and opportunities, not from wilfulness but from sheer blind stupidity of not appreciating how much they might mean and lots of things I thought I knew all about and didn't know there were worlds unknown that I was unaware existed.[85]

A trove of Dickson's personal papers, as well as medals and other artefacts, is held in RCSI Heritage Collections. In 2016 – marking the 150th anniversary of Dickson's birth – RCSI instituted the Emily Winifred Dickson Award to recognise women who have made an outstanding contribution in their field. The inaugural recipient was Prof Louise Richardson, first female Vice-Chancellor of the University of Oxford. The award itself is a specially commissioned piece in bronze by the sculptor Imogen Stuart RHA. Like her predecessor Mary Josephine Hannan, Dickson was also commemorated as part of the 2019 Women on Walls initiative. Her portrait, by Mick O'Dea PRHA, appropriately depicts her in her Fellow's gown. ∎

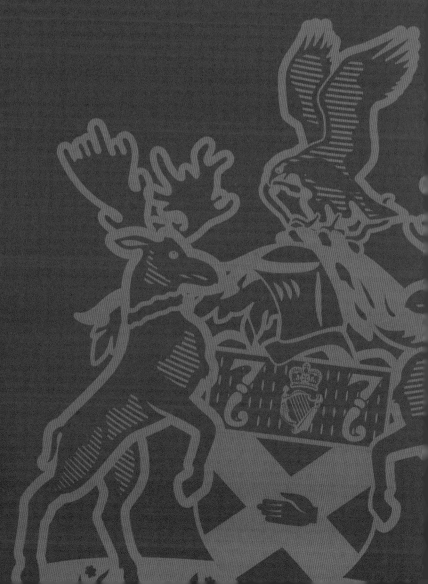

Chapter 5:
Revolutions, 1886–1923

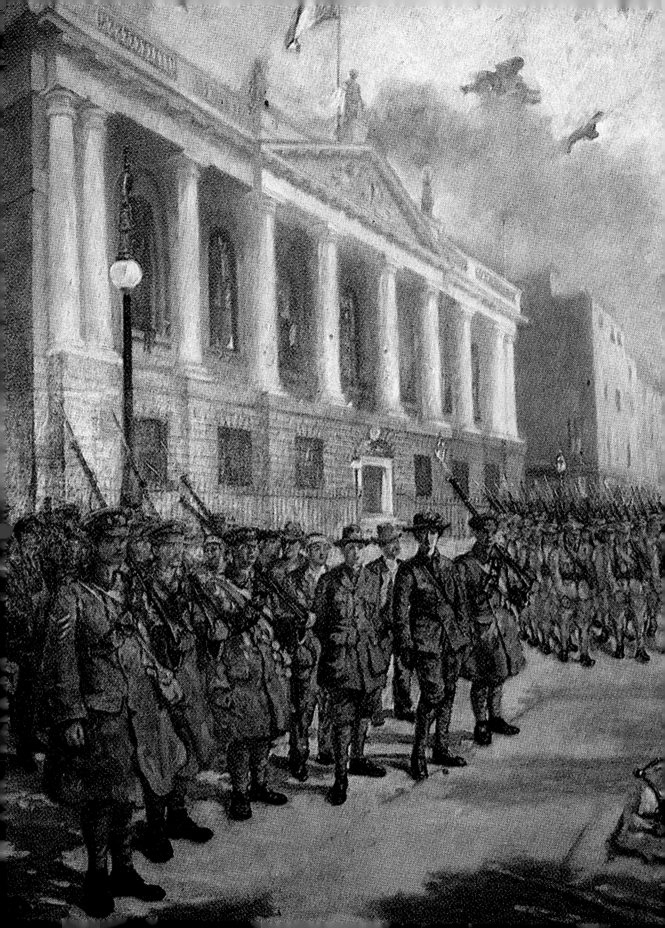

Chapter 5:
Revolutions, 1886–1923

PASTEUR, LISTER, HUXLEY AND KOCH

The generation of young men – and now women – who commenced at RCSI in the mid-1880s studied and practised in the midst of a medical Copernican revolution. Vast swathes of earlier thought were on the cusp of being junked ('if the whole *materia medica*, as now used, could be sunk to the bottom of the sea, it would be all the better for mankind,' said the American poet-physician Oliver Wendell Holmes (1809–1894), 'and all the worse for the fishes'.[1])

For twenty years, Darwin's theory of evolution had elicited excitement and disquiet, and now a focus on a microscopic realm – led by Louis Pasteur (1822–1895), Joseph Lister (1827–1912) and Robert Koch (1843–1910) – tilted the world even further. In April 1886, even as these new ideas were still being debated, RCSI awarded Honorary Fellowships to Pasteur, Lister and 'Darwin's Bulldog', Thomas Henry Huxley (1825–1895).[2] A little later, in 1891, as evidence of RCSI's commitment to this brave new world, the Council sent a deputation to Berlin to investigate and procure a supply of Koch's tell-tale protein, tuberculin. The name of Koch's assistant, Julius Petri, remains familiar to all laboratory-users.

Previous page:
The Arrest by
Kathleen Fox
(artist's copy of
the original).

SIR CHARLES CAMERON, RCSI'S RENAISSANCE MAN

Presiding over these honours was one of the larger-than-life figures of RCSI history, Sir Charles Alexander Cameron (1830–1921, Lic. 1868, FRCSI 1880, Prof of Hygiene or Political Medicine 1868–1920, Prof of Chemistry and Physics 1875–1920, PRCSI 1885–86). Born in Dublin, as a boy Cameron seemed destined to follow his Scottish father into the military, but Captain Cameron's death – Charles was 14 at the time – left the family in reduced circumstances. The military's loss was chemistry's gain ('my bedroom was practically a little laboratory,' Cameron later recollected[3]), and he was taken on by the apothecaries Bewley & Evans (later Hamilton & Long). He studied at a variety of institutions, including the Medical School of the Apothecaries' Hall and the 'Original' (later Ledwich) Medical School, and during a stint in Germany he studied organic chemistry under the 'father of fertilizer', Julius von Liebig (1803–1873); typical of Cameron's omnivorous mind, this sojourn also resulted in a later publication, *Short Poems Translated from the German* (1876).

Returning to Dublin, Cameron's zeal for chemistry was evangelical. In an attempt to bring the subject out from behind the closed doors of third-level institutions, he succeeded in getting himself elected 'Professor of Medicine' at the Dublin Chemical Society – which, as he later admitted, was a 'pretentious title' for a gathering of like-minded enthusiasts who gathered in a house in Capel Street; at

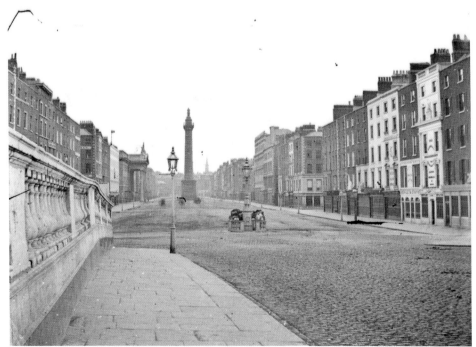

Sackville Street, with Bewley & Evans at nos. 3 and 4 (right-hand-side). Reproduced courtesy of the National Library of Ireland (STP-0049).

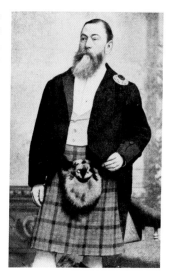

Photograph of Sir Charles Cameron, PRCSI 1885, in Highland dress.

the time, Cameron was still a 22-year-old med student and apothecary's assistant. But his enthusiasm turned it into something significant: his inaugural lecture was reported in the next day's paper, and future lectures (for which he never used notes) attracted and impressed an influential audience. Within a few short years, he was teaching at many of the same institutions where he had recently been a student.

Cameron had an uncanny knack for securing appointments ahead of parchments. From about 1857, he began to style himself 'Dr Cameron', but the origin of this doctorate is unclear – and in all his many writings, Cameron never made it any clearer. (Possibly he earned the degree in Germany; possibly he purchased it there, which was legitimate at the time, but not something one liked to advertise.) In any case, Cameron began his career as a public servant in 1862, when he was appointed Public Analyst for the city of Dublin. For the next six decades, he did more

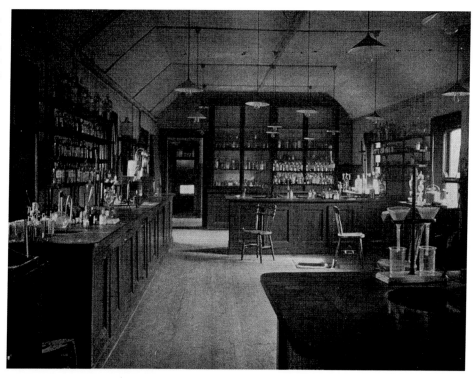

East End, No. 1, City Laboratory, Chatham Row, where Cameron carried out his analysis work. Dublin City Library and Archive. Courtesy of Dublin City Library and Archive.

than anyone else to improve public health in the city. Initially his primary role was the enforcement of the Adulteration of Food Act (1860), which many considered to be a Canute-like fool's errand.

In the era, all manner of food was regularly adulterated: milk was watered down, flour bulked with alum or sawdust, weak beer laced with strychnine to give it a kick; likewise, the sale of diseased meat was rife. In the face of powerful vested interests, Cameron enforced this hitherto apparently unenforceable law: he pursued unscrupulous traders, he analysed samples and he gave evidence in court to secure prosecution. (He took part in many trials, including on one occasion giving evidence for both sides: 'each paid my reasonable fee'.[4]) His role soon expanded to the point where he served as Public Analyst for twenty-three counties (his discovery of kaolin clay in Fermanagh led to the establishment of the celebrated Belleek Pottery Works[5]).

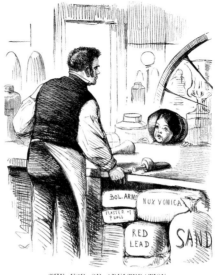

'The Use of Adulteration'. © Punch Limited.

THE USE OF ADULTERATION.

Little Girl. "IF YOU PLEASE, SIR, MOTHER SAYS, WILL YOU LET HER HAVE A QUARTER OF A POUND OF YOUR BEST TEA TO KILL THE RATS WITH, AND A OUNCE OF CHOCOLATE AS WOULD GET RID OF THE BLACK BEADLES'"

In 1874, Cameron was appointed Medical Officer for Health (MOH) for Dublin, rising to Superintendent MOH by 1879; it was under the auspices of this post, which also comprised Chief Sanitary Officer, that Cameron made his greatest contributions to the improvement of living conditions for the city's poor.[6]

Cameron's association with RCSI begins in 1868, when he succeeded Edward Mapother (1835–1908, Lic. 1854, FRCSI 1862, Prof of Hygiene or Political Medicine 1864–68, Prof of Anatomy and Physiology 1867–89[7]) as Professor of Hygiene or Political Medicine – a position he would go on to hold for an unrivalled fifty-two years.[8] 'For many years,' he recollected, 'I was connected with three medical schools which were practically rival institutions.'[9] Many of his RCSI lectures were open to the public and attracted standing-room-only crowds; to get a seat, one had to turn up an hour early. Chiefly, these lectures were concerned with food hygiene, disinfection and ventilation; he advocated throwing open all windows for several hours a day (the National Library holds a copy of one of his published lectures on the subject, in whose margin some contemporary hand has scrawled, 'Your own windows are never open!!'[10]).

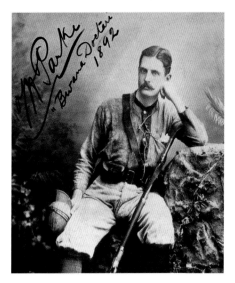

On another occasion, when he spoke on 'skin and hair', he feared the audience was more interested in how to maintain 'colour and quantity' than cleanliness. In passing, he mentioned that a well-diluted solution of phosphorus could be beneficial, only to discover later that one audience member took this advice, failed to adequately dilute the solution, and caused his hair to burst into flame. In 1875, Cameron was appointed to a second Chair at RCSI, that of Chemistry and Physics, and in 1892 he was elected Secretary to the College. A little earlier, he was instrumental in conferring an Honorary Fellowship (1889) on his former student, the colonial explorer Thomas Heazle Parke (1857–1893, Lic. 1878). (Reputedly the first Irishman to cross Africa, Surgeon-Major Parke brought a water sample from an African lake back to Dublin for Cameron to analyse. Cameron also spearheaded the erection of a statue of Parke outside the Natural History Museum on Merrion Square. Parke's diaries and other artefacts are now in RCSI Heritage Collections.[11])

Under Cameron's guidance, RCSI conferred its first American, John Shaw Billings (1838–1913), with an Honorary Fellowship (1892). Surgeon, librarian, architect and public health specialist, Billings' many interests came together when he developed the Surgeon General's Library, forerunner of the National Library of Medicine, now the world's largest medical library. By the time of Cameron's retirement (1920), his own many qualifications and honours comprised a lengthy litany.

RCSI'S FIRST HISTORIAN

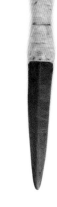
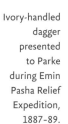

In 1884, RCSI marked its first centenary with a banquet attended by one hundred guests including the Lord Lieutenant. The correspondent from the *British Medical Journal* noted that 'the after-dinner speeches were brief, and above the average on similar occasions'.[12] The President, William Ireland de Courcy Wheeler (1844–1897, Lic. 1866, FRCSI 1874, PRCSI 1883–84), looked back at the College's early days:

... in the very first years of the centenary which they were now celebrating, the Government reposed confidence in the College, and from that early period, when its public duties first commenced, it had been continuously and efficiently engaged in providing for the surgical wants, not only of Ireland, but of Her Majesty's naval and military services.

Wheeler also looked to the School:

... and to the educational work performed by it; and alleged that the College had voluntarily, and at much sacrifice of its financial interests, occupied a foremost place amongst the licensing institutions of the kingdom, by the zeal for advancement which it had manifested, and by the improvement in the systems of education and examination which it had initiated, and in which it had forestalled other institutions.

The backward glance occasioned by the centenary caused Cameron to embark upon his magnum opus, whose full title – *History of the Royal College of Surgeons in Ireland, and of the Irish Schools of Medicine; including Numerous Biographical Sketches: also a Medical Bibliography* – gives a sense of the larger-than-life plenitude of both the author and his work. Running to some 760 pages, it is an invaluable source for the medical history of the period, all the more impressive when one learns that it was completed in a mere two years.

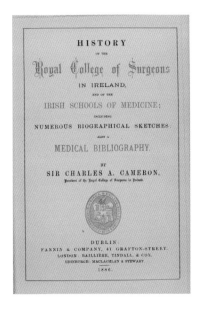 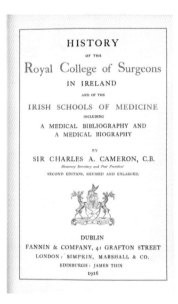

Title pages of the first (1886) and second (1916) editions of Cameron's *History of RCSI*.

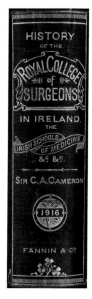

A labour of love - and grief.

If it has its flaws and errors, the sheer wealth of information, collected nowhere else, more than compensates. It is, quite obviously, a labour of love – but it is also, between the lines, an expression of channelled grief. Cameron's wife Lucie had died in 1883, after which he 'did not go into society for a year, and only to a slight extent during the following two years'. His time was devoted to the *History* – except, perhaps tellingly, when he emerged in 1885 to champion the admission of women to RCSI – and though the labour was demanding, he relished the work; when it was finished, he later wrote, 'a feeling of loneliness came over me'.[13] The couple had six sons and two daughters, and for the widowed Cameron more family sadness was to follow. A second, revised edition of the *History* was published in 1916.

A CONJOINT DIPLOMA

Ever since the passage of the 1858 Medical Act, the differences between RCSI and the College of Physicians as examining institutions were increasingly superficial. The requirements of various bodies – for example, the Poor Law Boards – that their employees should have both medical *and* surgical licences, led to the somewhat farcical situation whereby students would sit RCSI's exams one day, then troop down to Kildare Street to answer much the same set of questions to gain the Physicians' Licence – and vice versa.

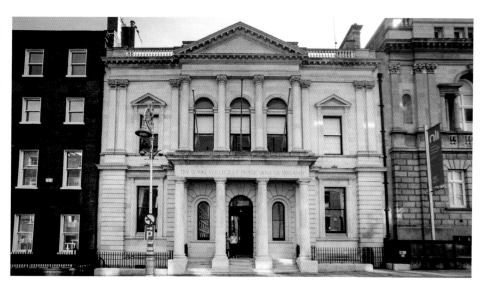

Sister college: the Royal College of Physicians' premises on Kildare Street. Courtesy of RCPI.

Over the course of nearly thirty years, many attempts to combine the respective licences came and went: sometimes it was RCSI who initiated rapprochement, sometimes Physicians; on occasion, Trinity College was in the mix, and on the rarer occasions when the Apothecaries were listened to, they too had their say. But negotiations invariably broke down – not least when it came to the vexed question of how to divide up students' fees.

In 1886, however, an amendment to the Medical Act put an end to this to-ing and froing. Henceforth, admission to the Medical Register required a 'triple qualification' in medicine, surgery and midwifery. The fact that these subjects were already taught and examined at RCSI was immaterial in the eyes of the law: the right postnominals were demanded. Representatives of RCSI and the College of Physicians swiftly formed the Irish Conjoint Board to come to a mutually beneficial arrangement. (From the start, RCSI was willing to admit the Apothecaries, but Physicians objected; later, RCSI and the Apothecaries' Hall came to a side arrangement between themselves, which Physicians unsuccessfully contested.)

Under the new terms, the College of Physicians now participated in the final medical exams at RCSI and successful candidates were awarded the Licence of both Colleges. The fee for this new Conjoint Diploma was fixed at 42 guineas, of which the slightly larger share, 25 guineas, went to RCSI. The first exam was held in May 1888,[14] following which the first cohort of successful candidates could see themselves styled in the Register as: 'Lic., Lic. Midwif. 1888, K. Q. Coll. Phys. Irel. Lic., Lic. Midwif. 1888, R. Coll. Surg. Irel.' Formerly rivals, the two bodies increasingly acted as 'sister colleges'.[15] In 1890, the King and Queen's College of Physicians of Ireland changed its name to the Royal College of Physicians of Ireland (RCPI).

AMALGAMATION OF THE LEDWICH AND CARMICHAEL SCHOOLS

In 1888, RCSI embarked on a further 'conjoint' initiative: it amalgamated with two private medical schools, the Ledwich and the Carmichael – the only surviving private schools in the city, having outlasted almost twenty others that had come and gone in the century.

The Ledwich claimed descent from John Kirby's school at 28 Peter Street, though in fact the connection was somewhat spurious. Kirby had closed his school when he was appointed RCSI's Professor of Medicine in 1832 – much to the annoyance of one of his employees, Andrew Ellis, who hoped to continue the enterprise. Unable to come to an arrangement with Kirby, Ellis opened his own school next door, at no. 27, to which he gave the exact same name as Kirby had

Amalgamation:
the Ledwich and
Carmichael
Schools.

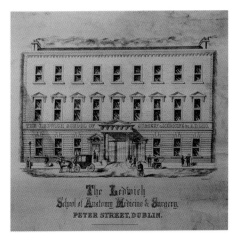

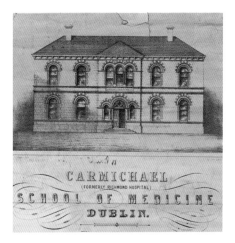

used, the 'Theatre of Anatomy and School of Surgery'.

Then, in 1834, a maverick figure called George Thomas Hayden (*c.*1798–1857) – he proudly advertised he was a Licentiate (1826) and *ex*-FRCSI (1845) – opened a medical school at Kirby's old address, no. 28. Brazenly, he called this 'the Original School' to steal a march on Ellis next door. (Twice bitten, Ellis moved on to the School of the Apothecaries' Hall and let the 'Theatre' slide into oblivion.) Hayden's 'Original School' flourished for a time, then struggled, then was reborn when Thomas Hawkesworth Ledwich (1823–1858, Lic. 1844, FRCSI 1845) was appointed Lecturer in Anatomy in 1849.

A pale, asthmatic man, he had taught Cameron, who remembered him being 'of studious habits, and though he rose early he sat up very late... and during the latter portion of his short life frequently spent the whole night in his chair, alternately dozing and reading – his large microscope always being placed in a convenient position, and ready for use'.[16] With his brother Edward (1817–1879, Lic. 1848, FRCSI 1852), he published a celebrated work, *The Practical and Descriptive Anatomy of the Human Body* (1852). Esteemed as a teacher, when Ledwich died in 1858 – aged just 35 – his students petitioned to have the school renamed in his honour; ten years later their wish was granted.

The Carmichael School began in 1826 as the School of Anatomy, Medicine and Surgery of the Richmond Hospital. It was founded by Colles' contemporary and sometime sparring partner, Richard Carmichael, whose prescient arguments back in 1841 ('there cannot be a good physician who has not the knowledge of a surgeon, or a good surgeon who has not the knowledge of a physician') were now belatedly vindicated by the 1886 Amendment to the Medical Act. Carmichael served as RCSI President three times, the last in 1845.

Four years later, in his 70th year, he set out to ride from the city centre to his summer residence in Sutton. Reaching the coast road, he saw the evening tide was out, and so took a short cut across the sands. Four days later, his drowned body was found, unmarked by any injury. In his will he created bequests for RCSI (£3,000 to fund the Carmichael Essay Prize[17]), the Medical Benevolent Association (£4,500) and the Richmond Hospital School (£10,000) – in honour of which the school was renamed 'the Carmichael'. The school buildings were handsomely revamped by the windfall – in fact, the edifice still stands – but in 1879 the Carmichael School relocated southside to the corner of Aungier Street and Whitefriar Street.[18]

The amalgamation of these two neighbouring schools had first been proposed four years earlier, in 1884, but was rejected at that time. The reasons for or against were unclear then, and not very much clearer in May 1888 when the reanimated proposal was passed. The resolution speaks of 'having regard to the interests of medical education in Dublin, it is desirable to diminish, as far as possible, the number of private schools'.[19] Reading between the lines, medical education was now an expensive endeavour requiring specialised equipment and facilities – long gone were the days of lectures in a repurposed house or hayloft – and the private schools were likely feeling the pinch of keeping up.

RCSI still aspired to accredit those students, however, so it was in everyone's interests that they could make the modern grade; if that meant amalgamation, so be it. The contractual details of amalgamation were worked out through the winter of 1888, so that the start of the following academic year – that is, 1889–90 – marked the launch of 'The Schools of Surgery of the Royal College of Surgeons in Ireland, including the Carmichael and Ledwich Schools'.[20] This extended title was employed for a time, until amalgamation revealed itself to be, in fact, wholesale absorption, and the Carmichael and Ledwich names faded from use.

'RECONSTRUCTION AND ENLARGEMENT': MAKING SPACE FOR THE SCHOOLS

From RCSI's point of view, the merger proved punitively expensive. In the preceding three years the average annual income of both the Ledwich (£2,527) and the Carmichael (£2,636) outstripped that of RCSI (£2,107).[21] Lacking space, RCSI was obliged to retain the Carmichael premises until 1902 – plus the ground rent and taxes that came with it (the Ledwich house, meanwhile, was taken over by the Adelaide Hospital). Before amalgamation, the combined income of the three schools amounted to £7,270; in 1890, the pooled income shrank to £4,837; and seven years later it was down to £3,434. Playing the long game with student fees was always going to be costly, but RCSI surely hoped for a better bargain than this. To ease the general financial embarrassment, certain day-to-day expenses – such as electricity, coal and advertising – were funded out of professors' own pockets.

All this time, as income fell, capital expenditure remained high – as outlined by a vividly informative article in the *Irish Times* in January 1892:

THE NEW SCHOOLS OF THE ROYAL COLLEGE
OF SURGEONS IN IRELAND

The reconstruction and enlargement of the schools of the Irish College which have been in progress since 1st July is now very nearly completed, and it has been arranged that they shall be opened on Monday, the 1st of February, by the President and Council of the College. Such of the Fellows of the College as desire to be present are also invited to attend. The chief work of re-construction has been the erection of a very fine and spacious dissecting room, capable of accommodating 300 or 400 students. Most of the old buildings which did duty for this purpose have been entirely removed, and the space on which they stood excavated. Fireproof floors and roof have been put in, and every requirement for anatomical study provided. Attached to this department is a bone-room, a ladies' dissecting room, and a suite of apartments for female students, as well as a workroom and private room for the professors. For the accommodation of the physiological department a new lecture theatre has been built, a laboratory for biological study, a room for physiological chemistry, and private rooms for the professors have been erected. The large histological laboratory which was constructed a few years ago still remains. The chemical laboratory has been enlarged to nearly double its previous size, and private rooms for the professors have been attached thereto. In the old part of the school, room has thus been made for a students' common room and other apartments. The lighting and heating of the school have been provided for by a complete new system of hot-water heating and by an electric light installation, which latter also extends to the college itself. The effect of this illumination will be to extend indefinitely the opportunities for anatomical study, which has heretofore been pursued, after nightfall, under difficulties. The electric installation has been put in by the Electric Engineering Company of Ireland. Pending the completion of these alterations in the college school, its work has been carried on under some disadvantages at the Carmichael College, but it will be transferred to its proper habitation on the 1st of next month.[22]

ESTABLISHING THE RULES OF THE GAME

In 1889, following amalgamation, the RCSI student population was 173. How much of a boost this represented is not known, as the figures for the previous four years are missing. The Ledwich and Carmichael students also brought their teachers with them – which was not an entirely smooth transition. Certain newcomers who had resisted the merger had to be placated with plum appointments – which irked some *in situ* staff (Anatomy, for example, temporarily reverted to a co-chair[23]). Amongst the new arrivals were many talented individuals, such as Sir John Moore (1845–1937, Prof of Medicine 1889–1916). In a welcome lecture to students at the Meath Hospital in his 87th year, he spoke of

> the noble and ennobling profession to which many of us have already the honour to belong to, or – as is the case of many whom I am now addressing – to which, as medical students, they aspire. And yet are not all of us in a very special sense still medical students? Not a day passes in our professional life that an opportunity does not offer of learning something new, of testing that 'something' and of making use thereof.[24]

Another notable newcomer was Hugh Alexander Auchinleck (1849–1929, Lic. 1879, FRCSI 1881, Prof of Medical Jurisprudence 1889–1920), formerly Lecturer on Forensic Medicine at the Carmichael. He made one of the great contributions to Irish sport in early January 1883, when he convened a meeting of the Dublin Hurling Club in his home at 35 York Street. There, with Michael Cusack in attendance, they drew up the rules of the game. Auchinleck was elected President of the Club, with Cusack as Vice-President; two years later, Cusack went on to found the Gaelic Athletic Association.[25] This RCSI-GAA connection was commemorated in 2002 by the Presidents of both institutions.

Also joining from the Carmichael was Ephraim McDowel Cosgrave (1853–1925, Lic. 1876, Prof of Biology 1889–1925). A new chair – that of Biology – was created for him, which he held for the next thirty-six years, during which time he was also President of RCPI (1914–16). A Knight of the Order of St John, his handbook for the St John Ambulance Association – *Hints and Helps for Home Nursing and Hygiene* (1915) – sold in the region of 400,000 copies. Outside of medicine, Cosgrave's fascination with photography – he was President of the Amateur Photographic Society – coupled with an interest in Dublin history, led to two remarkable illustrated books, *The Dictionary of Dublin* (1895) and *Dublin and*

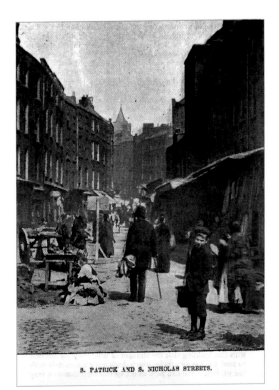

S. PATRICK AND S. NICHOLAS STREETS.

THE
DICTIONARY OF DUBLIN

Being a Comprehensive Guide to the City
and its Neighbourhood

BY

E. MacDOWEL COSGRAVE, M.D., Dub. Univ., F.R.C.P.I.
Member of Council, Photographic Society of Ireland

AND

LEONARD R. STRANGWAYS, M.A.
*Ex-Sch. and Senior Moderator, Dub. Univ.; Vice-President,
Photographic Society of Ireland*

*ILLUSTRATED BY NUMEROUS PHOTOGRAPHS
TAKEN BY THE AUTHORS*

DUBLIN: SEALY, BRYERS & WALKER
(A. T. & C. L.)
94, 95 AND 96 MIDDLE ABBEY STREET
LONDON: SIMPKIN, MARSHALL, HAMILTON, KENT & CO., LTD.
1895

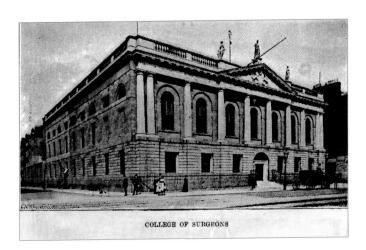

COLLEGE OF SURGEONS

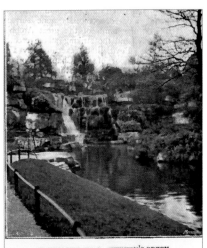

WATERFALL IN S. STEPHEN'S GREEN.

Co. Dublin in the Twentieth Century (1908).[26] Cosgrave's obituary in the *BMJ* also recorded that he was 'President of the Irish Chess Club, and was the first to play the game with living men as pieces... Dr Cosgrave's genial personality won him friends in all directions.'[27]

Facing page:
From Cosgrave's
*Dictionary of
Dublin* (1895).

SIR THOMAS MYLES: KNIGHT OF THE REALM AND GUN-RUNNER

Thanks to continental strides made by Virchow and others, pathology was now becoming a formal field of study in its own right. One of Virchow's pedagogic innovations was his 'Railway Course', described thus by one visiting RCSI Licentiate:

> The room in which the lectures are held is provided with a fixed table about two feet in width, running in a zigzag direction from one end of it to the other; on this a miniature railways is laid down for the conveyance of microscopes on little trucks from one part of the class to another...[28]

In 1889, RCSI established a Chair of Pathology – the first of its kind in Ireland – and Thomas Myles (1859–1937, FRCSI 1885, Prof of Pathology 1889–97, PRCSI 1900–02) was the inaugural appointee. He was one of the first Dublin surgeons to wear gloves while operating – the cotton ones advocated by Jan Mikulicz-Radecki (1850–1905).[29] As Koch advised boiling one's operating instruments, Myles took his to the hospital kitchens and dropped them in a fish kettle; so novel was this that the cook supposed he wanted to soften them. In addition to being an authority on French literature and a devotee of Shakespeare, Myles also had an impressive publishing record – but no biographical commentary fails to mention his 'magnificent physique'.[30] He is reputed to have sparred with John L. Sullivan, the heavyweight boxing champion of the world, when the 'Boston Strong Boy' toured Ireland in 1887.

Five years earlier, in May 1882, Myles was at work in Dr Steevens' Hospital when he received an emergency summons. Across the Liffey, in Phoenix Park,

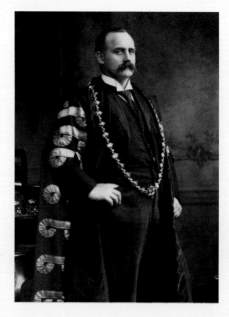

Sir Thomas
Myles,
PRCSI
1900–02.

two men had been attacked: Lord Frederick Cavendish, who had arrived that day as Irish Chief Secretary, and Thomas Henry Burke, the Permanent Under Secretary. Myles attempted treatment at the scene – a cross etched in the grass still marks the spot – but both men died of their wounds. This became one of the most notorious murder cases in Irish history, and since the weapons used were surgical knives, suspicion turned to the medical community. At a meeting on 11 May, RCSI passed resolutions expressing 'deep horror and indignation at the atrocious murders', and condolence letters were sent out.[31] A year-long investigation resulted in trials and executions; in the end, no medical personnel were implicated.

Politically, Myles was a moderate nationalist, in favour of Home Rule – which put him at odds with many of his RCSI colleagues. In 1893, the Fellows petitioned against Home Rule because they feared it would adversely affect RCSI; as it happened, the bill passed in the Commons but was defeated by the Lords. As the century wound to a close, Myles was considered a controversial candidate for RCSI presidency. One opponent declared that Myles would 'associate the College with the promotors of anarchy and discord'[32] – but in the event he was successfully elected.

His term as President (1900–02) witnessed the end of the Victorian era, when the Queen died on 22 January 1901. Eight seats were allotted to RCSI for the subsequent memorial service at St Patrick's Cathedral. As PRCSI, Myles was there – as was the loyalist Cameron – both in mourning black; the RCSI mace was also draped. At the end of his term, Myles was conferred with a knighthood, and shortly afterwards, he and Lady Myles received an invitation to the Westminster coronation of Edward VII. His successor as PRCSI, New Zealand-born Lambert Ormsby (1849–1923, FRCSI 1875, PRCSI 1902–04), complained: as sitting President, Ormsby said, the invitation was meant for him. 'Possibly,' replied Sir Thomas, 'but you can't take Lady Myles,' which apparently settled the matter.[33]

In every possible sense, Myles was a pillar of the establishment – and yet in 1914 he added another astonishing activity to his list of accomplishments: he became a gun-runner for the Irish Volunteers. A lifelong mariner, he sailed his yacht, the *Chotah*, to the coast of Wales in late July, where he collected 600 rifles and 19,000 rounds of ammunition that had been sourced in Germany. At the same time, a slightly larger consignment was collected by the writer Erskine Childers (1870–1922) aboard the *Asgard*; the *Asgard* reached Howth on 26 July, but the *Chotah* was delayed by a split mainsail. Its illegal load was eventually landed at Kilcoole, County Wicklow, through the night of 1–2 August. Amongst those who brought Myles' cargo ashore was Seán T. O'Kelly; the load was then hidden in

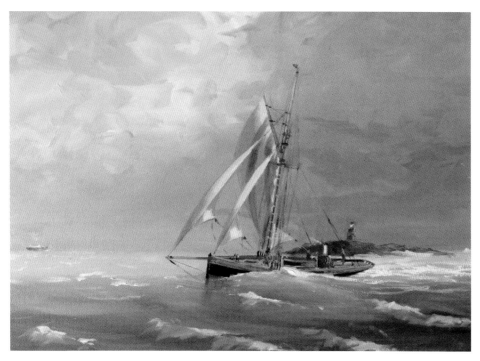

Myles' yacht, the *Chotah*, by Brian Byrnes.

the grounds of Pearse's school in Rathfarnham. Forty-four years later, in 1958, O'Kelly – by then President of Ireland, Seán T. Ó Ceallaigh – was conferred with Honorary Fellowship of RCSI.

After independence, Myles devoted much of his significant energy to sport: he was centrally involved in fundraising to send an Irish team to the 1928 Olympics in Amsterdam – where Patrick O'Callaghan (1906–1991, Lic. 1927) won the country's first gold medal. Myles also remained a lifelong sailor – not least as President of the RCSI Boat Club – and when, in his seventies, he shipwrecked his yacht, the *Sheila* (incidentally, a former Royal yacht) off the coast of the Isle of Man, he simply bought a new, bigger one and kept sailing. The fate of the *Chotah* is unclear – in fact, no known photographs of it survive. But a painting of it hangs in RCSI – in the Sir Thomas Myles Room.

THE FIRST CHARTER DAY DINNER

Outwardly at least, RCSI was in rude health under such charismatic leadership. From 1901, a celebratory Annual Dinner took place – from 1911 this event happened on or close to 11 February and was – and is – known as the Charter Day Dinner.[34] But behind the scenes, the demands of running a modern medical school caused much day-to-day stress. It is a measure of the pace of change that the reconstructed and enlarged facilities that were vaunted in the press in 1892 were deemed inadequate a little more than a decade later.

In 1905, a confidential internal report ran the rule over the various departments, and in general the findings were stark: 'it is hopeless to expect anything approaching to thorough efficiency in the School unless important structural alterations are made... In conclusion, your Committee regret to observe that, the condition of the School is very much more unsatisfactory than it need be, even taking into consideration its defective accommodation.' Noted too was a general dishevelment and absence of that orderliness which should serve as an object lesson for students. And the problem was not only with defective fixtures and fittings: 'Your Committee, too, find evidence that but little cohesion exists among the professors in the working of the School as a whole. No professor appears to do more than give his own lectures, and there is a total absence of supervision.'[35]

To remedy this last 'grave' defect, it was recommended that a Dean be appointed ('to be responsible for the efficient working of the School in general'); this appointment went to the Professor of Anatomy, Alexander Fraser (1853–1909, FRCSI 1895, Prof of Anatomy 1883–1909). While popular with students and respected by his colleagues, Fraser was not, alas, the new broom the School required.

A 'CONSTITUENT SCHOOL' OF THE NEW NATIONAL UNIVERSITY?

To make matters worse, an even greater, existential threat loomed over RCSI. This came in the form of the long-proposed Irish Universities Bill, which was set to expand third-level education – including, crucially, the teaching of medicine. The bill was part of a debate that had been rumbling for nigh-on fifty years, since the advent of the Queen's Colleges, but the new century brought new impetus. If new, rival bodies were about to receive state funding, RCSI wanted to know if it too would get a slice of the pie.

As early as 1903, Cameron urged RCSI to make its case to the Chief Secretary – but the answer, it turned out, was a flat no. For the next five years, RCSI repeatedly fought its corner, reiterating certain key points: as a regulatory body as well as a school, RCSI had responsibilities that mere teaching

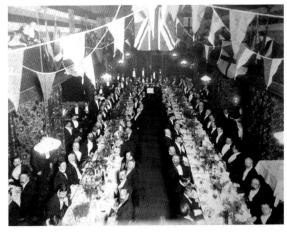

The Annual Dinner, 1903.

bodies did not have to worry about; RCSI's non-sectarian ethos already implicitly addressed a fundamental point of the bill (essentially, the bill was an attempt to address Ireland's endemic sectarianism); and, finally, there was historic precedence for aid ('In its early years [RCSI] was nursed into existence by the government of that

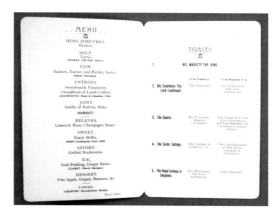

The Charter Day menu, 1913.

day. It should not now be helped out of existence by the government of this day'[36]).

But repeatedly, these appeals met rebuffs. Late in the day, in April 1908, RCSI made a final gambit: a grant of £5,000 per annum would keep the School open – but, failing that, the Council proposed (after 'anxious consideration') a daring alternative solution:

> We would be willing that the precedent of London University should be adopted, and that our School should be made a 'constituent school' of the new University. Provision would then be made in the Bill that our School be placed ceteris paribus [all else being equal] in the same position of the proposed School of Medicine with regard to equipment, endowment, scholarships, privileges, representation on Senate, Examining boards, etc.[37]

The School, in this vision, would continue to educate students for RCSI diplomas, 'as well as for degrees of the new University'. It would remain under RCSI management, but education would be under the University's supervision. The College, meanwhile, would remain independent. Thus, the dual remit of the original 1784 Charter ('to regulate the profession of Surgery, and to maintain a reliable and extensive system of surgical education in Ireland') could still be fulfilled. The signatories to this proposal were Swanzy, Cameron and Sir John Lentaigne (1857–1915, Lic. 1879, FRCSI 1886, PRCSI 1908–10).

Ingenious – perhaps even desperate – as this proposal was, the authorities were unmoved. RCSI received neither the grant nor the 'constituent school' status. There were many roads not taken in answering the so-called 'University Question' – Trinity, for its part, formed a Dublin University Defence Committee to resist any state meddling. But what did come to pass, in December 1908, was the Irish

Universities Act, which established two new universities, the Queen's University of Belfast and the National University of Ireland, which was comprised of three constituent colleges at Dublin, Cork and Galway. (The first honours graduate in Medicine of NUI was William 'Bill' Doolin (1888–1962, FRCSI 1912, PRCSI 1938–40).)

The 1908 act also empowered the NUI Senate to accredit courses of study in other institutions for the purpose of degrees. These were known as 'Recognised Colleges' – which to some extent was the status proposed by Swanzy *et al*. As it happens, RCSI would in time become a Recognised College of the NUI – but not until 1977. In the meantime, it was left – as it had been since 1811 – to its own devices. As the end-of-year report put it:

> The College must now look forward to a period of intense competition with State-endowed Institutions, supplied at the public expense, with the most costly equipment, with well-salaried officials, and with all the prestige of Government Institutions. Time alone can demonstrate whether our College will be able to hold its own against such competition...[38]

One tantalising future direction was outlined a little later by Thomas Myles:

> With the increasing competition due to the establishment of the National University, it will be necessary for us to seek outside Ireland for our due proportion of Medical Students.[39]

AUCKLAND GEDDES' NEW BROOM AND CLEAN SWEEP

The new Dean, Prof Fraser, died in July 1909 after a short illness. He was replaced in his professorship – first temporarily, then on a permanent basis – by Auckland Campbell Geddes (1879–1954, Prof of Anatomy 1909–13), a veteran of the Boer War. As soon as he arrived, Geddes implemented literally sweeping measures. Discovering that students were contracting tuberculosis, he arranged for the disinfection of the entire medical school. Then in August he produced a damning fourteen-page report on conditions in the Anatomy Department; the phrase 'swarming with flies and maggots' was liberally used.

A chastened Council acted upon every recommendation: in the end, the entire floor ('saturated with disease germs') was replaced, new ventilation and new tables were installed, and walls were cleansed and re-painted (total cost, £1,400).[40] Recent neglect notwithstanding, Anatomy was still considered by far the most

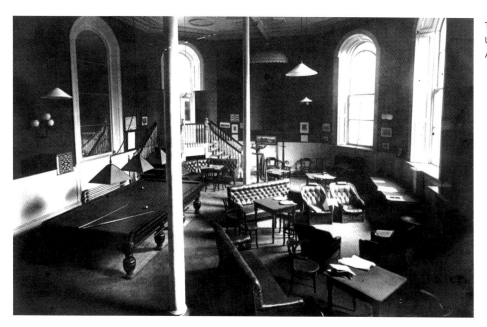

The Students' Union in the Albert Hall.

important department, and Geddes used his position to make many School-wide changes ('That the request of Prof Geddes be acceded to' becomes a refrain in the Council Minutes).

Geddes was particularly active on the students' behalf: under his influence, a Students' Union was set up (December 1909), with the Albert Hall furnished with a billiard table and newspapers. As a document on the objects of the Union declared, 'True Medical education does not consist merely of attendance at lectures, hospitals, &c. There is something wider and greater to be aimed at.'[41] Moreover, in the wake of the close call of the Universities Bill, the Union offered other, intangible benefits:

> Hitherto the School had been looked upon only as a place where the student obtained his education. [The Council now] wanted their students to feel, like those of a University, that they were members of an institution having an independent existence of its own; and that, when they became licentiates they should be able to look back with pleasant memories on the old days, and to feel pride in the body to which they belonged.[42]

At first open until 6 p.m., the Union was so popular that students successfully petitioned to have this extended until 10.30 (their argument was that junior students could be 'led astray' if they ventured into the city in the evenings). Led by Geddes, a Students' Athletic Club was started (July 1910) and RCSI leased its first sports ground (a seven-acre field in Terenure); not unconnected, in the run-up to war, Geddes also led the RCSI Officer Training Corps (1909), who used the field for their manoeuvres. The students had Geddes to thank too for the introduction of a bicycle shelter.

In 1913, after a little less than four years in his post, Geddes left for McGill University in Montreal. For all his improvements, it seems likely he was not greatly missed by his colleagues. By then he had clashed with the new Registrar, Alfred Miller (1874–1940), who had replaced George Blake in 1911.[43] (In fact, Geddes called Miller 'thoroughly incompetent', but the Council disagreed;[44] Miller was by all other accounts an extremely capable Registrar, serving for twenty-seven years, until 1938. He received an OBE for his work in 1920.)

Geddes was also – briefly – Dean, but stepped down when he found he did not have a free hand in hiring and (especially) firing. But his transformation of facilities – much of it, he claimed, from his own pocket – cannot be gainsaid. In 1912, in his independent assessment of the School, Prof G. Sims Woodhead of Cambridge declared:

> I know of no School in the Kingdom to be so well-equipped, in proportion to the number of students... There is evidence of great thoroughness and activity in the conduct of the School which gives good promises for the medical education of its students.

The 'Anatomical Department' in particular, he noted, 'gives the keynote to the work of the School'.[45]

Geddes went on to have a stellar political career: during the war, he was Director of Recruiting at the War Office, then an MP in Lloyd George's government; he was successively Director of National Service, Minister for Reconstruction and, from 1920, British Ambassador to the United States; he served again during World War II, when he was made Baron Geddes. His replacement as Prof of Anatomy was Evelyn John Evatt (1868–1951, Prof of Anatomy 1913–47), who would spend most of the war on active service, for which he was awarded the Distinguished Service Order.

Through RCSI in general, there were signs of new brooms coming in and dead wood going out (the rotten Library floor was fixed[46]). Out front, new granite steps were laid; inside, the flagstones of the Entrance Hall were levelled. The building was connected to the Corporation's electricity supply, replacing the old in-house dynamo. The museum continued its ignominious shrinkage: a report (1903) recommended that a committee be appointed to 'go through the contents... and to select the specimens they consider worth keeping, and to indicate those that may be destroyed or disposed of'.

In 1907, when it was belatedly discovered that RCSI had no Coat of Arms, that was remedied. A telephone was installed in the School ('Students not to be allowed to use the College Telephone any longer'). That year, PRCSI Swanzy attended the Vivisection Committee in London – this was in the aftermath of the so-called 'Brown Dog affair', when medical students clashed with anti-vivisectionists

TIME (Ireland) ACT, 1916.

On and after SUNDAY, the 1st OCTOBER, 1916, Western European Time will be observed throughout Ireland. All clocks and watches should be put back 35 minutes during the night 30th SEPTEMBER--1st OCTOBER.

The proper time to make the change is 3 a.m. Summer Time and the correction to the nearest second is 34 minutes 39 seconds.

BY ORDER OF THE LORD LIEUTENANT.

DUBLIN CASTLE.
12th September, 1916.

Time (Ireland) Act. Reproduced courtesy of the National Library of Ireland (EPH F252).

– and the Minutes record that RCSI considered such experiments to be 'absolutely essential to medical progress'. When daylight saving was introduced – and Dublin Mean Time abolished – RCSI approved of that too, 'both from a Hygienic and Economic perspective'.

The wider cultural revival did not go unnoticed either: in 1903, a delegation led by future President of Ireland Douglas Hyde visited RCSI to ask that the Irish language be added to the optional subjects of the Preliminary Examination; this was approved. Elsewhere, certain proposed reforms went a step too far: in 1908, Council-member Robert Woods (1865–1938, FRCSI 1893, PRCSI 1910–12) suggested that 'no one shall be eligible to hold a professorship of Surgery, Medicine, Midwifery, Forensic Medicine or Public Health in the College after he has passed the age of forty years or any examinership in those subjects after fifty'.[47] Unsurprisingly, this proposition received no support among the Council's greybeards.

THE GMC'S THREATENED GUILLOTINE

For all this concerted modernisation, RCSI found itself plunged into a fresh existential crisis in November 1910, when the General Medical Council (GMC) wrote – out of the blue – to say that, three years hence, from 1913, they would no longer recognise RCSI's Preliminary Examinations. In a reply to the GMC, signed by Sir Arthur Chance (1859–1928, Lic. 1880, FRCSI 1891, PRCSI 1904–06), RCSI's predicament was baldly stated:

> The 'elimination' of our Preliminary Examination in General Education, either by its non-recognition by the General Medical Council or by raising its standard to an impossible height, will reduce the number of our students to such an extent that the residue will not be sufficient to enable the School (practically without endowment) to be carried on.

Failure of the School means failure of the College.[48]

What particularly antagonised RCSI was the seemingly arbitrary actions of the GMC: first, because there had been no warning, but more crucially, 'that it had been arrived at... without any recent inspection or investigation of the methods or standard of the Examination'.[49] This Damoclean threat hung over RCSI for the next three years, as Chance – RCSI's representative on the GMC – pressed the case in London. Lengthy documents were compiled, attesting to the thoroughness of the exams in question – these featured sample papers, results and the names and qualifications of the various examiners. (In 1913, for example, the examiner in Irish was one 'E. de Valera B.A. R.U.I.' Curiously, too, another future rebel, Joseph Mary Plunkett, passed RCSI's entrance exams in 1911, but owing to ill health did not progress any further.)

Along the way, as clarification from the GMC was forthcoming, RCSI willingly made the minor modifications that were asked for, and by June 1913, Chance was able to give an early verbal report that disaster was averted: the GMC would 'continue to recognise unconditionally the Preliminary Examinations of the College'.[50]

If, in the end, this seems like a storm in a teacup, it is nonetheless likely that if Chance and RCSI had not defended their position, then the end result could have been very different. At the same time, with dark storms brewing over Europe, the revised priority for the GMC and everyone else was to keep open as many medical schools as possible.

HOW THE POOR LIVE (1904)

Beyond the precincts of RCSI, what was the city of Dublin like in the Edwardian era? One answer is in the pages of James Joyce's *Ulysses*, set on a single day in June 1904. Since Charles Cameron was ubiquitous in the city, it is no surprise that he appears in the novel – characteristically, in the context of society dining ('The annual dinner you know. Boiled shirt affair. The lord mayor was there, Val Dillon it was, and sir Charles Cameron...'[51]). After all, Cameron himself had once advised that one 'ought never to refuse an invitation to dinner, as pleasant dinners were conducive to longevity'.[52]

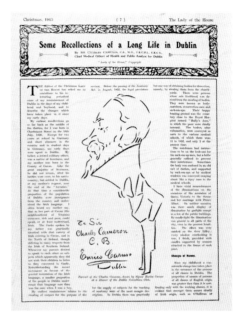

Sketch of Cameron by the tenor Enrico Caruso, 1909.

But Cameron also knew a darker Dublin than the one Joyce conjured up in continental exile. That city exists in the pages of a short, vivid, crusading volume Cameron published in 1904. Entitled *How the Poor Live*, from its first line it pulls no punches: 'There are probably no cities in the United Kingdom in which so large a proportion of the population belong to the poorest classes as is the case in Dublin.' Cameron brings the forensic (a three-page 'Table of Diet') together with the emotive ('No inconsiderable number of the poor get out of their beds, or substitutes for them, without knowing when they are to get their breakfast, for the simple reason that they have neither money nor credit').

Repeatedly, he returns to his two main – indeed, lifelong – concerns: the plight of underfed, underdressed children, and the blight of inadequate housing. By his count, 33.9 per cent of families in Dublin lived in a single room; in a survey of seventy-four tenements in Church Street the number of families per house ranged from two to fourteen. *How the Poor Live* ends by pointing the reader towards the various charities who could make a difference, because the authorities to whom Cameron reported and appealed – not least in his 100-plus-page *Annual Reports* – were incapable or unwilling to stir themselves to action.

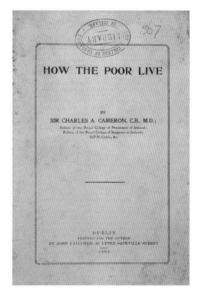

Cameron's pamphlet, *How the Poor Live* (1904).

Unlike so many of his class, Cameron knew the Dickensian squalor of Dublin intimately, not least as Superintendent Medical Officer of Health (for which he often used RCSI's laboratories). On one occasion, to bridge that chasm, Cameron insisted that the

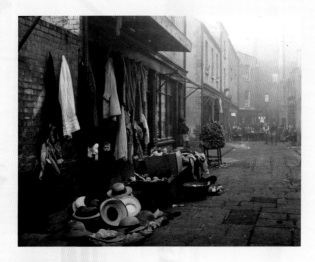

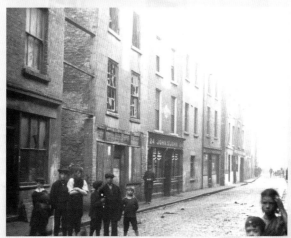

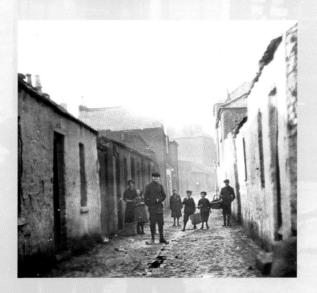

visiting Prince of Wales – later Edward VII – come with him for some first-hand experience ('as [he] had visited many model dwellings for the working classes, he ought to see some of the wretched dwellings in which the poor lived and which it was desirable should be replaced by healthy abodes'[53]).

The unscheduled detour – to Golden Lane, close to RCSI – caused consternation for the prince's handlers, but soon after Cameron was rewarded with a knighthood for his work. To some extent, the royal handlers were right to be concerned: working in tenements – to say nothing of living in them – was to put oneself in harm's way; a short time earlier, William Wilde had calculated that the lives of medical men who attended the poor were shortened, on average, by twenty years.[54]

'THIS TERRIBLE BLOW'

Cameron was well aware of the toll of lives cut short. In his public-facing guise, he was an energetic, indestructible, even bumptious, figure; his own *Reminiscences* (1913) and *Autobiography* (1920) paint that same portrait. But the four volumes of his private diaries – now in RCSI Heritage Collections – tell a different story, one of a more insecure, harried man engaged in a Sisyphean task. Poverty, overcrowding and unsanitary dwellings created conditions perfectly antithetical to public health. Disease – typhus, typhoid, smallpox, dysentery, tuberculosis and cholera – was rampant, and when outbreaks occurred, hard-won improvements could be wiped out overnight.

Cameron's diaries also record the hammer blows of personal tragedy. By the time his wife Lucie died, in 1883, the couple had already buried one child, William (8), who had contracted scarlet fever, in 1875. Lucie's death left the widowed Cameron, then aged 51, with five surviving sons and two daughters, ranging in age from 16 to 1. But death kept calling: Douglas (24) and Mervyn (23) both succumbed to pulmonary tuberculosis, in 1895 and 1898, respectively; his eldest son, Charlie (37), drowned in 1913; his youngest, Ewen (33), who joined the Royal Dublin Fusiliers at the start of the war, died by suicide in 1915 ('This terrible blow,' Cameron confided to his diary, 'will leave the little of life left to me joyless'[55]). It was all a far cry from

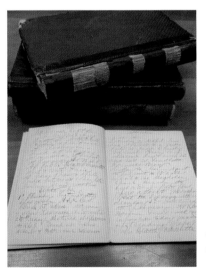

Facing page: Dirty old town: Mason's Market, Cooke Street and Rainsford Street. Courtesy of the Royal Society of Antiquaries of Ireland.

Cameron's diaries, 1880–1916.

the jolly pastimes ('attending musical and Masonic dinners') he listed for readers of *Who's Who*.[56]

In September 1913, a tragedy occurred in Church Street. The houses at numbers 66 and 67 collapsed, killing seven inside. This caused an outcry – not least as tensions were already high owing to recent industrial unrest – this was the year of 'the Lockout'. An inquiry into *The Housing Conditions of the Working Class in Dublin* was instituted. In giving evidence, Cameron reiterated the points he had been making for thirty-five years, but with Home Rule on the horizon, the authorities did not want to own up to their neglectful record. Instead, with selective findings and distorted interpretations, the octogenarian Superintendent MOH was made a convenient scapegoat: the disaster, after all, had struck on his watch.

Cameron defended himself in a book called *A Brief History of Municipal Public Health Administration in Dublin* (1914), but his reputation was damaged. Only recently have the inquiry's 'facts' been examined and Cameron's record vindicated. On his essentially singlehanded watch, after all, the death rate per 1,000 of the city's inhabitants was 37.5 when he began as MOH, coming down to 17.5 in 1920.[57]

THE OUTBREAK OF WAR: 'FOR YOU THE ONLY ENEMIES ARE DISEASE AND PAIN AND DEATH'

After Myles' *Chotah* unloaded its cargo of guns and ammunition, it sailed up the coast and weighed anchor at Kingstown (Dún Laoghaire). After a few days lying low, one of the crew rowed ashore for provisions on the morning of Wednesday, 5 August. On dry land, he found that all the newspapers were reporting the same thing: at 11 o'clock the night before, war with Germany had been declared.

The conflict was not unexpected. Europe had been simmering with tension for many years, the effects of which were already felt at RCSI. As early as 1909, an Officer Training Corps had been set up in RCSI at the students' request (as part of wider military reforms, OTCs appeared across British and Irish educational institutions from 1907; Trinity College, Dublin, followed suit in 1908[58]). Led by Prof Geddes, based on his Boer War experience, within weeks some seventy 'cadets', as they were known, had joined the RCSI OTC. They were drilled and received special lectures and brought on fortnight-long camping excursions. A rifle range was set up in the basement, beside the embalming room. The *Irish Times* reported bemused pedestrians on Nassau Street watching the cadets on parade, noting too: 'Professor Geddes reckons that not more than two hours a week of the student's time is taken.'[59]

RCSI's strong military connections dated back to the Napoleonic Wars. More recently, many RCSI Licentiates had served in Crimea (1853–56) and the two Boer Wars (1880–81, 1899–1902). From the 1860s on, Irish medical schools graduated more doctors than the country needed, so emigration to Britain and, in particular, enlistment in the armed forces was to some extent expected.[60] In 1898, for example, 124 of 892 Navy medical officers – close to 14 per cent – were Licentiates of RCSI.[61]

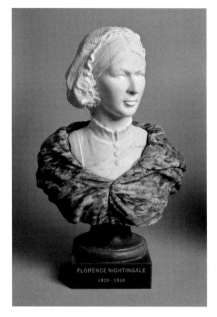

Bust of Florence Nightingale by John Rainey (2022). Commissioned by RCSI's Faculty and School of Nursing and Midwifery.

Medically speaking, Crimea represented a painful eye-opener to the military authorities. Putting actual combat aside, after little more than six months in the region, 36 per cent of the army's 28,000 men had died of disease.[62] (This was the conflict that led Florence Nightingale to push for reform of the profession of nursing, particularly in relation to hygiene.[63]) The South African campaigns were not much more successful: there were shortages of medical personnel, poor sanitation practice and widespread outbreaks of disease (22,000 soldiers suffered curable wounds, but 78,000 required treatment for dysentery and typhoid[64]).

As the military began to take medicine seriously, a new body was set up, the Royal Army Medical Corps (RAMC). At RCSI, the Boer War divided opinion: 'Why,' asked Thomas Myles, with more care for rhetoric than anatomy, 'should Irishmen stand with their arms folded and their hands in their pockets when England calls for aid?'[65] But at the end of hostilities, RCSI declined to contribute to the commemorative Fusiliers' Arch at the entrance to St Stephen's Green. That said, RCSI was proud to honour one of its own, Thomas Joseph Crean (1873–1923, Lic. 1896).

An international rugby player, Crean (not to be confused with his near-contemporary and namesake, the Antarctic explorer) was awarded the military's highest honour, the Victoria Cross, in December 1901; he received Honorary Fellowship of RCSI some months later. Previously, in 1899, John Crimmin (1859–1945, Lic. 1879) was the first RCSI recipient of the VC. RCSI was also quick to honour another Boer veteran, Sir Alfred Keogh (1857–1936), the Dublin-born Director-General of the Army Medical Services, awarding him an Honorary Fellowship in 1906. His successor, the Limerick-born Sir William Launcelotte Gubbins (1849–1925), was likewise honoured in 1913.

RCSI'S ROLL OF HONOUR – AND ITS OMISSIONS

At the outbreak of the war, some 210,000 Irish personnel enlisted in the British Army. They joined up for a wide spectrum of reasons: some were heeding the appeals of politicians who promised that victory for the British forces would usher in Irish Home Rule; some felt they were fighting for the rights of similarly small nations like the overrun Belgium; some were escaping poverty and lack of opportunity; some joined for the adventure, expecting to be home by Christmas. Whatever their motivations, they were largely written out of Irish history for much of the rest of the century.

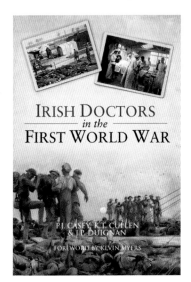

Irish Doctors in the First World War (2015) by Casey, Cullen and Duignan. Courtesy of Merrion Press.

The same may be said of the 3,336 Irish medics who enlisted (some 30 per cent of the entire RAMC) – though their stories likewise have been retold lately.[66] These were physicians, surgeons and general practitioners – and, indeed, medical students who had yet to obtain their qualifications. Their personal motivations were as various as any other cohort, but with the added impetus of the nature of their training. On 3 December 1914, Thomas E. Gordon (1867–1929, FRCSI 1895, PRCSI 1928–29), then a surgeon at the Adelaide Hospital, emphasised this point in an address delivered to the RCSI Students' Union. 'For you,' he urged,

there is a call to join a band of men to whom are entrusted the highest use of science; whose duty it is, not to destroy life, but if possible, to save it, to relieve the suffering and to heal the wounded... With the soldier you are called to a work of self-sacrifice – it may be to acts of heroism; you must share with him the dangers of battle, but unlike him, you must in your work, see no difference between friend and foe; for you the only enemies are disease and pain and death...[67]

By the end of the war, enlistments from RCSI comprised 180 students, 247 Fellows and 839 Licentiates. The RCSI Roll of Honour records the 1,266 names of those who served – but even that list is incomplete. Many of the women who enlisted – a call went out in spring 1916 – were never given the rank, grading, uniforms or even the ration and billeting allowance of their male counterparts, and so did not appear in the Roll.[68] Two such women from RCSI were Mary Josephine Ahern (1889–1976, Lic. 1913) and Nora Williams (Lic. 1911), both of whom served in Malta.[69]

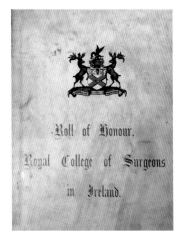

RCSI's World War I Roll of Honour.

'AS SPEEDILY AS POSSIBLE': JOINING UP

Conscription was not introduced in Ireland, so all medical enlistment was overseen by the self-governing Irish Medical War Committee. In the chair was RCSI photographer, live chess enthusiast and Prof of Biology, Ephraim Cosgrove. He was aided by committee members Frederick Conway Dwyer (1860–1935, FRCSI 1898, PRCSI 1914–16, Professor of Surgery 1901–12) and William Taylor (1871–1933, Lic. 1893, FRCSI 1898, PRCSI 1916–18). In March 1915, Dwyer, as both PRCSI and IMWC committee member, found it especially easy to give career advice to that year's graduating class:

> Graduates should enter as speedily as possible the Royal Army Medical Corps to place their professional skill and knowledge at the disposal of their King and country. Of the absolute propriety and necessity of that choice from every point of view there can be no question. In giving their services to the Empire in her hour of supremest need they were fulfilling the paramount duty of every citizen.[70]

The new Licentiates did as they were told; in that particular year, 87 per cent of the class enrolled in the RAMC and duly shipped out.[71] Few, by then, would have had any illusions that the war was a lark. The previous December, Sir Alfred Keogh — he had come out of retirement for the conflict — forbade medical students from enlisting. All the signs were that war would now be a protracted affair, so only the fully qualified were required. Indeed, some students were sent home to finish their studies — in some cases to their annoyance. Charles Brennan, an RCSI student who had enlisted early on, complained in March 1915 that

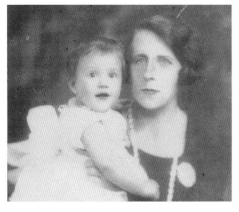

Mary Josephine Ahern with her daughter Adele, 1927. Courtesy of Antonia Lehane.

on the 8th August last [I] was equipped and thought I would be called on immediately, but the war office changed their minds and alas, sent me home to get qualified. Since then I have been working hard and hope to get qualified in the minimum time next June (with luck). Also I have to sit near some dear old lady in a tram or theatre, who settles her spectacles on her nose, and looks at you, and sniffs, as much to say 'Are you funky?' I know at least a score of men in the same position, most of whom, including myself, have done their three or four years in an Officers' Training Corps. They have to look at fellows in uniform and on duty who have never seen an Officers' Training Corps in their lives.[72]

Brennan did indeed qualify (Lic. 1915), whereupon he returned to the front. In 1917, he won a Military Cross.[73]

'THEIR NAME LIVETH FOR EVERMORE'

RCSI staff, students, Licentiates and Fellows served in all theatres of war, on land, sea and in the air. In some respects, the responsibilities of medical personnel were the inverse of the other combatants: they treated wounds, as opposed to causing them, and they evacuated casualties away from the frontlines while the larger ob-

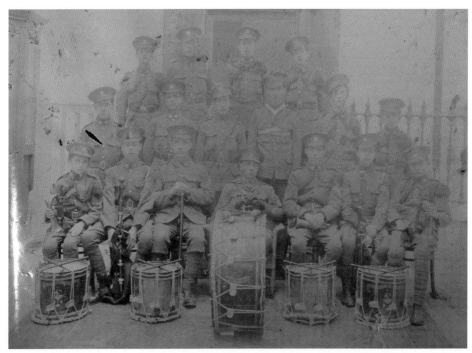

RCSI's Officer Training Corps.

jective was to advance. Even so, both activities were fraught with danger: of the 3,336 Irish doctors and students, 261 died in the war; of the 1,266 named individuals in the RCSI Roll of Honour, a cross is printed next to eighteen names, including that of Lieutenant Colonel Charles Dalton (Lic. 1888). Hit by shrapnel in September 1914, he was the first Irish doctor to die in the war. His is the sole military grave in the Vieil-Arcy Communal Cemetery. Many fellow RAMC doctors attended his burial, even as shells fell around them.[74]

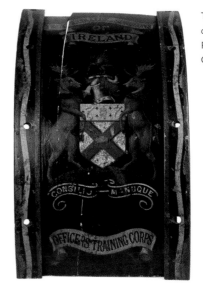

The OTC drum, now in RCSI Heritage Collections.

To quote the famous inscription, RCSI names 'liveth for evermore' on memorials across the map of the conflict: there is Joseph Patrick Pegum (Lic. 1916), no known grave, whose name may be read on the Tyne Cot Memorial; there is John Dauber (FRCSI 1899), drowned at Gallipoli and commemorated on the Helles Memorial; there is Pierce Power (Lic. 1910), buried at Kemmel Chateau Cemetery; there is George Adams (Lic. 1917), interred in Dar Es Salaam War Cemetery.

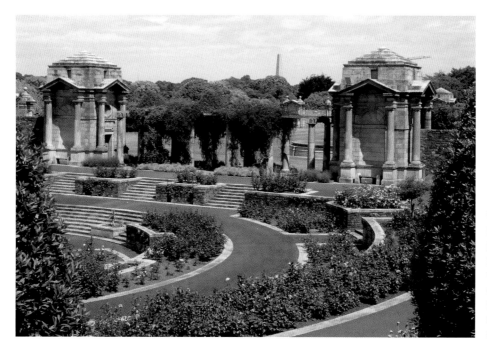

'Their Name Liveth For Evermore'. The Irish National War Memorial Gardens at Islandbridge. © Creative Commons.

The drowning of Digby Burns recorded in RCSI's copy of the Medical Register.

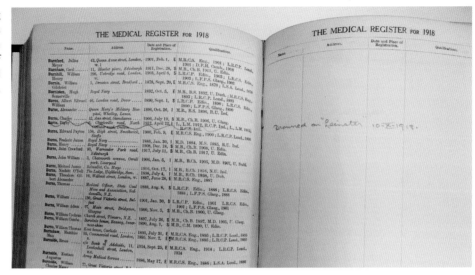

These few names may stand for the fallen many. But names and graves only convey so much; it is another matter to visit RCSI Heritage Collections and take down a century-old copy of the Medical Register and find that a clerkly hand once took a moment to record the fate – and to cross out the name – of Digby Burns (1884–1918, Lic. 1912), from Phibsboro. In the last weeks of the war, Burns was one of 569 soldiers and civilians drowned in the Irish Sea when RMS *Leinster* was torpedoed by a German submarine.

'IT'S NOT SURGERY, IT IS PACKING': AT THE FRONTLINE

Technological advancements meant that human suffering during the war had no precedent in history. Large-calibre shells could literally pulverise a body, leaving no identifiable remains[75] – except in the traumatised minds of witnesses. And yet for the first year of the war, soldiers on both sides did not even have steel helmets; they wore cloth or leather caps. Survival rates from injury were probably higher sixty years earlier in Crimea.

The majority of RCSI volunteers were stationed along the Western Front, where the medical chain worked as follows: stretcher-bearers collected the wounded, bringing them to a Regimental Aid Post, often in a shell crater; from there, they were brought to an Advanced (that is, frontline) Dressing Station where some received minor treatment; others continued the journey to a Casualty Clearing Station. These were busy places: 'it's not surgery,' one visitor told RCSI's Students' Union, 'it is packing'.[76]

The more seriously wounded were then conveyed by road or rail to base hospitals along the Normandy coast. Generally speaking, these base hospitals were

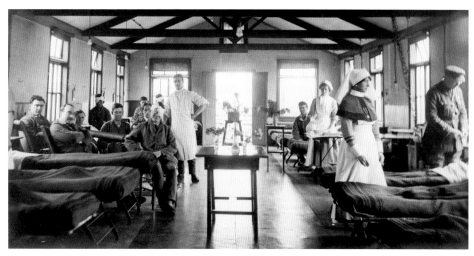

The 83rd (Dublin) General Hospital, Boulogne. © Crown copyright. Imperial War Museums.

temporary establishments, albeit well-equipped ones, staffed by senior doctors who were considered too old for the frontline. RCSI would have been represented at every stage of this journey, but was probably most associated with the 83rd (Dublin) General Hospital at Boulogne. This had opened in 1914 (as the 13th Stationary Hospital), earning its Dublin moniker in May 1917 when the first of four detachments of Irish doctors arrived. Leading that first detachment was the serving PRCSI, William Taylor. He had enlisted at the outbreak of the war, thereby earning the moral authority to urge students and alumni to do the same.

For the 83rd Hospital, he recruited his colleagues and peers to come with him – one stipulation he was given was that doctors had to be 'over 40 years of age, and only to exceed 50 by a small margin'.[77] Many senior figures were apparently disappointed (at least publicly) by this. Later, as recruitment became more difficult for Taylor, the rules were bent; for example, Arthur Wyndoe Baker (1852–1924, FRCSI 1888) was 65 when he shipped out. (It was not surprising that Taylor increasingly had his work cut out: within weeks of his arrival at Boulogne, the massive losses of life at Ypres and Messines occurred, significantly altering public sentiment back home. And this is to say nothing – yet – of the change in attitude that had already followed the Easter Rising.)

Amongst those who served at the 83rd General Hospital were seven RCSI Presidents: Thomas Myles; Edward Henry Taylor (1867–1922, FRCSI 1896, PRCSI 1920–22); William de Courcy Wheeler (1879–1943, FRCSI 1905, PRCSI 1922–24 – he was a son of William Ireland Wheeler, PRCSI 1884); Charles Maunsell (1872–1930, FRCSI 1900, PRCSI 1924–26); Andrew Fullerton (1867–1934, FRCSI 1901, PRCSI 1926–28, 1929–30[78]); Thomas Gordon; and

William Taylor. Other RCSI staff who completed rotations include Thomas Gillman Moorhead (1878–1960, Prof of Medicine, 1916–17, PRCPI 1930–33), who had already served at Gallipoli; George Jameson Johnston (1866–1926, FRCSI 1896, Prof of Surgery 1912–26) and Robert Rowlette (1873–1944, Prof of Surgical Pharmacy 1921–26).

Many Fellows and alumni served too, including Alexander Joseph McAuley Blayney (1870–1925, FRCSI 1898) – Blayney enjoys the distinction of being described by James Joyce when the novelist was considering a medical career: 'A florid athletic looking, balding man with striped trousers and expensive, highly-polished shoes';[79] and Maurice R.J. Hayes (c.1878–1930, Lic. 1906, FRCSI 1908), the Mater Hospital's first full-time radiologist or, as he was titled, 'Medical Electrician'.[80]

The many hospitals in Boulogne provided a great font of knowledge for RCSI personnel to bring home. Close by, at the 13th General Hospital, were the bacteriologists Sir Almroth Wright (1861–1947), who had been an Honorary Fellow since 1906 (and, incidentally, the inspiration for G.B. Shaw's play *The Doctor's Dilemma*), and Alexander Fleming (1881–1955), yet to discover penicillin. At this time, Fleming became a lifelong friend of future PRCSI Thomas Ottiwell Graham (1883–1966, FRCSI 1912, PRCSI 1942–44); Graham won the Military Cross for bravery in October 1918. Distinguished visitors operated at the 83rd too, including the American neurosurgeon Harvey Cushing (1869–1939); in 1918, he would travel to Dublin to accept RCSI's Honorary Fellowship.

'WE SHALL EACH AND EVERY ONE DO HIS SHARE': ON THE HOME FRONT
From the base hospitals, soldiers were either sent back to the front or, if too badly injured, returned to Britain and Ireland on hospital ships. Indeed, by the end of the war some 20,000 soldiers (mostly Irish) were brought back to Ireland – where of course they were in need of further treatment. The RAMC already ran the King George V Hospital (now St Bricin's) at Arbour Hill, where, for the war period, three surgeons – all RCSI Presidents: Conway-Dwyer, William Taylor and Henry Stokes (1879–1967, FRCSI 1907, PRCSI 1940–41) – undertook some 4,000 operations.

With bed-space at a premium, many auxiliary hospitals were also set up. Again, RCSI input abounded, whether on a small scale – William Wheeler turned his private nursing home over to wounded servicemen – or much larger: the hospital most associated with RCSI personnel was the Red Cross Hospital in Dublin Castle (1915–18), founded by Ephraim Cosgrave. The vice-regal consort, Lady Aberdeen, who was a leading fundraiser, joked that the Castle was suddenly about to

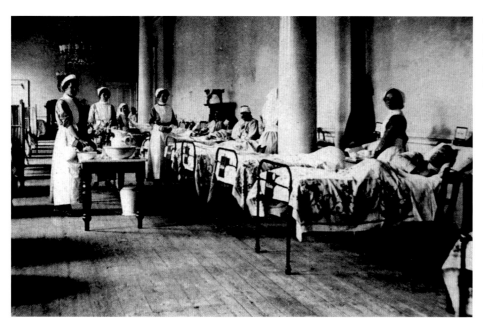

The Red Cross
Hospital, Dublin
Castle. Courtesy
of *History
Ireland*.

become popular for the first time in its history,[81] but in fact her involvement – and her nationalist sympathies – caused some controversy.

Early on – in November 1914 – it fell to Thomas Myles (who knew a thing or two about complicated loyalties) to urge Dubliners to see the bigger picture:

> Let us no longer be Montagues or Capulets, but let us think only, on these cold, wet and stormy nights, of our brave soldiers, heroes, name-less too often, lying in the frozen sludge of the trenches, giving their lives for us without a murmur, enduring with stoical fortitude atrocious suffering; and let us all pledge ourselves that, with God's help, we shall each and every one do his share.[82]

When the hospital closed at the end of the war, RCSI received as a thank-you gift the valuable X-ray machine that had been *in situ*.[83] Before that, however, the hospital's medics found they were suddenly treating injuries received closer to home. Bullets were flying in the surrounding streets, it turned out. It was April – and Easter – 1916.

'OUR PARTY ENTERED THE COLLEGE': EASTER MONDAY, 1916

Monday, 24 April was a bank holiday, and many Dubliners decamped early to the seaside or to Fairyhouse Racecourse for the Grand National (won, as it happens,

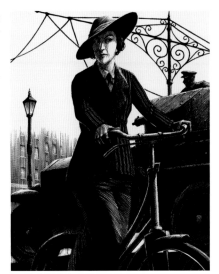

Margaret Skinnider by David Rooney. © David Rooney.

by a horse called All Sorts; also running was Civil War, though it did not place). The morning quiet of the city centre was broken by an insurrection that would change the course of Irish history – but in the first few hours, most bystanders thought it was just another common-or-garden riot. 'Riots are not rare,' wrote Margaret Skinnider (1892–1971), a Glasgow-born schoolteacher and rebel, 'and this might well seem to many of them only rioting on a large scale, with some new and interesting features.'[84]

Amongst these new and interesting features were bullets whizzing past the elderly head of Dr John Freeman Knott (1853–1921, Lic. 1877, FRCSI 1880). He had ambled in from Ranelagh to do some research in the quiet of RCSI's Library. Nothing – including close-range gunfire – seemed to bother Knott very much. Half a century earlier, at the age of 21, married and in charge of a forty-five-acre family farm in Roscommon, Knott decided to launch himself into a medical career, and so he left his wife in charge of the farm (and his elderly parents) and enrolled at RCSI. A brilliant undergraduate career followed, much influenced by his teachers, Cameron and William Stokes (1839–1900, Lic. 1862, FRCSI 1873, Prof of Surgery 1872–1900, PRCSI 1886).

After a stint on the continent, Knott returned to Dublin to establish a private practice at 34 York Street. This practice proved less successful than Knott's 'sideline' as a private tutor – otherwise known as a 'crammer', whereby medical students were drilled on the bare essentials of how to pass their exams (in the era, such crammers were plentiful, their services prominently advertised in national newspapers). Failing to secure either an academic or clinical position, Knott supplemented his crammer income by writing articles and reviews; across a forty-year freelance career, he would go on to produce some 2,000 such articles, often on medical arcana, including spontaneous combustion, death masks, matted hair specimens, the pathologies of figures such as Napoleon and Lord Byron, or the curative efficacy of mistletoe and kissing ('the claims have been utterly discounted in the light of modern science'[85]). Knott was also the ghost-writer of Thomas Heazle Parke's memoirs, *My Personal Experiences in Equatorial Africa* (1891) and *Guide to Health in Africa* (1893) – a scheme they hatched to-

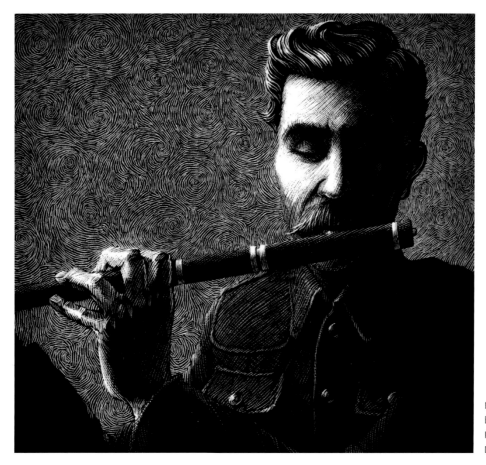

Michael Mallin
by David
Rooney. ©
David Rooney.

gether to cash in on Parke's celebrity.[86] Knott's apparent obliviousness to the gunfire he walked through made one rebel wonder if he was drunk. But no, he just had his mind on higher things.

In fairness to Knott, the early aspects of the Rising were confusing to many of the rebels themselves. The authorities in Dublin Castle had been warned of an insurrection as far back as September 1914 — England's difficulty, as the phrase went, being Ireland's opportunity. Life during wartime was so martialised that Dubliners got used to displays of marching and drilling in plain sight. As Easter 1916 approached, more confusion reigned: Sunday was due to be the day of the Rising, but this was called off the night before: rank and file rebels read about the change of plans in an advertisement in the *Sunday Independent*. This meant that when the postponed rebellion went ahead on Easter Monday, there were far fewer rebels than might previously have been expected. Some, indeed, had headed off to Fairyhouse instead.

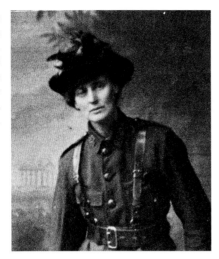

Countess Constance Markievicz. Reproduced courtesy of the National Library of Ireland (NPA POLF206).

While Pearse and Connolly took over the General Post Office, Michael Mallin (1874–1916) led his contingent of the Irish Citizen Army (ICA) – about 120 men and women (of the various nationalist groups, only the ICA accepted women members) – to St Stephen's Green at midday, where, in a curious emulation of the Western Front, they began digging trenches. Mallin had extensive military experience, having served twenty-one years in the British Army, particularly in India (this period shaped his politics; he wished 'it was for Erin I was fighting and not against these poor people'[87]).

Of all those later executed, Mallin probably came from the humblest socio-economic background. By contrast, his second-in-command was Countess Constance Markievicz (1868–1927), born to the aristocratic Gore-Booth family. In some respects, she travelled farther than most: in 1887, she made her society debut and was presented to Queen Victoria; by 1911, she was arrested while protesting the visit of George V. To the rank and file under her command, she was known as 'Madame'.

The rebels cleared the Green of civilians; in the process, an unarmed constable was shot dead for refusing to leave his post; barricades made of seized carts and motor cars were erected along the streets (one car belonged to Dr Kathleen Lynn (1874–1955, FRCSI 1909), chief medical officer to the ICA based at City Hall; one of the carts belonged to an elderly theatre-worker, Michael Cavanagh, who was shot dead for trying to retrieve it). Strategically, the Green made sense as a nexus of wide roads leading into the city; on the other hand, with reduced rebel numbers owing to the confusion of Saturday's countermand, the area swiftly proved impossible to hold. Crucially, the rebel who was supposed to occupy the commanding position of the Shelbourne Hotel found himself redeployed at the last minute to the GPO. Towards three o'clock, Mallin detailed a group including Markievicz and two other women and a young man called Frank Robbins (1895–1979) to enter RCSI to hunt for rifles or ammunition belonging to the College's OTC.

This is where Knott comes in – or, at least, where he tries to get in, as RCSI was already closed by the time he reached it. This was not simply because there were no classes, being a bank holiday, but because the Registrar, Alfred Miller, had telephoned at about 1 o'clock to say that trouble was afoot in the city and the premises should be secured. The beadle — that is, the Head Porter — James Duncan, who lived on-site with his wife and daughter, duly locked the front and back doors. Duncan, who had been in RCSI's employ since 1890, left a record of what then unfolded (he refers to himself as 'the Petitioner'):

> … your Petitioner observing from his bedroom window in the College Dr Knott a Fellow of the College (who was in the habit of arriving every day at the College) coming to the College door at which he knocked he (your Petitioner) opened the door slightly telling Dr Knott at the same time that the College was closed for the day…

In his own record of events, Robbins called Knott's appearance 'an early stroke of luck':

> When we approached the gate of the Green we saw the caretaker of the College engaged in animated conversation with another man in the doorway. As he was about to open the gateway Mallin told us to saunter quietly across as if going straight up York Street. He was afraid that the caretaker would 'smell a rat' and shut the door in our faces… I had every intention of obeying Mallin's instructions but when we were half-way across the road, the man in conversation with the caretaker seemed to be having trouble. In fact, the caretaker was using some force to get him out of the doorway and was succeeding fairly well. Too well, indeed, for my liking. I took the shortest cut, dashed across the road and shouted to the others to follow. The caretaker gave his companion a push and slammed the door. I jumped from the pathway to the top step. As I did so a shot rang out and a bullet whizzed by my ear and entered the top-right-hand side of the door. While it was a remarkably close shave for me it helped to save the situation. It must have unnerved the caretaker because he failed to shoot the lock home on the first attempt. With the full force of my weight and strength I crashed against the door. It gave a few inches, enough for my foot to jam it from being closed…[88]

This is Duncan's version of the same moment:

> Before your Petitioner could close the door the Countess Markievicz with two other Rebels presented themselves at the Hall door, one of the Rebels firing at close range a rifle at your Petitioner. The shot broke

the glass of the inner door. They then forced their way in, the Countess Markievicz covering your Petitioner with a revolver saying at the same time 'where is the roof' and also 'if you hesitate I will shoot you dead'...

Back to Robbins:

He [Duncan] abandoned resistance very promptly when I shoved the muzzle of my revolver against his throat. There was no further obstruction and our party entered the College. It was to prove a very useful headquarters for the St Stephen's Green area.

Duncan was forcefully questioned ('Had not Madame Markievicz intervened he would certainly have had a very rough time'), but apart from pointing the way to the roof, he gave nothing away. OTC? Rifles? Ammunition? 'We tried a few threats but this poor "innocent" knew nothing.' Apparently, Duncan did not even know where the keys to front and back doors were... For being so uncooperative, he was locked in his bedroom with his wife and child.

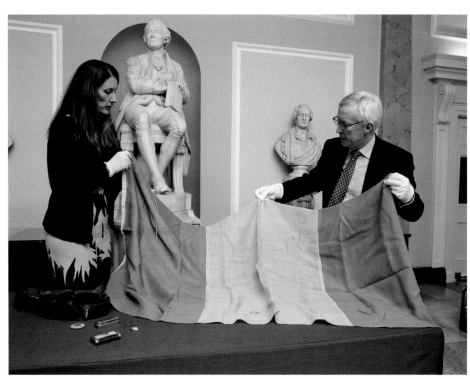

Janet Wilkinson, grand-niece of Margaret Skinnider, presenting to Declan Magee, PRCSI 2014-16, the tricolour believed to have flown over the College in 1916.

While Knott wended his way home, his day's research thwarted, Robbins went up to the roof with a tricolour under his arm – Margaret Skinnider had brought it by bicycle from the GPO. Up there, Robbins had Asclepius' view of the tree-clothed Green: it was quiet, the sky clear, the streets seemingly empty, but now and then he caught a glimpse of his comrades' activity behind the railings. In the distance, around the city, there was the crackling of rifle-fire. No marksmen threatened Robbins where he was, but this was still a dangerous spot: the roof was slippery beneath his boots and the flagstaff, loose in its mount, swayed alarmingly over the pavement below. Robbins shinned halfway up the flagpole in an effort to disentangle the halyards ('probably after long disuse,' he was still complaining sixty-one years later), but it was too risky; a lighter rebel, Daithi O'Leary, took his turn and succeeded. 'Soon it was up,' Robbins recalled, 'and fluttering bravely in the slight breeze.' One hundred years later, what is believed to be the same flag revisited RCSI – this time brought from Australia by Margaret Skinnider's grand-niece.

Markievicz and others had meanwhile returned to the Green. There were isolated skirmishes, but generally the St Stephen's Green garrison busied itself with bedding in. As night fell, rain did too. The first-aid nurses and dispatch girls sheltered in the wall-less summer-house, the men had their trenches, while Markievicz, unimpressed with either option, slept under a rug in Kathleen Lynn's car in the barricade. 'Almost everything was going our way,' was Skinnider's chipper interpretation;[89] others, such as the Cumann na mBan member Nora O'Daly, were less sanguine. 'Even to a mind untrained in military matter,' she recollected, the Green 'looked like a death trap.'[90] Under cover of the dark, soldiers slipped into the Shelbourne Hotel and made their way to the roof and set up machine guns, and at four o'clock on Tuesday morning, they opened fire. Soon enough, Mallin gave the order to evacuate the Green and head for RCSI. They did so in twos and threes, under a hail of gunfire from the British on one side, and rotten vegetables and curses from the locals on the other.

Not everyone made it, as one witness saw:

> … inside the Green railings four bodies could be seen lying on the ground. They were dead Volunteers. Some distance beyond the Shelbourne I saw another Volunteer stretched out on a seat just within the railings. He was not dead, for, now and again, his hand moved feebly in a gesture for aid; the hand was completely red with blood. His face could not be seen. He was just a limp mass, upon which the rain beat pitilessly, and he was sodden and shapeless, and most miserable to see.[91]

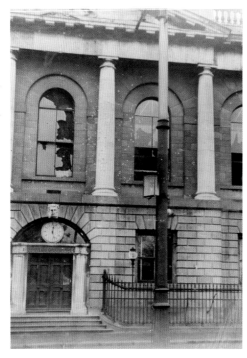

RCSI's 'peppered' façade. Reproduced with the kind permission of the National Museum of Ireland.

'THE MACHINE-GUN BULLETS... MIGHT HAVE BEEN DRIED PEAS': INSIDE RCSI DURING THE RISING

By Tuesday afternoon, there were more than one hundred men, women and, indeed, children – boys of the Scout-like Fianna Éireann – inside RCSI. In addition to the Shelbourne, soldiers were now firing at closer range from the United Services Club. Up with the Greek gods on the parapet was the most dangerous place to be: Michael Doherty (1879–1919) caught a strafe of bullets ('he hung there, head and arms dangling over the street, his blood staining the face of the building'[92]); Robbins thought his comrade was 'a goner' (and indeed told him so). In the end, Doherty lost an eye and the use of a hand, but he lived – only to succumb later to the 'Spanish flu'.

But downstairs, inside, after the debacle of the Green, the rebels could legitimately feel safe. 'For all the impression they made,' said Skinnider, 'the machine-gun bullets with which the British soldiers peppered it for five days might have been dried peas.'[93] The evidence of that 'peppering' can still be seen in the stonework; it can be seen, too – and, indeed, felt – in the bullet-dimpled fingerplate of the Board Room's door, from whose windows the rebels returned fire. Portraits in this room were also perforated, including that of Colles.

But the room next door, College Hall, was 'impregnable', thanks to architect William Murray's three blind windows. This was where the rebels slept and where Madeline ffrench-Mullen (1880–1944) set up a first aid station behind a screen previously used for projecting medical slides.[94] Elsewhere, the rebels did their best to make themselves at home in what was to them an alien environment ('The classrooms of the College seemed huge and draughty. Everywhere were huge glass cases filled with objects for students, pebbles and specimens. In an adjoining room the jars had parts of human bodies preserved in liquid'[95]). Barricades were built in the Entrance Hall using furniture and a steady supply of books from the Library ('as a book lover,' Robbins said, 'I was saddened' – but needs must). A makeshift mortuary was set up in the space

Facing page: A bullet's lasting impression in the Board Room's fingerplate.

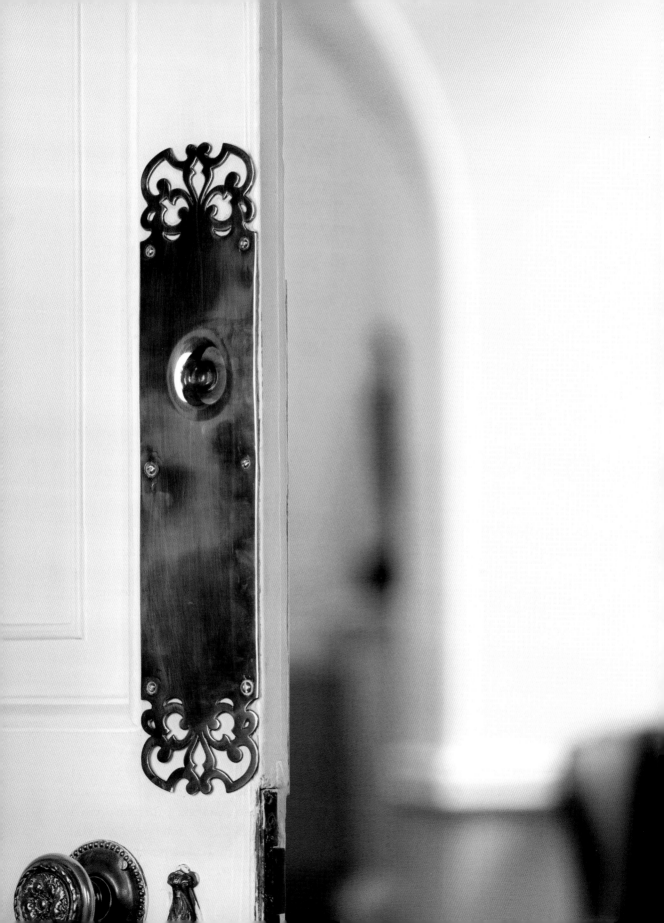

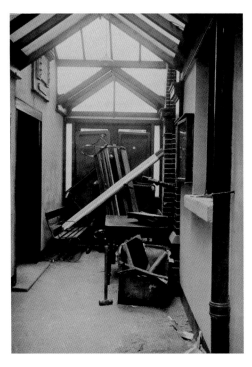

One of
the rebels'
barricades.

beneath the seats of the Chemistry theatre; the actual Anatomy Room, presumably, had too much dangerous glass overhead.

RCSI'S CASUALTIES: JOHN O'DUFFY (1836-1916, LIC. DENT. 1878) AND CHARLES HACHETTE HYLAND (1887-1916, LIC. DENT. 1907)

For the rest of the week, all around the city RCSI staff and alumni treated civilians, soldiers and insurgents with equal care. Passing City Hall as the rebels attempted to take the Castle, Sir Thomas Myles found himself tending to the very first person shot on Easter Monday. This was James O'Brien, a constable of the Dublin Metropolitan Police. Despite Myles' efforts, O'Brien's wound was fatal. Anticipating further casualties, Myles hurried on to the Richmond Hospital, where he found that the rebel commandant of the Four Courts area wanted beds for his wounded men.

Myles' wards were already full of Western Front casualties, so he arranged for an improvised medical depot around the corner on Church Street. Despite his own history, Myles considered the Rising a foolish move, but when Captain Éamon Martin of the Irish Volunteers was brought in with a serious chest wound, Myles' actions told their own story. He knew Martin from the Kilcoole episode and did not want to see him arrested; as soon as the wound was stabilised, Myles donned his full RAMC uniform, called for his chauffeur and he and Martin drove out of the Richmond to a convalescent home in Blackrock. Martin subsequently escaped to the US, again with Myles' help.

At Mercer's Hospital, two future RCSI Presidents, William Wheeler and Charles Maunsell, treated approximately 200 casualties during Easter Week. (Wheeler, incidentally, had had his own St Stephen's Green skirmish; as a student, an encounter with a spiked railing left him blind in one eye — hence his invariably side-profile poses.[96]) At the Eye and Ear on Adelaide Road, the first female ophthalmic surgeon in Ireland, Euphan Montgomerie Maxwell (1887–1964, FRCSI 1914), treated a steady flow of casualties. The matron on duty on Thursday recorded the admission of '42 soldiers... 13 of them convalescents and the remainder Sherwood Foresters who had come in the night before, some suffering from shock but three or four with fairly serious wounds'.[97] In August 1916, Maxwell was amongst the first contingent of female doctors who shipped out to Malta.

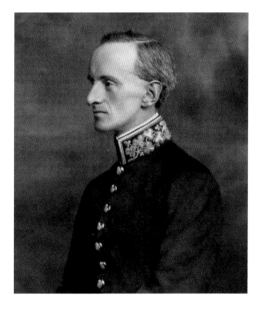

Sir William Ireland de Courcy Wheeler, PRCSI 1922-24.

Wednesday saw the 'Battle of Mount Street Bridge', where a small band of rebels inflicted heavy losses on the troops – raw recruits, mostly ('untrained, undersized products of the English slums' was one military man's verdict[98]) – who had only lately landed at Dún Laoghaire; some, apparently, thought they were in France. The activist Sighle Humphreys, who witnessed the conflict, called them 'rank and file cannon fodder for their imperial masters'.[99] On Northumberland Road, Emily Winifred Dickson's aunt's house was searched ('nice boys,' she wrote to her niece, 'but very new to their work – one of them confided that he had never had a real rifle before'[100]).

When the fighting began in earnest, the dead, dying and injured piled up on the bridge. At intervals there were ceasefires, allowing medical staff from Sir Patrick Dun's Hospital – just around the corner – to come and collect the wounded. Amongst the hospital's staff were Sir Charles Arthur Ball (1877–1945, FRCSI 1905), Charles Molyneux Benson (1877–1919, FRCSI 1906) and Sir Robert Henry Woods. Between them, they treated some seventy-nine casualties, regardless of whether they were rebels or soldiers. (Seeing the uniforms, Woods was likely thinking of his own son, William Thornley Stoker Woods, then stationed in France; in fact, he would be killed by a shell in October, aged 19.)

Also providing medical assistance in his white coat was 29-year-old Charles Hachette Hyland (Lic. Dent. 1907); the next day, Thursday, as the sniping continued, a bullet struck him as he stood outside his parents' house on Percy Place. He was one of 184 civilians to be killed that week, and the first RCSI Licentiate. The second was also a (retired) dentist, John O'Duffy (Lic. Dent. 1878), hit by a stray bullet on Beresford Place on Sunday, 30 April, making him one of the Rising's last civilian casualties.

Some of the injured from Sir Patrick Dun's were transferred to St Vincent's Hospital, then on the east side of St Stephen's Green. On duty at St Vincent's were two RCSI Licentiates with known nationalist sympathies, Michael Francis Cox (1852–1926, Lic. 1875, PRCPI 1922) and John Stephen McArdle (1859–1928, Lic. 1879, FRCSI 1884). The authorities wanted all suspicious wounds reported, but Cox and McArdle refused to comply. Cox – father, incidentally, of the solicitor Arthur – ranked his allegiances as follows: 'I am first an Irishman, secondly a member of the medical profession and other matters only follow those.'[101] McArdle, for his part, was a 'vigorous, fiery legend in his lifetime', probably Myles' only surgical rival in popular opinion. 'He's dead but I'll do what I can' was an entirely fictional line attributed to him by Oliver St John Gogarty[102] – but in a way it speaks volumes of his ebullient optimism.

The 86-year-old Charles Cameron was busy, too, sending his Sanitary Officers to collect the bodies of those killed. 'The City Morgue presented a gruesome sight,' he wrote in his *Autobiography*:

> I found nearly 40 bodies lying on tables and floor. I recognised the body of The O'Rahilly, he was a handsome man of fine physique... I went about very much during Easter Week and had some exciting experiences. Whilst speaking to a lady in Ely Place an explosive bullet fell quite close to me.[103]

'WE DID NOT FEEL WE WERE DOING ANY WRONG'

Back on the west side of the Green, hails of lead continued to be traded over the treetops. Mallin had the idea that if fires could be started in houses close to Grafton Street, then smoke would obscure the enemy's view. A company of twenty men left RCSI by the back door and made their way to the back of no. 127, which was a Turkish bathhouse. Here they collected towels and sheets and mattresses to bring back to the first aid station in the College Hall; then, with seven-pound sledgehammers, they began the arduous job of breaking holes in stout Georgian walls to crawl on hands and knees from house to house.

Within the garrison, Mallin maintained strict discipline – 'no noise or hilarity was allowed,' one rebel recalled.[104] When Mallin heard that someone had slashed the life-size portrait of Queen Victoria by Stephen Catterson Smith (1806–1872, PRHA) that hung in the Board Room, he was furious and threatened to shoot the vandal – but when it turned out the perpetrator was a small boy ('who should not have been there at all,' according to Liam Ó Briain, who was on guard at the time[105]), Mallin let him off with a pair of boxed ears. Margaret Skinnider had a slightly different version: 'At the College of Surgeons we had destroyed nothing except a portrait of Queen Victoria. We took that down and made puttees [leg bindings] out of it. We did not feel we were doing any wrong.'[106]

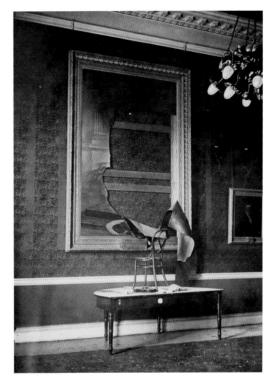

The damaged portrait of Queen Victoria in the Board Room.

Poking through the Chemistry lab, Thomas O'Donoghue gathered jars of chlorine with a view to lobbing them at armoured cars. He also found a set of bagpipes, but Mallin would not let him play them because that would be 'tantamount to looting'.[107] Such compunction did not apply when the OTC cache was finally discovered on Wednesday: the rebels helped themselves to some sixty-four rifles with bayonets – all more modern than what they had already – and ample supplies of ammunition.[108] As Skinnider pointed out, 'All this... would have been used against us had we not reached the building first'. Whether Mallin knew about it or not, there was some singing in the lecture theatres to keep spirits up; likewise, there were nightly rosaries for those who wished to consider the spiritual implications of their actions.

Generally, however, the garrison's chief concern was more corporeal: they had next to nothing to eat. The only sustenance Robbins found on the first day were two eggs and some loose-leaf tea. By Wednesday, this was a major problem (in marked contrast to their enemies, well-fed in the United Services Club, the Shelbourne and the Russell Hotel on the south-west corner of the Green). William Oman remembered contemplating the execution of a horse stabled behind RCSI.

Meanwhile, still locked away in his bedroom was the beadle and his family, 'suffering much from hunger and thirst'; on the third day, he managed to attract a York Street neighbour's attention and succeeded in getting three cuts of bread and butter delivered up to him on the end of a rope made from torn sheets. On Wednesday night, the Duncans were transferred to the basement, where they would remain for the rest of the week 'upon scanty rations'. All this time there was another hostage on the premises, a man called Laurence Kettle, chief of Dublin Corporation electricity department, whose car had been commandeered on

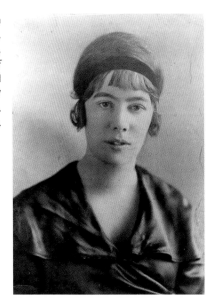

Helen Ruth 'Nellie' Gifford, Boston 1917, Courtesy of Kilmainham Gaol Museum/OPW (KMGLM. 2012.0143).

Monday. Frank Robbins recalled that Kettle's first experiences as a prisoner 'were not very pleasant', but later he became much more comfortable, passing the time by adding books to the barricade.[109]

Meanwhile, the hungry men tunnelling towards Grafton Street reversed their exertions, on the hunt now for a French patisserie rumoured to be near (it was at number 125, between the baths and Glover's Alley). The food situation improved when supplies were delivered from the garrison in Jacob's biscuit factory, close by on Bishop Street. Shooting apart, two Citizen Army women, Helen 'Nellie' Gifford (1880–1971) and Chris Caffrey (1898–1976), probably did more of practical use for the garrison than anyone else. Both made forays under fire to gather supplies – Caffrey wore a Fusilier's pin and widow's weeds in case she was stopped (which she was, swallowing the communiqué she carried in her mouth). Gifford was a domestic economy instructor and Markievicz later remembered the near loaves-and-fishes manner in which Gifford produced 'a quantity of oatmeal from somewhere and made pot after pot of the most delicious porridge which kept us going'.[110]

On Friday, to great joy, the patisserie was discovered ('everything that went to the making of pastry was there in large quantities'[111]); by this time, too, a quantity of bacon had been confiscated from somewhere and the plan was to eat it on Sunday – but that was not to happen.

SURRENDER: 'A GREATER CALAMITY THAN DEATH ITSELF'

Friday saw renewed heavy shooting from the army positions and Mallin and Markievicz suspected an assault was imminent. The walking wounded left RCSI for treatment in local hospitals (Skinnider, who had been shot four times on a foray outside, refused to leave). Communication with the GPO had

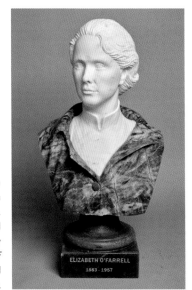

Bust of Elizabeth O'Farrell by John Rainey (2022). Commissioned by RCSI's Faculty and School of Nursing and Midwifery.

been cut off, so no one knew about its evacuation on Friday night; but up next to Asclepius, the vista of the burning city was eloquent enough.

The assault did not come that day, though the shooting continued to fray nerves; nor did it happen on Saturday, when the first rumours of surrender began to filter through; indeed, some civilians took it upon themselves to gather at the College end of York Street to shout the news to those inside. Instead, the end of the St Stephen's Green garrison came with the arrival on Sunday morning of the Cumann na mBan member and nurse Elizabeth O'Farrell (1884–1957).[112] She brought confirmation that Pearse had surrendered the day before. Rosie Hackett remembered the sight of Markievicz at this moment: 'sitting on the stairs, with her head in her hands'.[113] Mallin walked around shaking hands with his troops; some wanted to fight on, but he said no, orders were orders, all guns and ammunition were to be discarded immediately.

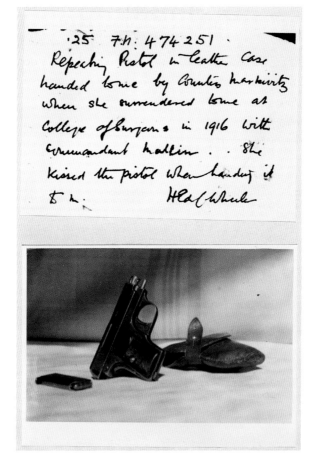

'Repeating pistol in leather case handed to me by Countess Markievicz when she surrendered to me at College of Surgeons in 1916 with Commandant Mallin. She kissed the pistol when handing it to me. H.E. de C. Wheeler'. Reproduced courtesy of the National Library of Ireland (MS 15 000/8/5).

As Robbins recollected:

> Strong, brave, upstanding men and women, all of whom had taken risks of one kind or another during that week, not knowing and not caring whether they would forfeit their lives, were now broken-hearted. It was apparent that at that moment the act of surrender was to each one a greater calamity than death itself. Men and women were crying openly with arms around each other's shoulders.[114]

The tricolour that had been so effortfully hoisted was now lowered, replaced by a white flag. A single army rifle-shot acknowledged the transition, and this was the signal for the Crown representative to approach the front door. This was Captain Henry de Courcy Wheeler (1872–1956), brother and son of the two Williams who were RCSI Presidents; his wife was also a first cousin of Markievicz. Mallin and Markievicz stepped out to offer the formal surrender.

Later, Mallin expressed his gratitude for Wheeler's 'kindness and consideration'.[115] Markievicz kissed her revolver before handing it over. She declined the offer to be driven to the Castle. 'No,' she said, 'I shall march at the head of my

The Arrest by Kathleen Fox (artist's copy of the original).

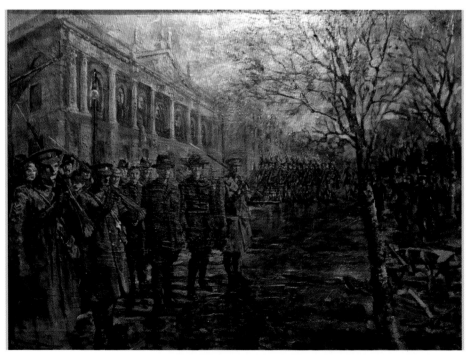

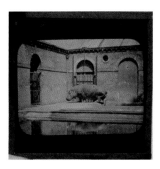 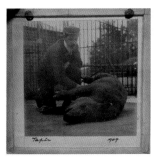 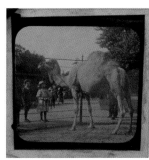

Prof Scott's photographs from Dublin Zoo.

men as I am second in command, and I shall share their fate.'[116] The artist Kathleen Fox (1880–1963) happened to be passing at this moment and later captured the scene on canvas. As the rebels were marched away, a small number of onlookers were sympathetic, but the vast majority was openly and vociferously hostile.

THE AFTERMATH

From that date – Sunday, 30 April – until 27 May, some 400 soldiers remained in occupation of RCSI. Stepping between them, the College authorities surveyed the week's damage. The scenes they found were captured by Prof John Alfred Scott (1854–1926, Lic. 1881, FRCSI 1886, Prof of Physiology 1889–1926). Formerly of the Carmichael School, Scott was a photography enthusiast (his extensive collection of colour plates of animals in Dublin Zoo – another enthusiasm – are in the RCSI Heritage Collections). Scott's images show the general disarray that the rebels left behind, but compared to sites elsewhere in the city, RCSI escaped very lightly indeed. There was the scarification of bullets, but nothing by way of structural harm. A subsequent insurance claim, prepared by Registrar Alfred Miller, estimated the entire cost of the damage at £764. Individual staff members also made claims for lost or damaged property – microscopes and the like.

After the ordeal of his incarceration, the beadle James Duncan was to suffer further misfortune. Released at the surrender, he found his old rooms – occupied, apparently, by Markievicz – in 'the greatest disorder and confusion':

> There were two beds in the dining room and there were strewn about a motley assorted of looted articles such as ladies jackets, dresses, boys and mens [sic] shoes, flannel cricket trousers. In the sitting room upstairs there was sugar, currants, raisins, candles, soap, different articles of male and female wearing apparel and also a number of hammers and chisels, etc.

Prof Scott's photographs of the aftermath in the College Hall.

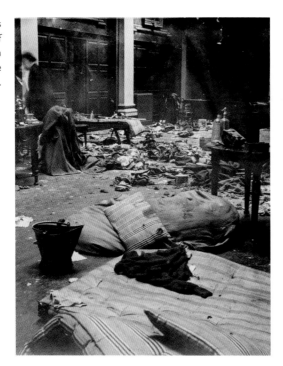

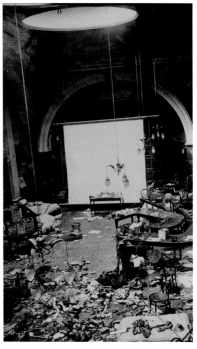

For a week, he did not disturb the scene, 'the Petitioner [i.e. Duncan] being desirous of letting the College Authorities see the place before he interfered with it'. When the authorities showed up — Miller, Prof Scott and a military man — they came across two silver-backed ladies' hairbrushes stowed under loose floorboards in the room. A professor's attaché case was also lying in plain sight; by the initials 'W.B.' on it, Duncan suggested it belonged to the Professor of Pathology, William Boxwell. Very shortly afterwards, for the supposed theft of these items, the axe fell on Duncan and he was dismissed from his post. He appealed, writing a lengthy 'petition' — the document quoted herein — that gave his eyewitness account of the week, from Dr Knott's attempted entry on Monday to the surrender on Sunday, all of which tallies with accounts by Robbins and others.

Left: Prof Scott's compensation receipt for damaged instruments. Right: The Registrar, Alfred Miller, prepares the College's claim.

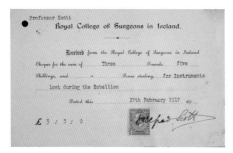

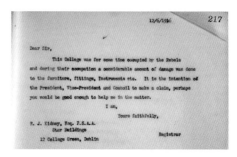

The first page of James Duncan's 'humble petition'.

As Duncan put it, 'if he were being tried by a jury of his fellow citizens he would be unhesitatingly acquitted on the evidence'. 'Your Petitioner's case is very hard,' he concludes,

> as he and his wife and child are thrown upon the world without a penny after his 26 years faithful service to the College and without the pension which doubtless he would receive on retiring for good conduct. He therefore earnestly and respectfully begs the Council of the College of Surgeons to reconsider his case.

But it was to no avail. Duncan's own property loss claim, submitted later that year, amounted to £44-worth of effects and £14 in cash. The state adjudicators recommended he receive £41 compensation. He never returned to RCSI, and little is known of his fate thereafter.

More collegiately, in early June, the Registrar of RCPI wrote to RCSI to say that the President and Fellows 'heard with regret of the damage done to the Royal College of Surgeons during the recent rebellion... [we] trust that if necessary the President and Council of the Royal College of Surgeons will avail themselves of

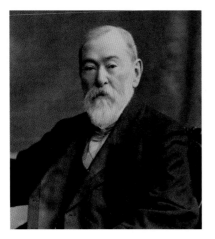

'Snowy-bearded' Cameron in his later years.

the hospitality of this College'. Council Secretary Charles Molyneux Benson replied with 'cordial thanks', but said there was no need.[117] Indeed, by the end of May, RCSI students were once again sitting exams in the College Hall.

'Some of the leaders like myself will very probably be shot, but I can't say what will happen to the rank and file.'[118] So said Mallin as he went around shaking hands. He was right: he was executed by firing squad a fortnight later, on 8 May. A few days earlier, when Áine Ceannt visited her husband Éamon in jail – he had commanded the garrison at the South Dublin Union, now St James' Hospital – he urged her to contact Charles Cameron in the hope he could intervene. She duly called on Cameron at his home on Raglan Road, where Cameron said he would 'do his best'.

In the event, Ceannt was shot the same day as Mallin. Meanwhile, in Dublin Castle, Richard Francis Tobin (1843–1919, Lic. 1864, FRCSI 1882) was treating James Connolly for injuries sustained in the GPO. They struck up an immediate rapport, the rebel calling the surgeon 'a wonderful man', and after Connolly's execution – on 12 May – Tobin arranged financial assistance for the impoverished Connolly family (perhaps because his own son Paddy, a Trinity medical student, had been killed at Gallipoli, he took a fatherly interest in Connolly's son Roddy; interestingly, one of Connolly's daughters, Moira Elizabeth Connolly (1899 – 1958) earned her Licence from RCSI in 1925). Markievicz, too, had been sentenced to death, but this was commuted.'

Many of the 'rank and file' Mallin had wondered about were interned in a prison camp at Frongoch in Wales – whither, in December 1916, Charles Cameron travelled to inspect conditions. He spent two days there, tramping over the snow-covered ground and asking searching questions. One internee remembered him as a snowy-bearded, immensely old man, bent over his walking-stick:

> Entering the dormitory he went straight over to the two latrines in the corner. Although his voice was sharp and strong we could not distinguish what it was he was saying; but we gathered that he was not quite satisfied with the arrangement. He also made down one of the beds and got into it. He looked a most comical sight in the bed, with his tall silk hat still on his head...[119]

Another internee recalled Cameron's sharp criticism of the camp doctor, who refused to treat prisoners until they had given their names: 'this was no business of a doctor,' Cameron pointed out. 'Complaint too, apparently, was made to the British Medical Council'.[120] Many — Cameron included — believed that his subsequent report ('almost wholly in favour of the prisoners'[121]) led directly to the camp being closed soon after. This was Cameron's 'last official assignment' — but his life's work was not yet done. In fact, he was about to face a final great test.

From February 1918, an influenza virus began to sweep around the globe; because of the war, censorship repressed much reporting of it, but in neutral Spain it was covered extensively, giving the world the erroneous impression that this was 'the Spanish flu'. And when it arrived in Ireland, all eyes turned to the 88-year-old Medical Officer of Health.

'THE EPIDEMIC OF INFLUENZA IS NOW VERY GENERAL THROUGHOUT THE CITY'

Across three waves of the global influenza pandemic of 1918–19, approximately one billion people were infected and probably 60 million died.[122] In Ireland, about one fifth of the population was infected, and at least 20,000 people died. A century on, the exact origins of the disease are still debated, but its global spread — in three near-simultaneous waves — was certainly facilitated by the upheaval of the war: viruses go where people go.

Influenza is an acute and sometimes life-threatening viral infection of the respiratory tract. To this day, it is not easily diagnosed; laboratory tests are required to distinguish it from other respiratory infections. In 1918, however, it was not even clear that influenza was a viral infection — indeed, until the early 1930s, the prevailing thinking was that it was a bacterium. But even at the outset of the pandemic, it was not obvious to the medical community that the disease in question was in fact influenza. Previously, influenza outbreaks exhibited high morbidity but not high mortality — but now death could be terrifyingly sudden, with victims collapsing in the street. (This was often via uncontrollable haemorrhages, such as nosebleeds. Familiar, too, was a tell-tale bluish tinge to the skin — helio-

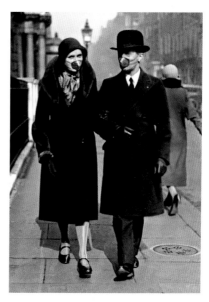

Mask-wearing during 'the Spanish Flu', 1918. © Vintage_Space / Alamy Stock Photo.

trope cyanosis – caused by a lack of oxygen to the extremities as the sufferer's lungs became clogged.) Moreover, those dying were an unusual cohort: healthy young adults (as opposed to the very young or elderly, as might have been expected). And the time of year of the initial outbreak – the summer months – was unusual too. By the time of the second, much more devastating wave – mid-October to December – the verdict that this was influenza was generally accepted, albeit in an extreme form.

Throughout, there was a near-complete absence of leadership from the authorities in Dublin Castle or the Local Government Boards, so response – if not responsibility – devolved to individuals, especially the frontline of the Poor Law (essentially, public) system. The statistics show that Medical Officers of Health worked more or less around the clock, paying 100,000[123] more home visits during the pandemic than in the previous year (infection was common amongst physicians and nurses – as it was amongst all public-facing roles, such as pharmacists, police, shop and tram workers, bank officials and the religious – though deaths appear to have been rare[124]).

Owing to his public profile, Cameron was regularly consulted by reporters, and his response from the start has been characterised as 'clear, cautious and practical'.[125] As the pandemic spread, he too worked tirelessly, visiting hospitals to conduct an audit of available beds, and he asked the military authorities not to send any more wounded soldiers to public beds. As the second wave hit, he appealed to school managers to close schools. He wrote to the *Irish Times* on the subject:

> Sir –
> The epidemic of influenza, as it is termed, is now very general throughout the city, and I earnestly entreat the managers of closed schools not to open them until Monday, 4th November, 1918. I would again urge the desirability of avoiding crowded assemblies...[126]

For these measures, he was accused of overreaction by some, underreaction by others, who wanted to see theatres and cinemas closed too. Such places of entertainment were disinfected between shows, but in any case attendance was much reduced. Elsewhere, trade practically ceased: 'One leading grocer remarked that the great bulk of his customers were sending in written orders by messenger rather than coming to collect them themselves.'[127]

About the only traders who thrived were the undertakers – and the timber-merchants who supplied them. Not since the cholera outbreak of the 1830s had the cemeteries been so busy, as the *Irish Times* (31 October) reported:

Yesterday, from early morning till well after midday, cortège after cortège reached Glasnevin Cemetery, sometimes as many as three corpse-laden hearses being seen proceeding up Sackville Street at the same time. Close on forty orders for interment were issued at the Cemeteries' Office yesterday, and, inclusive of the remains brought for burial on the previous day, which had been temporarily placed in the vaults overnight, there were close on one hundred bodies for sepulture...

The same article reported Cameron's optimism that 'the epidemic is now at its height, and that this week it will begin to abate'.[128] But the end of war on 11 November occasioned many of the 'crowded assemblies' he had warned against – enabling, amidst the celebrations, a worldwide resurgence of infection.

THE RESEARCH RESPONSE: 'URGENCY AND EXCITEMENT'

The pandemic largely stumped the scientific community, who had lately grown more accustomed to announcing breakthroughs. In the absence of antibiotics, no one's advice was any better than Cameron's: 'go to bed and stay there until well after the attack had passed, in order to prevent a relapse'.[129] But researchers got to work, including William Boxwell (1875–1943, Prof of Pathology 1918–43, PRCPI 1937–40). Boxwell was based at the Meath Hospital, where he was assisted by Dorothy Stopford Price (1890–1954).

Price vividly recalled the 'urgency and excitement'[130] the new illness provoked. Her interest in post-mortems, she wrote,

> was inculcated in my student days by Professor William Boxwell. He was mad on post-mortems and I was acting as his clinical clerk in the November 1918 influenza epidemic. He tried to get a portion of lung from each victim of the 'black' influenzal pneumonia, and at 10 p.m. every night I biked down to the Mortuary, and with or without the aid of a night porter carried in about three corpses into the p.m. room, and stripped them ready and put them tidy afterwards; these were all surreptitious p.m.s and once or twice we got a fright when someone came to the door which was locked. I well remember nights when the rain came pelting down on the glass roof, and I alone inside trying to get the corpse into its habit and back to its bench; he often helped but was run off his feet and frequently had to leave at midnight on a call. He said the results of microscopic examination of the lung were disappointing, engorgement with blood obscured the picture...[131]

Price would later gain fame for her contribution to the eradication of tuberculosis. Boxwell, for his part, took a great interest in the incipient vaccine debate. He was generally unpersuaded by the claims of efficacy that some were making, not least because of the rapid evolution of the infection (in fact, it was not until the 1930s that the first generation of live-attenuated vaccines were developed).

Meanwhile, in the streets and theatres, and on trams and trains, people hopefully held to their noses handkerchiefs soaked in eucalyptus oil – which one medic believed 'was about as potent to repulse influenza as a black beetle would be to halt a steamroller'.[132] For those who met 'the Spanish lady' – the parlance of the day – the most effective widely available treatment was a dose or two of whiskey with hot water and sugar; it was 'probably no less worthless than any of the other nostrums,' opined a doctor at the Mater, 'and at least its customers had a merry spin to Paradise'.[133]

The third wave came in mid-February 1919, lasting until mid-April. Cameron's own *Annual Reports* give the following statistics for Dublin:

Period *13 weeks to*	Deaths *Number*	Death Rate *Per 1,000 living*	12 months before
End Jun 1918	1,554	20.4	21.4
End Sep 1918	1,662	21.8	16.0
End Dec 1918	2,756	36.1	16.9
End Mar 1919	2,923	37.7	21.7
End Jun 1919	1,496	19.3	20.4

It is likely that Dublin did not fare as badly as other major cities thanks to the 'prompt and effective measures of Cameron and his office'.[134] Ironically, the Public Health Committee had decided in late 1918 that Cameron should be 'relieved from the active work of the Department, and confine himself to consultative duties and analytical work in the City Laboratory...'[135]

In fact, Cameron was granted a year's leave of absence in October 1918 – just prior to the apex of the pandemic – but he remained at his post because the Corporation did not adopt the recommendation until the following March. What he himself thought of this remains unknown – he was no longer keeping his diary – but in his later *Autobiography* he pays tribute to his assistants during the period, Dr Matthew Russell (1874–1956, Lic. 1898, FRCSI 1902) and Bernard Fagan (1888–1959). Russell succeeded Cameron in 1921, becoming the first full-time MOH in the new state, a position he held until 1947. Fagan succeeded Cameron as Public Analyst from 1921 to 1956. (In 1920, Fagan organised the first annual Liffey Swim, deeming the water cleanest at high tide; an entrant himself, he came third.[136])

If there is little in Cameron's writings about the pandemic, there is nothing in the RCSI muniments either. This may seem surprising at first – as the Registrar General, Sir William Thompson (1861–1929, Lic. 1888) put it, 'Since the period of the Great Famine with its awful attendant horrors of fever and cholera, no disease of an epidemic nature created so much havoc in any one year in Ireland as influenza in 1918'[137] – but in fact RCSI was no different to other institutions in this regard.[138]

One explanation is that, for all its havoc, the influenza pandemic had little effect on institutions as institutions – certainly not in the way the war had (or, in Ireland, the Rising, or the upheaval before and after independence). The pandemic killed thousands, but it did not particularly change politics or social structures. Its many tragedies, then, were essentially private tragedies, its griefs and ghosts confined to families, and when it passed, it fairly cleanly passed from public memory too.[139]

Cameron was almost ninety when he finally bowed out of public service in 1920. He also retired from his two RCSI professorships that year, at which point he became the first Professor Emeritus. When he died a short time later – on 27 February 1921, at the age of 91 – his sole surviving son, Ernest, wrote to RCSI's Registrar, Alfred Miller:

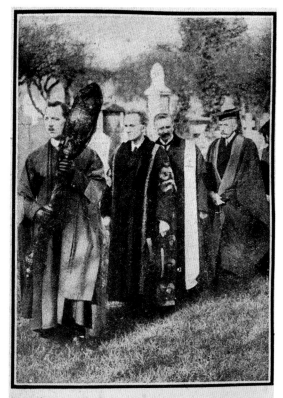

The mace draped for Cameron's funeral in Mount Jerome Cemetery.

DOCTORS' TRIBUTE.—Sir W. de Courcy Wheeler, preceded by the mace, represented the Royal College of Surgeons at the funeral at Dublin of Sir Charles Cameron, the public analyst.

… my Father was so long connected with the College and had such a deep and strong interest in its work that the very building itself would have a sentiment almost akin to an old friend. You can have no idea of the bitter disappointment he felt last Summer at not being able to give the full number of his lectures – I think that his heart was greatly bound up in the old College.[140]

AFTER THE WAR: 'OTHERS WAKE UP TO CONSCIOUSNESS AND MISERY'

The war was over by now – but that did not mean the suffering ended, especially for those with 'shell shock'. The term first appeared in *The Lancet* in 1915, but for the first two years of fighting, there was little understanding of the concept. At the time, doctors were asked to assess physical fitness only, and perhaps 300-plus shell shock sufferers were, as a tragic result, court-martialled and shot as cowards. In Ireland, Francis Carmichael Purser (1876–1934, Prof of Medicine 1917–26) took a pioneering interest in the subject, publishing a paper on it in 1917.

English, Scottish and Irish soldiers were equally susceptible, he wrote, with younger men more frequently affected:

Many of the men know of the origin of their trouble only by hearsay: they remember, perhaps, an explosion, and then a blank, which may represent any length of time of unconsciousness. Some do not develop any symptoms until some days after the shock… Others wake up to consciousness and misery… It is a state of depression, mental and physical; a state of silent hopeless inability…[141]

Purser himself had served in the war – he held the rank of major in the RAMC and was consulting neurologist to the forces in Ireland. Accordingly, he could attest to seeing genuine cases of shell shock in soldiers who 'had never been nearer the war than the south of England'.[142] He also refused to accept that shell-shocked men lacked courage, as was the widespread suspicion. 'On the contrary, I know that many have behaved with conspicuous bravery.'[143]

Another notable advocate for shell shock survivors in Ireland was William R. Dawson (1864–1950, Lic. 1896), who had formerly been a demonstrator in the Pathology Department; in 1911, he was appointed HM Inspector of Lunatic Asylums in Ireland and from 1915 was a specialist in 'nerve disease' to the troops in Ireland. Both Purser and Dawson received OBEs for their work.

RCSI'S AMERICAN FRIENDS

For his frontline work, the pioneering American neurosurgeon Harvey Cushing (1869–1939) received an Honorary Fellowship from RCSI (1918). He travelled to Dublin to accept it, later publishing his impressions in *From a Surgeon's Journal, 1915–1918*. Ireland was an 'inscrutable and incomprehensible country which the Irish, if possible, seem to understand even less well than anyone else'. He admired RCSI's 'fine old Georgian building' – flying the Stars and Stripes – and mused on the RCSI's connection to the recent 'half-baked rebellion... which chose as its fortress and chief scene of operations the one place in Dublin which boasts that neither politics nor religion concerns its affairs'.

He had heard the story of the damaged portrait of Victoria, too, noting 'the frame is still empty':

> The ceremony in the afternoon was most elaborate, and amusingly disproportionate to the occasion – viz., me. There was a guard of honor drawn up in the lower hall – the students' O.T.C., which I had to inspect. Then tea in the council room for the elect... I was put in a robe with blue stripes, surrounded by four proctors, male and female – it's a co-educational school – and some hitch occurred, for old Sir Chas. Cameron forgot that he was to escort me... we walked in rather belated – applause – and I sank... into a large carved chair in which, as I was told later, Daniel O'Connell once died or did something equally foolish. As a matter of fact, I should have stood, but too late now.
>
> Then they began tormenting me – the Vice President read slowly the names of former Honorary Fellows – 66 I believe... Then they told other things about the College and finally, coming to me, read dates out of an ancient Who's Who, about someone I vaguely recognized as having met... Then, horrors! I was given the opportunity of making a public acceptance!! It was pretty bad, but they cheered me along... I was permitted to sit again in the lap of Daniel O'Connell's chair and wished I too might also die there – but no, I had to sign the roll – a slippery parchment containing signatures if anything less legible than mine... So we filed out again with the help of the band and went down and had more tea – the elect, that is... Meanwhile, the students tea'd in the Library, where I should greatly have preferred to be.[144]

Cushing's honour was most likely led by then-President William Taylor, both men having worked together at Boulogne. RCSI's American relations were further

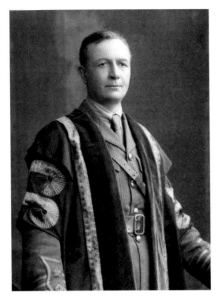

Sir William
Taylor, PRCSI
1916–18.

strengthened after the war when, in 1918 and 1920, respectively, Myles and Taylor were conferred with Honorary Fellowship of the American College of Surgeons.

By way of thanks, Taylor organised the gift of an Irish elk's head and antlers to the ACS (the remains, at least 11,000 years old, had been excavated in Leitrim in 1832). Warming to the transatlantic theme, in 1921, PRCSI Edward Taylor (1867–1922, FRCSI 1896, PRCSI 1920–22) led a delegation to Philadelphia to confer RCSI Honorary Fellowships on eight American surgeons including William and Charles Mayo of the eponymous clinic, and George W. Crile of the Cleveland Clinic. On that occasion, Robert Woods travelled onwards to Chicago, where he became the third Irish Honorary Fellow of the ACS.

THE WAR OF INDEPENDENCE AND THE GUN IN THE FRONT HALL

It made sense to look across the Atlantic at this time, not least as Ireland's political relationship with Britain was being radically revised. The date 21 January 1919 marks both the beginning of the War of Independence and the sitting of the first

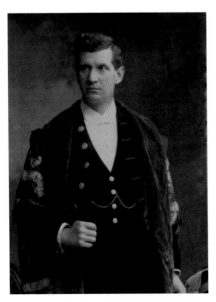

Sir Robert
Woods, PRCSI
1910–12.

Dáil – that is, a parliament for the Irish Republic. Two of the elected representatives that day were RCSI Licentiates: Patrick McCartan (1878–1963, Lic. 1910, FRCSI 1912) and Richard Francis Hayes (1882–1958, Lic. 1905). All Irish MPs, regardless of political persuasion, were invited to attend the breakaway parliament, but of those who preferred to continue to sit at Westminster, only Robert Woods (MP for Dublin University) wrote to decline the invitation.[145]

The escalating War of Independence can be glimpsed in RCSI's Council Minutes, where, for example, William Wheeler is recorded negotiating with the military authorities on the 'desirability of exhibiting a red cross on the screen and right hand lamp of motor cars used by Doctors whilst the Curfew Order was in force'.[146] Another curfew in early 1921 caused the Charter Day dinner to be postponed.[147] Then there was a more alarming development: Crown forces issued an order requiring doctors to 'furnish daily particulars of wounded persons under their care in hospitals' – that is, essentially, to inform on combatants ('the names and descriptions of all persons... suspected to be suffering from wounds caused by bullets, gun fire or other explosives'[148]).

Failure to comply, they said, 'would render the medical practitioners liable under the Restoration of Order in Ireland Regulations'. A number of RCSI Licentiates and Fellows asked the Council to intervene to prevent this 'breach of professional confidence'. All this was reported in the *BMJ* – including the information that 'the Republican Army in Ireland have countered the military Order' and any doctors obeying the order 'will be treated as spies'.[149]

William Wheeler responded on behalf of the Council, forwarding a copy to the Irish Medical Secretary:

> The Council are of the opinion that it is contrary to the public interest that medical men should break their professional tradition and, without the consent of their patients, disclose information which they have obtained in the discharge of their professional duties. If any instance is reported to the Council in which one of the fellows or licentiates of the College is pressed to break confidence, such specific case will be considered by the Council, and representations made to the authorities if such be thought necessary.

The *BMJ* noted that this position 'will be much appreciated by the profession generally'.[150] (As the Minutes record, the Council was in fact sharply split on the issue: the resolution passed by seven votes to six.[151]) As if to illustrate the point, one house surgeon at the Mater – John O'Shea (1898–1976, FRCSI 1934) – refused to let a squad of 'Black and Tans' see a patient, even when they threatened to shoot him.[152] Less fortunate was RCSI student Louis Darcy (1897–1921), who was shot dead by this Auxiliary force at Merlin Park, Galway, on 24 March 1921. The Chief of Intelligence at Dublin Castle called Darcy 'the Michael Collins of the West'.[153]

As the unrest continued, more RCSI names appear in reports of arrests, such as Thomas Higgins (Lic. 1879, FRCSI 1887), septuagenarian coroner for Queen's County (Laois) and his son, Thomas Francis (1890–1953, Lic. 1914), 'interned for some months without being brought before a court-martial'.[154] On 7 July –

that is, mere days before the Truce – the Minutes record 'the desirability of affecting an insurance to cover the College building and contents against damage from Riot, etc'.[155] In October, as the Treaty was being negotiated in London, tensions were still high in Dublin as 'Lambert Ormsby drew the attention of Council to the unsuitable position of the gun in the front hall...'[156]

RCSI WELCOMES THE IRISH FREE STATE

The Treaty led to the Civil War, more bloodshed and civil unrest: on 20 July 1922, the following letter from Registrar Miller was entered in the Minutes:

> Gentlemen,
>
> I beg to report that, on the 30th June, acting on the advice of Sir William Taylor, I called on the Minister of Defence and asked him to place a Guard in charge of the College as I feared that the premises might be taken by Irregulars. The Minister of Defence kindly sent a Guard [that is, a unit or brigade, not a lone policeman] at once and, within one hour of the arrival of the Guard, an attempt was made by the Irregulars to get possession of the College. The Guard remained in possession until 11th July. I am happy to report that no damage was done and that the Guard were most considerate and did not put us to any inconvenience...'[157]

A letter of thanks was duly sent to the Minister of Defence.

At the funerals of Arthur Griffith and Michael Collins – both in August – RCSI was represented with its ceremonial mace (it is not clear who held it). Both men had been embalmed by Oliver St John Gogarty (1878–1957, FRCSI 1910). The unclear circumstances of Collins' death in particular seem to have been muddied further by Gogarty. The embalming took place in St Vincent's Hospital, on the far side of the Green, where Gogarty is also said to have carried out a post-mortem.[158] (The post-mortem certificate was apparently placed in a safe in RCSI, but it has not been found – if it ever existed.) Gogarty was, amongst his many talents, a successful ENT surgeon, a senator and a prolific author. He was a friend of Joyce in his youth (he is the model for Buck Mulligan in *Ulysses*) and Yeats in his maturity. His portrait (1911), by Sir William Orpen – which also features an impressive bill from London's Café Royal – hangs in the Colles Room.

In October, the Incorporated Law Society held their lectures and exams in RCSI, their own premises having been damaged during the siege of the Four Courts. Elsewhere, there was legal nation-building: in accordance with Article

Facing page:
Oliver St John
Gogarty by
William Orpen,
1911.

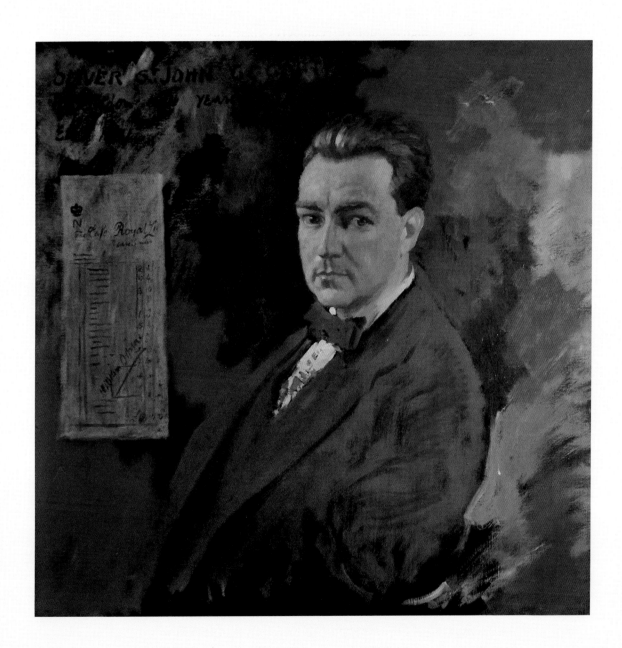

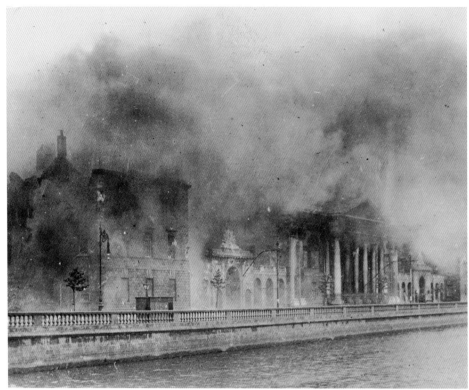

The shelling of the Four Courts, June 1922. Reproduced courtesy of the National Library of Ireland (HOG57).

82 of the new Constitution, the Seanad (Senate) was to feature members of bodies not otherwise represented in the Dáil, and RCSI was named as one such body in the debates.[159] The Council put forward the names of William Wheeler and Arthur Chance (1889–1980, FRCSI 1915, Prof of Surgery 1929–46), though neither were subsequently elected. Perhaps it was just as well: of the sixty new Senators, thirty-six would have their houses burned by Anti-Treaty forces.

Wheeler would later express his sense of alienation with the new State; he spoke of being 'tired of the turmoil, bewildered at the outlook, [and] anxious for the safety of our families'. (There is reason to believe, too, that this world-weariness was prompted at least in part by Chance's recent appointment as RCSI Professor of Surgery. Wheeler himself had prepared an application, but at the last minute decided not to submit it.) Wheeler left for England – and various prestigious posts – in 1932. Once, on a return visit, an old woman in the Liberties told him: 'Ah, Sir William, when you left Dublin the whole place shook.'[160]

Before all that, however, on 1 May 1923, as PRCSI, Wheeler led a deputation to Phoenix Park to present an address of welcome on behalf of RCSI to the new Governor-General of the Irish Free State, T.M. Healy:

We, the President, Vice-President, and Council of the Royal College of Surgeons in Ireland, wish to greet you on your appointment... We can assure your Excellency that the services of our College will on all occasions be placed loyally and whole-heartedly at the disposal of the Government of the Irish Free State whenever questions arise affecting public health or the welfare of the people.[161]

The Civil War ended soon after, on 24 May. Amongst its recent victims was an RCSI student, Eugene McQuaid (1899–1923) – son of Dr E.W. McQuaid (Lic. 1890) of Cootehill, Co. Cavan, and brother of the future archbishop of Dublin, John Charles McQuaid – who died of his wounds after an ambush near Newport, Co. Mayo. The *Freeman's Journal* reported that McQuaid was unarmed and wearing a Red Cross badge.[162] ∎

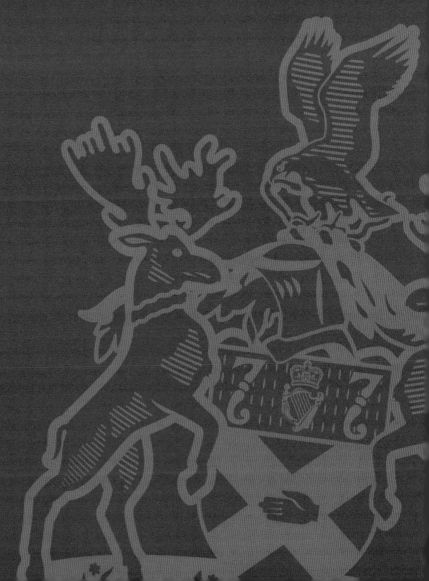

Chapter 6:
In Adversity, 1924–61

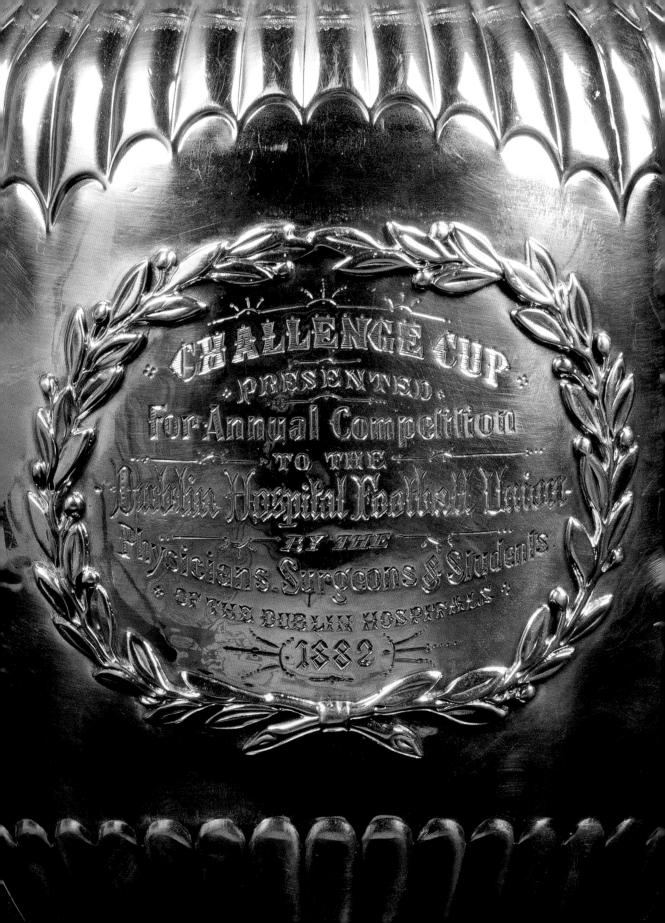

CHALLENGE CUP
PRESENTED
for Annual Competition
TO THE
Dublin Hospital Football Union
BY THE
Physicians, Surgeons & Students
OF THE DUBLIN HOSPITALS
1882

Chapter 6:
In Adversity, 1924-61

'ONE OR TWO GREAT PROBLEMS REMAIN'

'The last twenty-five years have shown a greater advance in medicine and surgery than the previous twenty-five centuries.' This is what PRCSI Wheeler told students at an assembly in December 1923. No doubt Wheeler meant to be inspiring – the occasion was, after all, a prize-giving ceremony. But while the claim was largely correct, it somewhat glossed over the fact that the Irish medical student experience – in all schools, not just RCSI – had hardly changed since the 1880s.[1]

This did not impinge upon Wheeler's optimism. 'One or two great problems remain to be solved,' he admitted, 'but the probability is that before you have reached your zenith, cancer will be well under control, and will have taken its place, subdued and conquered, alongside of diabetes, syphilis and smallpox...'[2]

THE ROCKEFELLER FOUNDATION AND THE IRISH MEDICAL REGISTER

Previous page:
The Dublin
Hospitals Cup.

Wheeler was likely thinking of the gleaming medical world he had seen on the far side of the Atlantic, where the future seemed already present at Baltimore's Johns

Hopkins Hospital and University at Baltimore. Here was a hospital, a medical school and a laboratory-based research institute under one roof, to the mutual benefit of all. Funded from the deep pockets of the Carnegie and Rockefeller Foundations, this flagship endeavour led to a complete reform of American health sciences education.[3]

The Rockefeller Foundation aspired to spread this good work worldwide. When its representatives first visited Ireland, the political turmoil they found – it was 1922 – suggested they wait a while before investing. As the situation calmed, further visits followed – resulting in scathing reports: there were too many students, too many schools; teachers were practitioners, not academic specialists; clinical experience was barely supervised, with students wandering from one hospital to another as the mood took them ('Dr A at such a hospital, and on Tuesday Mr B at another').

Sniffily, the reviewers opined that Irish students cleared a low bar, 'no more than the ordinary general practitioner would need of the various preliminary and essential disciplines such as physiology, bacteriology and pathology'.[4] (This perhaps missed the salient point that the vast majority of Irish students were, in fact, destined for general practice.) Over time, the Americans discovered that 'Medical education in Ireland... is no simple educational matter but one involving some of the deepest and most sensitive and most maltreated emotions and sympathies of the Irish people.'[5]

The complication of denominational hospitals was duly noted, as was the rivalry between Trinity and UCD (the latter was expected to benefit from its 'close relationship with the Free State Government'[6]); Queen's was 'the best of its kind',[7] though no more than a respectable provincial school; Galway, it was predicted, 'would die', while Cork was 'doomed to slow extinction'. And RCSI, for its part, was 'futile... continuing entirely on students' fees... but not doing much harm'.[8]

Adding insult to these injuries, when a leading Rockefeller thinker produced a comprehensive comparative survey of American and European medical schools, Ireland was left out entirely (even Graves and Stokes were referred to as English). Ideally, the Foundation wanted to see a single medical school in the Free State, born of a union of TCD and UCD, and attached to a hospital untethered from religious control. (For a time, the two universities conspired in the fiction that this was possible, but they never had any intention of amalgamating, only of splitting the funds.[9]) In this regard, the Foundation was to be sorely disappointed.

The prospect of a Rockefeller windfall diminished further when the Free State Government proposed the establishment of a separate Irish Medical Council and Register for Ireland, severing the historical connection (since 1858) with the General Medical Council in London. On one level, this was as simple as painting red pillar boxes green: after all, why should Irish doctors be answerable to a foreign body? If this ruffled some medical feathers along the way, so be it – as W.T. Cosgrave put it, 'we must be prepared to face whatever minor and temporary disadvantage may accrue from the cessation of this previous arrangement'.[10]

But members of the profession saw things differently: to them, sudden ineligibility for the GMC Register was a potential disaster, not least as Irish doctors were essentially reared for export, generally to the UK and its colonies; indeed, for the 400-odd doctors qualifying annually in the period, only about fifty could expect to find posts in Ireland.[11] Without that escape valve, Irish students would enrol either in the North or in Britain, thereby impoverishing the Free State schools.

This was deeply disconcerting to all of the third-level institutions concerned: at this time, medical students comprised the single biggest cohort of university students in the country, and so to weaken one's medical school was to undermine the finances of the entire university. For the likes of RCSI, unsupported by other means (as the Americans had discerned), any precipitous diminution of fees looked distinctly fatal. It was little wonder, then, that RCSI personalities such as Thomas Myles were amongst the most vociferous opponents of the measure. 'If the worst happened,' he warned, 'the loss to the Free State would be very considerable. It would be a financial, moral and social loss – a loss in sport, a loss in everything.'[12]

In some respects, the registration controversy lifted a lid on other long-simmering tensions. 'Greater issues are at stake than even the future of the Free State's medical schools,' said the *Irish Times* (itself an Anglo-leaning organ). 'Two ideals are at war in this country. One is that ideal of international culture which admits no barrier to the march of science... The other is the parochial ideal which would put on our country a double bereavement of brain and soul.'[13] In the opposite corner was the likes of *The Leader*, which pulled no punches:

> With the inevitable exceptions we never thought much of the medical doctors in Ireland from an Irish point of view or of those that Ireland produced for exportation. In the lump they are a poor Anglicised, shoneen lot, mostly recruited from the first generation of gombeen or other parents who wanted a doctor in the family...[14]

For those who wanted a 'self-sufficient' Ireland, the end of the practice of doctors-for-export – that is, RCSI's bread-and-butter – was entirely to be welcomed.

The incoming RCSI President, Charles Maunsell (1872–1930, FRCSI 1900, PRCSI 1924–26), accepted the inevitability of the Irish Medical Register. After four years of disputation, it was his plan of 'reciprocal registration' that settled the matter — essentially, a 'both/and' solution, as opposed to 'either/or'. By the Medical Practitioners Act of 1927, the Irish Medical Council would oversee the regulation of Irish doctors and all ancillary disciplinary matters; at the same time, Irish doctors could still automatically register in London, while UK practitioners had the right to practise in the Free State (should any want to). The Irish schools had representatives on both Councils (initially, RCSI was expected to share its nominee with RCPI, but both Colleges insisted on separate representation). When the Irish Medical Council convened for the first time, in 1928, it was in RCSI's College Hall, with Maunsell at the table as the home team's spokesman.

Relatively soon after the registration matter was settled, the Rockefeller Foundation returned — but warily this time. It surveyed the scene, and decided on a course of piecemeal action that would fund individuals and institutions through the decade ahead. But its earlier ambition to kickstart a secular, research-driven revolution in Irish medical education — in other words, to foster the expansive, expensive, near utopian vision Wheeler had invoked for his prize-winners — that was gone for good.

'CONSIDERABLE ANXIETY': THE COST OF LIVING

After the unrest of recent years, the Charter Day Dinner was revived in 1923; on that occasion Sir Harold Stiles (1863–1946), President of the Edinburgh College, was made an Honorary Fellow. But within a year, belts were being severely tightened: for the 1924 Dinner, the number of guests was more than halved from its heyday; afterwards, the Dinner Committee was relieved to report that 'expenditure was kept below the pre-war level. The price of the Dinner, including smokes and wines, amounts to 30/- per head. The total cost was approximately £68, as compared with £76: 6: 0. in 1914.'[15] (Perhaps illustrating priorities, when it was reported that the Library's bookstock was 'inadequate', the only suggested recourse was to apply to the Carnegie Trust for assistance.)

Also in 1924, a Report from the Special Finance Committee claimed that RCSI was 'just living within its income', but warned — in light of the registration controversy — of leaner years to come.[16] The auditors' report for that year shows a modest excess of expenditure (£2,499 7s 10d) over income (£2,436 3s), but then there was also a significant annual debt carried over (£2,208 15s 8d). Mere figures clearly did not explain enough: in 1926, the Council asked the auditors to 'include in their report a statement, so that the Council may fully understand the financial position of the College'.[17]

Whatever the nature of this statement, a year later the negative balance had deepened further, to £3,480 11s 1d — which gave rise to 'considerable anxiety'.[18]

After a hiatus of several years, an Honorary Fellowship was again awarded in 1927. The recipient, Hugh Hampton Young (1870–1945), an American urologist, recalled the 'small private session... followed by a delightful little dinner in the spacious rooms of the college'. The 'informality' he approved of was likely a virtue made of financial necessity.[19]

A ROYAL COLLEGE IN A FREE STATE

The spacious rooms of RCSI – in particular the College Hall – were central venues for the social and scientific life of Dublin in the period, frequently hosting events for the Royal Dublin Society, the Zoological Society, the National Society for the Prevention of Cruelty to Children (it became the ISPCC in 1956), the Women's National Health Association and the children's holiday charity Sunshine House. The Irish Cancer Research Board met at RCSI from 1926 to 1929, until it folded 'for want of funds'.[20]

Such difficulties of funding and finance were endemic in the period, and RCSI invariably offered its facilities without charge. (One of the few non-charitable bodies they allowed in for an annual dinner was the Bank of Ireland, which was probably prudent.) When the Eucharistic Congress came to Dublin (1932), RCSI declined the proposal that the College Hall be used as some sort of refectory – but when this was revised to a 'high-class' restaurant ('serving meals at first class hotel prices'), the hungry faithful were catered for.[21]

Despite its long non-confessional history, RCSI was strongly associated with the old, Ascendancy order. In some respects, it fell between two stools: in the nineteenth century, it had fought to establish itself as a pillar of Protestant

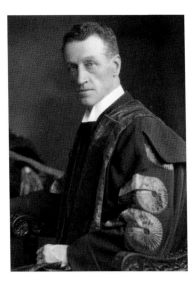

Andrew Fullerton, PRCSI 1926-28.

society, but it also educated Catholic doctors and recognised Cecilia Street's teaching, and never recorded students' religions; now, in the Free State, the Royal moniker alone rendered it suspect, to say the least. Even attempting to sidestep such confessionalism, it was easy to put a foot wrong.

In 1926, when Andrew Fullerton was elected PRCSI, much was made of his being Professor of Surgery at Queen's University, Belfast. At his first Charter Dinner, the newspapers reported that 'Good-will between North and South was the keynote',[22] and from 1928 Primary Fellowship exams

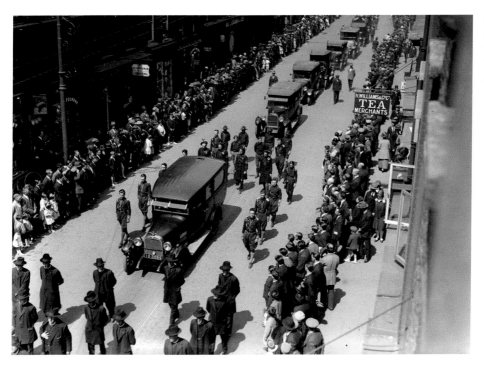

Funeral cortège of Countess Markievicz, 1927. © RTÉ Archives.

were held annually in Belfast. But when Fullerton declared 'In the field of surgery there should be no border,' this was reported by a Belfast newspaper as 'Famous Belfast surgeon says there should be no border.'[23] This scuppered the knighthood he might have expected.

Ever-vigilant observers watched for errors on both sides: once, at a dance in RCSI in 1934, when Amhrán na bhFiann was not played, a complaint was swiftly received, necessitating a grovelling apology – in Irish ('the omission to play the National Anthem on the occasion of the Dance was not by direction, or with the knowledge of, the President, Vice-President and Council of the College, nor does such omission meet with their approval...'[24]).

In the era, one sees RCSI constantly treading a fine line, trying to stay on good terms with everyone: sympathies were sent to the Queen in February 1936 on the death of George V; a month later, sympathies went to President de Valera, whose son died following a riding accident in Phoenix Park. Likewise, when Minister Kevin O'Higgins was assassinated, RCSI expressed 'horror at this appalling crime'.[25] Notably, though, in 1927, when Countess Markievicz died (she had been operated on, not successfully, by William Taylor) and thousands lined the streets for her cortège, which detoured via York Street and the Green to acknowledge her finest hour – RCSI had nothing to say.

ATTITUDES TO RESEARCH – OR, THE THREE TYPES OF SPECIALIST

Academically, there was a changing of the guard at RCSI, too. The death, after long service, of Alfred Scott (Physiology 1889–1926) caused much sadness ('it is difficult for the members of the Council to think of the College of Surgeons without the name of Professor Scott being associated with it'[26]); within weeks, George Jameson Johnston (Surgery 1912–26) died too (or *mortis ankaŭ*, as he – a keen Esperantist – might have said). That same year, both Ernest Hastings Tweedy (1862–1945, Prof of Obstetrics and Midwifery 1917–26) and Francis Carmichael Purser (1877–1934, Prof of Medicine 1917–26) retired; Robert Rowlette (Materia Medica 1921–26) took up a post in Trinity. A short time later, William Caldwell (Prof of Chemistry and Physics 1915–29) also retired. To fill the absences, various rounds of musical Chairs followed – notably including Victor Millington Synge's move from Medical Jurisprudence (1923–30[27]) to Medicine (1930–34).

Admired for his clinical acumen, Synge (1893–1976) – a nephew of the playwright John Millington Synge – was 'very conservative in outlook'[28] and inclined to look askance at research ('there is a feeling that anything which can be dubbed "research" puts the author in the seats of the mighty, and makes him feel that he is one of the elect who are advancing medicine'[29]). Synge considered Dublin too small for postgraduate teaching ('Let foreigners come here to study midwifery and let our graduates go abroad to study medicine and surgery'[30]), and he divided 'specialists' into three groups: first, 'those who know something about everything and a little about something' – they were the old-fashioned kind; second, 'those who know everything about something and nothing about anything else' – a group on the rise; and finally, 'those who know something about everything and everything about something'[31] – to Synge's mind, the most useful kind.

There was a seriousness behind this tongue-twisting humour. Synge was essentially taking sides in an ongoing debate about the place of specialisation in Irish medicine. This particularly centred on the future of hospitals: should the country's many small voluntary hospitals be supported, or was the time right for their amalgamation? Within RCSI opinion was divided: there were those like Wheeler who declared that 'Specialisation is the order of the day';[32] others – Myles, Moorhead and now Synge – argued that the profusion of hospitals allowed 'virtually every student who desired it... a three or six months course as a resident in a hospital... a doctor with a Dublin qualification... received a practical education such as he could receive nowhere else'.[33] How could a single hospital, they asked, no matter how modern, accommodate all those students?

One area of common ground was on the need to do something about how Irish hospitals were funded. For generations, many hospitals had relied on the charity galas, balls and bazaars that had been fixtures of the Irish high society calendar – but that moneyed world was more or less a casualty of the struggle for independence, and now the Free State did not have the means to meet the sudden shortfall. The religious ethos in the various hospitals complicated matters further. But the point later made by PRCSI Adams McConnell (1884–1972, FRCSI 1911 Prof of Surgery 1926–29, PRCSI 1936–38) was generally unarguable. 'The Dublin medical schools were inseparable from the Dublin hospitals,' he said, 'and if the latter were not first rate, the high standard of the former must be lowered'[34] – and no one wanted that. In the meantime, as the debate over amalgamation and specialisation continued, the hospitals were able to keep their doors open thanks to the establishment (1930) of a lottery that would become world-famous (and, in time, notorious): the Irish Hospitals' Sweepstake.[35]

PROF J.D.H. WIDDESS, THE BIOLOGICAL SOCIETY (1931) AND THE GRADUATES' ASSOCIATION (1932)

The limited research culture at RCSI was addressed not from the top down, but from the bottom up. In 1931, two recent students, Joseph Lewis (Lic. 1930) and J.D.H. Widdess (1906–1982, Lic. 1931, Prof of Biology 1960–73, Hon FRCSI 1975), founded the Biological Society of the Royal Colleges of Physicians and Surgeons in Ireland. 'The Society has been formed to enable students to give papers and addresses on medical and surgical subjects of a specialised nature,' the *Irish Times* reported, 'and it strives to fill a want which was felt in the College.'

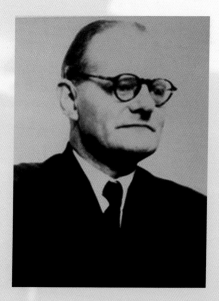

J.D.H. Widdess, co-founder of the Biological Society and RCSI historian.

There had been a handful of RCSI student societies before this – one in the 1790s, then the 'Junior Surgical Society' in the 1860s – but these sputtered out. The 'Bi', however, has been running continuously since its launch. Its value was recognised immediately by the authorities, who sponsored a gold medal ('of three to five guineas') for annual competitions. The inaugural address, delivered by the Society President, A.B. Clery (1899–1979, Lic. 1920, FRCSI 1923, PRCSI 1956–57), was on 'Rhinoplastic Surgery Through the

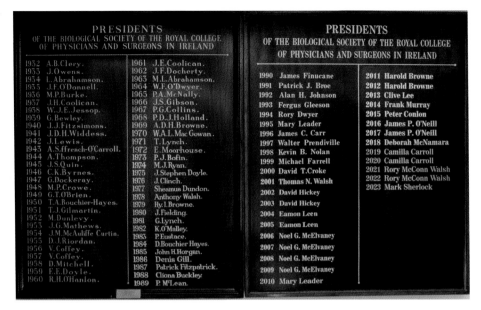

Presidents of the Biological Society from 1932.

PRESIDENTS
OF THE BIOLOGICAL SOCIETY OF THE ROYAL COLLEGE
OF PHYSICIANS AND SURGEONS IN IRELAND

1932	A.B.Clery.	1961	J.E.Coolican.
1933	J.Owens.	1962	J.F.Docherty.
1934	L.Abrahamson.	1963	M.L.Abrahamson.
1935	J.F.O'Donnell.	1964	W.F.O'Dwyer.
1936	M.P.Burke.	1965	P.A.McNally.
1937	J.H.Coolican.	1966	J.S.Gibson.
1938	W.J.E.Jessop.	1967	P.G.Collins.
1939	G.Bewley.	1968	P.D.J.Holland.
1940	J.J.Fitzsimons.	1969	A.D.H.Browne.
1941	J.D.H.Widdess.	1970	W.A.L.MacGowan.
1942	J.Lewis.	1971	T.Lynch.
1943	A.S.ffrench-O'Carroll.	1972	E.Moorhouse.
1944	A.Thompson.	1973	P.J.Bofin.
1945	J.S.Quin.	1974	M.J.Ryan.
1946	C.K.Byrnes.	1975	J.Stephen Doyle.
1947	G.Dockeray.	1976	J.Clinch.
1948	M.P.Crowe.	1977	Sheamus Dundon.
1949	G.T.O'Brien.	1978	Anthony Walsh.
1950	T.A.Bouchier-Hayes.	1979	Hy.I.Browne.
1951	T.J.Gilmartin.	1980	J.Fielding.
1952	M.Dunlevy.	1981	G.Lynch.
1953	J.G.Mathews.	1982	K.O'Malley.
1954	J.M.McAuliffe Curtin.	1983	P.Eustace.
1955	D.J.Riordan.	1984	D.Bouchier Hayes.
1956	V.Coffey.	1985	John H.Horgan.
1957	V.Coffey.	1986	Denis Gill.
1958	D.Mitchell.	1987	Patrick Fitzpatrick.
1959	E.E.Doyle.	1988	Cliona Buckley.
1960	R.H.O'Hanlon.	1989	P.McLean.

PRESIDENTS
OF THE BIOLOGICAL SOCIETY OF THE ROYAL COLLEGE
OF PHYSICIANS AND SURGEONS IN IRELAND

1990	James Finucane	2011	Harold Browne
1991	Patrick J. Broe	2012	Harold Browne
1992	Alan H. Johnson	2013	Clive Lee
1993	Fergus Gleeson	2014	Frank Murray
1994	Rory Dwyer	2015	Peter Conlon
1995	Mary Leader	2016	James P. O'Neill
1996	James C. Carr	2017	James P. O'Neill
1997	Walter Prendiville	2018	Deborah McNamara
1998	Kevin B. Nolan	2019	Camilla Carroll
1999	Michael Farrell	2020	Camilla Carroll
2000	David T.Croke	2021	Rory McConn Walsh
2001	Thomas N. Walsh	2022	Rory McConn Walsh
2002	David Hickey	2023	Mark Sherlock
2003	David Hickey		
2004	Eamon Leen		
2005	Eamon Leen		
2006	Noel G. McElvaney		
2007	Noel G. McElvaney		
2008	Noel G. McElvaney		
2009	Noel G. McElvaney		
2010	Mary Leader		

Ages'. Immediately upon qualification, Widdess was appointed as an assistant in the Physiology Department; in 1938 he was made lecturer in Biology, later advancing to the Chair and holding it until 1973. As Librarian of the College (1940–73), he made that long-neglected resource 'a living tool' and introduced the Dewey Decimal System. Amongst many works on medical history, he was the author of the second history of RCSI (first edition, 1949; second edition, 1967; third edition, 1984). He was conferred with Honorary Fellowship of RCSI in 1975, and the reading room of RCSI Heritage Collections is named in his honour.

Another important society followed soon after the 'Bi': in 1932, the past students' Association of the Royal College of Surgeons in Ireland, which in time became the Association of Medical and Dental Graduates (from 1978, RCSI *licenciates* would also be university *graduates*, putting an end to the historic semantic distinction that had long-bedevilled alumni). Again, the authorities recognised the value of this body and allowed them to meet in-house. The original objects of the Association were: (a) 'To forward the interests of the College, its institutions, and any of its members'; (b) 'To encourage intercourse between members'; and (c) 'To keep and circulate a register of its members'. Sir William Taylor served as the Association's first president.

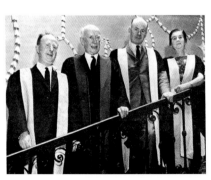

Four Fellows in one family: (from left) J.V. Clery, A.B. Clery (PRCSI 1956-57), A.P. Clery and Mary Gabriel (Gay) Clery, née Hogan.

'THE PHYSICAL AS WELL AS THE MENTAL FACULTIES': THE RISE OF SPORTS AT RCSI

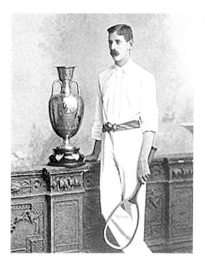

Joshua Pim, Wimbledon champion.

As far back as 1868, Prof Mapother (Anatomy and Physiology) had commented on the importance of training 'the physical as well as the mental faculties, which are closely interdependent' – not least, as he warned, because medical students were regularly exposed to contagious diseases. He advised that every medical school should provide sports facilities and that students' spare time should be spent in the 'ball-court, gymnasium or cricket field', rather than 'smoking at the dissection room fires, or in the taverns to which want of occupation will tempt them'.[36] (Smoking in dissection rooms, incidentally, lasted well into the 1950s.)

In truth, this was lip service only; not until Geddes came along did RCSI provide such facilities – but there were sporting heroes before that: there was Joshua Francis Pim (1869–1942, Lic. 1891, FRCSI 1896), who won the Wimbledon Men's Doubles title in 1890 and 1893, and the Men's Singles title in 1893 and 1894. In rugby, there was Sir William Watson Pike (1860–1941, Lic. 1880,

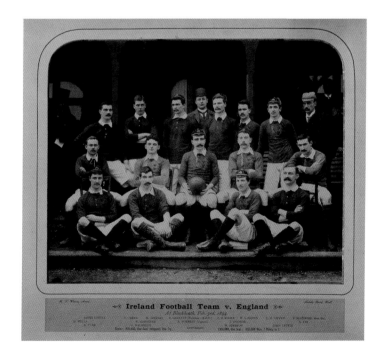

Ireland Football Team v. England
At Blackheath, Feb. 3rd, 1894

Thomas Joseph Crean (back row, second from left) and teammates, 1894.

The Dublin
Hospitals Cup.

FRCSI 1888), multi-decorated for his military career – he rose to the rank of Major-General – who played rugby for Ireland from 1879 to 1883; and – noted earlier – Thomas Joseph Crean (1873–1923, Lic. 1896, Hon FRCSI 1902). Crean was in fact a hero from his teens, when he saved a man from drowning at Blackrock. As a student at RCSI, he played for Wanderers Rugby Football Club, progressing to represent Leinster and Ireland (1894–96, nine caps, two tries).

In 1896, Crean captained the British and Irish Touring Side – the Lions Tour – that visited South Africa, where he stayed on to work in Johannesburg Hospital. For bravery during the Boer War, he was awarded the Victoria Cross (1901), and was decorated again during the First World War. He continued his life-saving exploits after the war as Medical Officer at Ascot Racecourse: on one occasion he performed a successful, if rudimentary, trepanning operation on a thrown jockey with a hammer and a chisel. He died in 1923, aged 49, having struggled with his health (and his finances) for some years. His medals are on display at the Museum of Military Medicine at Aldershot.[37]

Across all schools, rugby was the sport of choice for the medical fraternity (and *fraternity* it was: in the era, women students were largely excluded from sport, except when invited to fundraise). The affinity was elevated to tradition with the advent of the Dublin Hospitals Cup, founded in 1881. This still-running competition sees the city's various teaching hospitals vying with each other for 'the oldest trophy in world rugby'.[38] School and hospital authorities were happy to foster such competition, as it promoted 'traits of duty, solidarity and service'[39] and cemented collegiality. Senior students would tour dissecting rooms to try to enlist good rugby players to join particular hospitals. And there were cultural and class connotations too: in Ireland, rugby was seen as being a game for the professional classes in general (a trend bucked in the Limerick region).

There were times when medicine and rugby seemed barely distinguishable – as RCSI President Philip Crampton Smyly (1838–1904, FRCSI 1863, PRCSI 1878) declared:

Similar laws and training, similar earnestness and self-control, ensure similar results. The bodily training must be perfect; too much at once or too little is futile. It is the same with the mind. You would not have your cup this year had you trained your bodies as some of you try to train your minds for your examinations. Give something of the same training to your hands and minds as you do to your feet and bodies. You will then be successful, and win, not only the hospital challenge cup, but you will be successful men – men of the hand – surgeons.[40]

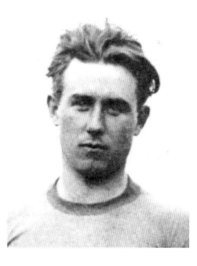

Pat O'Callaghan, Olympic champion. Courtesy of *History Ireland*.

Despite Hugh Auckinleck's connection with the rules of hurling, Gaelic sports made little inroads into the medical world in the era, due in part to the GAA's ban (1905–71) on its members participating in 'foreign games'.

With RCSI's acquisition of the Terenure grounds in 1909, the choice of sports widened. Thereafter, RCSI fielded women's and men's hockey teams, and athletics flourished, introducing RCSI's first athletics hero, Pat O'Callaghan (1906–1991, Lic. 1927). A hammer-thrower, he won gold at the 1928 Olympics in Amsterdam, the first competitor to do so under the Irish tricolour. 'I am glad of my victory,' he later said, 'not for the victory for myself, but for the fact that the world has been shown that Ireland has a flag, that Ireland has a National Anthem, and, in fact, we have a nationality.'[41] Four years later, he took home gold again, from the Los Angeles Games.

In 1936, owing to an internal dispute, Ireland did not send a team to Berlin – but O'Callaghan was there nonetheless, personally invited by Adolf Hitler (who was a hammer-throw enthusiast; the winner that year threw two metres short of O'Callaghan's personal best). In later life O'Callaghan turned down Louis B. Mayer's invitation for him to play the role of Tarzan in Hollywood; he opted instead for a quiet life in Clonmel. In 1988, he was the recipient of the inaugural RCSI Distinguished Graduate Award. A statue in his honour stands in Banteer, Co. Cork.

In October 1932, RCSI opened a new sixteen-acre sportsground at Bird Avenue in Clonskeagh, with pavilions for both men and women. 'The dressing-rooms,' reported the *Irish Times*, 'are claimed to be the most up-to-date in Dublin.'[42] The extensive grounds allowed for tennis courts to be added, while a disused quarry pit was considered for a swimming bath. In his ribbon-cutting speech, PRCSI Frank Crawley (1871–1935, FRCSI 1900, PRCSI 1932–34) credited the Registrar, Alfred Miller, as being 'almost entirely responsible for the idea'. Crawley also made the point that sport played a valuable role in fostering an RCSI identity (which was more difficult to create in a non-residential college).

In December, a memorial to the late Prof Scott was unveiled in one of the pavilions (perhaps reflecting Scott's pragmatism, the memorial took the form of a first aid cabinet). A notable student in this period was Bert Healion, another hammer-thrower, who broke the world record at Bird Avenue in 1939 – but owing to Ireland's non-membership of the International Amateur Athletic Federation this did not count in official records. (Healion did not complete his medical studies, opting instead for professional wrestling in the US; he won further Irish athletics championships in the 1950s.) Also from this period, Leo Leader (1918–2014, Lic. 1942) was a notable high-jumper.

In rugby between the wars, the prominent RCSI names are: James Daniel Clinch (1901–1981, Lic. 1936), who won thirty caps for Ireland;[43] Paul Finbarr Murray (1905–1981, Lic. 1929), who won nineteen caps; and Morgan Patrick Crowe (1907–1993, Lic. 1931), thirteen caps. The RCSI Boat Club was launched in 1930 (with Thomas Myles as President, naturally), while the Swimming Club held its annual gala at the nearby Iveagh Baths – which was calmer water than Dr Theodore Ashmore Cronhelm (Lic. 1924) experienced in July 1933, when he swam across Dublin Bay, from the Baily to Dún Laoghaire, in 4 hours 20 minutes. RCSI golf, soccer and cricket teams appear in newspaper fixtures from the early 1940s. In 1942, the Table Tennis Club was given permission to play in the Anatomy Room – 'provided that no outsiders other than Medical Students were admitted'.[44]

'THE OTHER SIDE OF LIFE': MUSIC AND DRAMA

Away from sport, the RCSI Literary and Dramatic Society thrived during these years, putting on an annual performance every Christmas; they also cheered up patients in nearby hospitals who were bedbound for the season. Established by Prof Evatt (Anatomy) about 1920, the Society provided 'an opportunity for self-expression in writing, and to cultivate imagination, so that in his engrossment in his work and his examinations [the student] would not forget the other side of life'.[45]

The plays staged were usually light comedies, such as *The Courting of Mary Doyle* by Abbey dramatist Edward McNulty; but there was an awareness of wider trends too. Noting an outbreak of 'suburban neurosis' on the British stage, one Society member wondered if a strain of that affliction would spread to Ireland – and the Abbey in particular – in the form of 'The Neurosis That Does Be On The Bog'. (In a related connection, RCSI Licentiate and politician Richard Francis Hayes was appointed Director of the Abbey Theatre in 1934 and subsequently, in 1940, official Film Censor – putting him simultaneously at the helm of the country's least and most censored public media.) Prof Evatt was also a prime mover in the College Choral Society – the Minutes record his request to use an organ in the

Facing page: The Presidents of RCSI, 1784-1935.

The Presidents of
The Royal College of Surgeons
IN IRELAND.

1784-5 Samuel Croker King	1835 Alexander Read (II)	1885 Sir Charles Alex. Cameron
1786 John Whiteway	1836 Francis White	1886 Sir William Stokes
1787 Robert Bowes	1837 Arthur Jacob	1887 Anthony H. Corley
1788 Philip Woodrooffe	1838 William Henry Porter	1888 Henry Fitzgibbon
1789 William Dease	1839 Maurice Collis	1889 Austin Meldon, D.L.
1790 Ralph Smyth O'Bré	1840 Robert Adams	1890 Henry Gray Croly } First Biennial
1791 Francis M'Evoy	1841 Thomas Rumley	1891 Henry Gray Croly } President
1792 George Stewart	1842 William Tagert	1892 Edward Hamilton (II)
1793 George Renny	1843 James O'Beirne	1893 Edward Hamilton (III)
1794 Solomon Richards	1844 Sir Philip Crampton, Bart (III)	1894 William Thornley Stoker
1795 Gustavus Hume Clement Archer	1845 Richard Carmichael (III)	1895 Sir William Thornley Stoker
1796 Francis L'Estrange	1846 Samuel Wilmot (III)	1896 William Thomson
1797 William Hartigan	1847 James William Cusack (II)	1897 Sir William Thomson
1798 Robert Moore Peile	1848 Robert Harrison	1898 Robert L Swan
1799 George Stewart (II)	1849 Andrew Ellis	1899 Robert L Swan
1800 Sir Henry Jebb	1850 Thomas Edward Beatty	1900 Thomas Myles
1801 Francis Rivers	1851 Leonard Trant	1901 Thomas Myles
1802 Abraham Colles	1852 Edward Hutton	1902 Lambert H Ormsby
1803 Solomon Richards (II)	1853 William Hargrave	1903 Sir Lambert Ormsby
1804 Francis M'Evoy (II)	1854 Charles Benson	1904 Arthur Chance
1805 Robert Hamilton	1855 Sir Philip Crampton, Bart (IV)	1905 Sir Arthur Chance
1806 Gerard Macklin	1856 Robert Carlisle Williams	1906 Henry Rosborough Swanzy
1807 Francis M'Evoy (III)	1857 Hans Irvine	1907 Sir Henry Rosborough Swanzy
1808 Solomon Richards (III)	1858 James William Cusack (III)	1908 John Lentaigne
1809 Richard Dease	1859 Christopher Fleming	1909 John Lentaigne
1810 John Armstrong Garnett	1860 Robert Adams (II)	1910 Robert H. Woods
1811 Philip Crampton	1861 William Jameson	1911 Robert H. Woods
1812 John Creighton	1862 Thomas Lewis Mackesy	1912 R. Dancer Purefoy
1813 Richard Carmichael	1863 William Colles	1913 R. Dancer Purefoy
1814 Cusack Roney	1864 Arthur Jacob (II)	1914 F. Conway Dwyer
1815 Samuel Wilmot	1865 Samuel G. Wilmot	1915 F. Conway Dwyer
1816 Robert Moore Peile (II)	1866 Richard G. H. Butcher	1916 William Taylor
1817 Andrew Johnston	1867 Robert Adams (III)	1917 William Taylor
1818 Solomon Richards (IV)	1868 George Hornidge Porter	1918 John B. Story
1819 Thomas Hewson	1869 Rawdon McNamara	1919 John B. Story
1820 Philip Crampton (II)	1870 Albert Jasper Walsh	1920 Edward H. Taylor
1821 Charles Hawkes Todd	1871 James Henry Wharton	1921 Edward H. Taylor
1822 James Henthorn	1872 Frederick Kirkpatrick	1922 Sir W. I. de C. Wheeler
1823 John Kirby	1873 John Denham	1923 Sir W. I. de C. Wheeler
1824 John Creighton (II)	1874 Jolliffe Tufnell	1924 R. Charles B. Maunsell
1825 Alexander Read	1875 Edward Hamilton	1925 R. Charles B. Maunsell
1826 Richard Carmichael (II)	1876 George Hugh Kidd	1926 Andrew Fullerton, c.b. c.m.g.
1827 James William Cusack	1877 Robert McDonnell	1928 Thomas E. Gordon
1828 Cusack Roney (II)	1878 Philip Crampton Smyly	1929 Andrew Fullerton, c.b. c.m.g.
1829 William Auchinleck	1879 Edward Dillon Mapother	1930 Richard Atkinson Stoney.
1830 Abraham Colles (II)	1880 Alfred Henry McClintock	1931 Richard Atkinson Stoney.
1831 Rawdon McNamara	1881 Samuel Chaplin	1932 Frank Crawley
1832 Samuel Wilmot (II)	1882 John Kellock Barton	1933 Frank Crawley
1833 James Kerin	1883 William I. Wheeler	1934 Seton Pringle
1834 John Kirby (II)	1884 Edward Hallaran Bennett	1935 Seton Pringle

College, which was granted ('but not before 5 o'clock in the afternoon'[46]). The Hibernian Catch Club – a musical society founded in 1680 – celebrated its 250th anniversary with a concert in RCSI. For many years its president was the late PRCSI Robert Dancer Purefoy (1847–1919, FRCSI 1879, PRCSI 1912–14). He was probably the last Dublin surgeon to wear a top hat in the operating theatre.[47]

By the time RCSI marked its 150th year – 1934 – its finances had finally turned a corner, as ever based on student fees. That year saw forty-eight students earn the Conjoint Licence, the highest number since 1926 and twice the number of four years earlier; five candidates passed the Fellowship exam; eleven earned their Dental Licence; no one sat for the Diploma in Public Health, while six obtained a Conjoint Diploma in Psychological Medicine, the highest number since its inauguration in 1927.

Back in the black, RCSI was able to spend again, albeit modestly: a typewriter was bought, wiring was upgraded, and some seating in lecture theatres was refurbished. But there was no such investment in the vestigial museum. With every relocation of its rickety cases, it disintegrated further. In 1937, arrangements were made for a near-total transfer to Trinity's School of Zoology as a permanent loan.[48] (Certain anthropological specimens, meanwhile, were retained, a number of which were ceremonially interred or repatriated for burial in the early 1990s.[49]) But as the 1930s drew to a close, the single most pressing issue for the medical schools of Ireland was a shortage of subjects for dissection.[50] In retrospect, this may be seen as bitterly ironic in view of the fact that the world was preparing to go to war again.

RCSI PERSONNEL IN WORLD WAR II AND THE ABSENT ROLL OF HONOUR
Everyone knew the war was coming. As early as 1935, the Irish Army was augmented by a reserve force, the Regiment of Pearse, drawn from third-level institutions; RCSI's company within the Regiment comprised some fifty volunteers. During the summer of 1939, there were demonstrations of Air Raid Precautions (ARP) in the Iveagh Gardens, where William Doolin (1888–1962, FRCSI 1912, PRCSI 1950–52) was one of those who oversaw the 'grim realism'[51] of the occasion.

War broke out on 3 September, and from the start, records of the Irish medical contribution were scattered. Unlike in the previous war, Ireland was now a neutral country, so there was no nationwide effort. Recent research suggests that at least 2,003 Irish doctors and surgeons served on the Allied side, of whom 44 were killed in action or died of their wounds, while 28 more lost their lives in active service from a variety of medical causes. At least 185 of those who served were

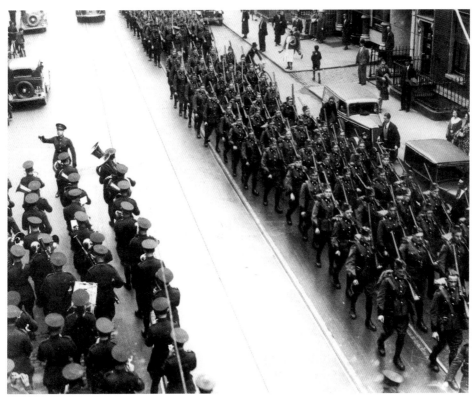

RCSI Regiment of Pearse (*foreground*) marching to Amiens Street Station, July 1939. From *A History of The Pearse Battalion, 1946-1959* (2005) by Louis O'Brien.

Licentiates or Fellows of RCSI.[52] Part of the difficulty in ascertaining numbers is owed to the fact that, unlike Trinity and Queen's, RCSI did not compile a Roll of Honour for the conflict. Neither did the NUI, but this was unsurprising: it was reflecting the ideology of its Chancellor, Eamon de Valera. For RCSI, however, in its financially vulnerable position, the decision not to go against the grain of government policy was perhaps considered the better part of valour.[53] Amends of a sort followed in 1947, when the Ex-Forces Association received permission to erect a memorial plaque to the fallen in the Anatomy Room – such as, to name but one, Henry Hurst (1895–1941, Lic. 1917), Surgeon Commander on HMS *Hood*, sunk in the Battle of the Denmark Strait.

Amongst those who saw service and lived to tell the tale were three future RCSI Presidents. Ian James Fraser (1901–1999, FRCSI 1926, PRCSI 1954–56) served in West Africa and with Montgomery's Eighth Army in

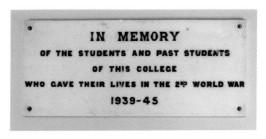

IN MEMORY
OF THE STUDENTS AND PAST STUDENTS
OF THIS COLLEGE
WHO GAVE THEIR LIVES IN THE 2ᴺᴰ WORLD WAR
1939-45

In lieu of a Roll of Honour.

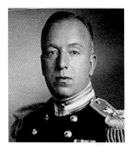

Henry Hurst of HMS *Hood*. Courtesy of HMS Hood.org.

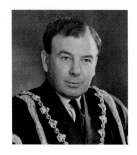

Sir Ian James Fraser, PRCSI 1954-56.

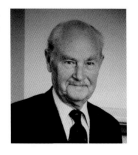

Nigel Kinnear, PRCSI 1961-63.

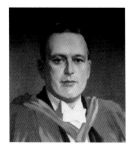

From Fort Wayne, Indiana, Douglas Wellington Montgomery, PRCSI 1968-70. Artist unknown.

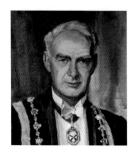

Self-portrait by Thomas George Wilson, PRCSI 1958-61.

North Africa, and he took part in the Allied advance north through Sicily and Italy, being present for the Battle of Salerno; soon after D-Day, he landed on the beach at Arromanches in northern France. He directed the RAMC team that pioneered the use of penicillin 'in the field'. Awarded the DSO and OBE, as President of the BMA (1962–63), he was also knighted. Nigel Kinnear (1907–2000, FRCSI 1934, PRCSI 1961–63) was one of the first medics to enter Bergen-Belsen concentration camp; his memory of the horrors he witnessed there 'stayed with him all his life'.[54] He spoke on the subject at the 'Bi' in November 1945, insisting that his comments were neither pro-British nor anti-German, but, simply, 'against war'.[55]

Lastly, there was American-born Douglas Wellington Montgomery (1913–1974, FRCSI 1943, PRCSI 1968–70), the first Allied surgeon to land at Normandy on D-Day, where the first patient he treated on the beach was an injured German. Montgomery damaged his back wading ashore – under his 36kg pack – and so his military career was cut short. For his work with the St John Ambulance he was made a Knight of the Order of St John.

A fourth PRCSI played his part, too, though not in uniform – nor, indeed, within the law. This was Thomas George ('T.G.') Wilson (1901–1969, FRCSI 1927, PRCSI 1958–61), who breached Irish neutrality by aiding some stranded British servicemen to escape north to Belfast. He was arrested, charged, found guilty and sentenced to twelve months' imprisonment (later suspended). He was defended by John A. Costello, the future Taoiseach. Wilson's portrait as PRCSI is, uniquely, a self-portrait.[56]

A fifth PRCSI, Thomas Ottiwell Graham (1883–1966, FRCSI 1912, PRCSI 1942–44), deserves mention for volunteering for service. He was initially accepted, but upon closer inspection of his record the War Office told him he was six months too old to enlist (or, more accurately, re-enlist: he had won the Military Cross for gallantry during the First World War). Instead, he became a driving force behind the St John Ambulance Brigade, gave lectures on first aid, and conducted 'manoeuvres' on his forty-acre estate on the Stillorgan Road (his house, Whiteoaks, is now University Lodge, the UCD President's official residence). In 1961, Graham gifted to RCSI a stained-glass window of the Colles family coat of arms by Catherine O'Brien; it is located in the Colles Room – that is, the President's Office – where it completes a diptych with the College coat of arms, also by O'Brien, gifted by the Association of Graduates in 1960.[57]

From the teaching staff, Robert F.J. ('Jack') Henry (1901–1970, FRCSI 1927, Prof of Surgery 1938–52) enlisted and found himself present for the mass evacuation from Dunkirk in 1940. Post-war, he returned to Baggot Street Hospital, where he was renowned for his clinical teaching, one student recalling:

> Teaching rounds with Jack Henry were excellent and stood me in good stead when doing my internship at a Hopkins-associated teaching hospital in Baltimore – I may not have been the most academic of interns but outshone the American interns when it came to examining a belly or a hip. In final year he took us on a 'lumps and bumps' round at Steevens. He had enormous time for students.[58]

During the 1950s, the reorganisation of clinical teaching in Dublin aligned Baggot Street with Trinity, at which point Henry left RCSI for that institution. His successor in the Chair was John Seton Pringle (1909–1975, FRCSI 1935, Prof of Surgery 1952–61),[59] who spent much of the war as a medical officer on the *Queen Mary*, ferrying troops across the Atlantic. He was also in Normandy for D-Day +1 and at Arnhem for the operation that inspired the film *A Bridge Too Far* (1977).

Finally, amongst the countless civilian deaths during the war, there is the random tragedy that occurred in Salford in December 1940. A parachute mine (aka a 'factory flattener') was released over the tank- and airplane-producing Trafford Park Industrial Estate – but the wind took it and it hit a house, killing the family who lived there: they were Edward

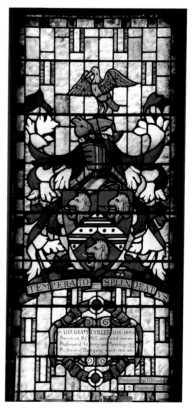

Colles family coat of arms by Catherine O'Brien, 1961.

D'Arcy McCrea (FRCSI 1922), a urologist and tennis Olympian, and his wife Edith Willcock McCrea (FRCSI 1925), a pioneering female paediatric surgeon – and their two children, Patrick (12) and Gillian (9). In fact, the McCreas were hosting a party that night, and their guests all perished too.

THE WAR'S REVERBERATIONS AT RCSI

The Charter Day Dinner – as ever, a mood-barometer – was suspended in 1940, and in October the Council Minutes record:

> The Registrar reported on the Air Raid Shelters constructed in the College basement, air raid precautions taken in the College and Schools, and that a request for the use of lecture rooms for A.R.P. lectures had been received.[60]

This basement shelter was not just for RCSI, but for public use; in the immediate vicinity there was another in Mercer Street, as well as overground shelters in Kevin Street and trench shelters in St Patrick's Park.

When President de Valera inspected RCSI's shelter in September, he was likely shown around by the new Registrar, William Norman Rae (1886–1964). From 1938, when he took over from Alfred Miller, until his retirement in 1962, Rae combined his Registrar duties with his Professorship of Chemistry and Physics (1934–61). Before coming to RCSI, Rae had been a government analyst in Sri Lanka (then Ceylon) at the outbreak of the Great War, whereupon he brought his chemical expertise to the Royal Gunpowder Mills at Waltham Abbey in Essex.

After the war, Rae returned to the east, serving in the Ceylon Light Infantry, and beginning an academic career at Colombo. With Joseph Reilly and Thomas Sherlock Wheeler (later chemistry dons at UCC and UCD, respectively), both of whom he met during the war, Rae authored *Physico-Chemical Methods* (1926; 5th ed. 1954), for many years the standard work on practical physical chemistry.[61] Away from RCSI, Rae cultivated asparagus and bred Jersey cattle at his home in Enniskerry, Co. Wicklow. A student prize is awarded annually in his name.

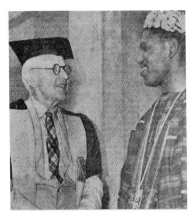

Norman Rae, Registrar, greets Chief Akitoye Coker, Commissioner for Western Nigeria, 1960.

Teaching at RCSI was generally unaffected throughout the war (or 'the Emergency', as the period was locally known). Nevertheless, there were some innovations, such as the introduction of new Conjoint Diplomas in Child Health (1940), Ophthalmic Medicine and Surgery (1941) and Anaesthetics (1942; amongst the first to qualify was Sheila Kenny (DA 1942, FFARCSI (Foundation Fellow of the Faculty of Anaesthetists) 1960.[62] Succeeding Doolin, the PRCSI in the first years of the war was Henry Stokes (1879–1967, FRCSI 1907, PRCSI 1940–41), a descendant of Whitley and William Stokes. He had a particular interest in blood transfusion and in 1946 RCSI was mooted to administer a national blood transfusion service (in the event, 'the structural impossibility of housing the laboratories required' put paid to this idea[63]).

Unlike many of his surgical contemporaries, Stokes was not wealthy: he was 'too kind' to charge the poor and 'too grand' to charge his friends.[64] He was also exceedingly modest, addressing the Biological Society one year on the subject of 'Some mistakes of Henry Stokes'. This was so successful that he returned the next year with 'More mistakes of Henry Stokes'.[65] By way of more typical contrast, the post-war PRCSI William Pearson (1882–1976, FRCSI 1910, PRCSI 1950–52) once declared: 'The only time I was wrong was the time I thought I was wrong, but events proved me to be right.'[66]

The war had a greater impact on extracurricular activities: in February 1942, Group Captain PC Livingston delivered that year's Montgomery Lecture on 'Studies in Night Vision and Night Vision Judgement as it Concerns the Ophthalmology of Flying'.[67] The Literary and Dramatic Society staged a new play, *Until We Die* (1940), in aid of the Red Cross. Set 'Somewhere in Europe today', it tells the story of a hostile airman who is shot down but treated with kindness by the locals who find him. The author was RCSI student John St Patrick Cowell (1912–2008, Lic. 1942), who went on to enjoy a distinguished double career as a medic (a lifelong anti-TB campaigner, he was appointed Director of the National BCG Committee in 1950) and as an author (his novel *The Begrudgers* (1978), about a returning emigrant doctor, was an Irish bestseller for several months).

In December 1944, RCSI donated 100 guineas to the Royal College of Surgeons in London 'for restoration and development',[68] the sister College having suffered extensive damage during the Blitz. Intriguingly, on 8 March 1945, RCSI's Compassionate Guild was given permission to show 'war films', the exact nature of which is unclear – censorship was in place until May, at which point newsreels of the horrors of the concentration camps were allowed to be shown in cinemas – but certainly they were not jingoistic tales of derring-do.

'A RIVER OF POVERTY' AND THE SCOURGE OF TUBERCULOSIS

Set up in late 1943, the Compassionate Guild was a student-led charitable initiative, whose primary concern was local poverty and its concomitant nutritional deficiencies. The guild had about fifty active members, who bicycled about the city visiting the needy. A typical visit was reported in the *Irish Times* in December, when a student paid a call on 'a family of six, living in a room twelve feet by fifteen'.[69] (In 1942, it was estimated that some 20,000 Dublin families lived in single rooms.[70]) Yet again, the College authorities followed the students' lead; within a year, former PRCSI Adams McConnell could be heard broadcasting an appeal on Radio Éireann on behalf of the Guild. 'Many people,' he said, 'were still perishing in "a river of poverty" in this country'.[71]

Inextricably related to poverty, the scourge of the nation at this time was tuberculosis (TB). TB rates rise on a long, slow curve – it takes perhaps fifty years for an epidemic to peak, as it had done in Ireland circa 1904; thereafter it began to fall decade by decade, but not fast enough, and in the 1940s Irish mortality remained higher than elsewhere in Europe. South of the border, mortality was in fact higher in 1947 than it had been at the outbreak of the war.[72]

For campaigning figures such as James Deeny (1906–1994) – whose papers are held in RCSI's Heritage Collections – the fight against TB was inextricably linked to social reform, and as such there was much resistance from both church and state. Indeed, when the Beveridge Report (1942) was published in Britain, paving the way for the NHS, Irish authorities were so alarmed by the costs involved that they swiftly set about lowering expectations that such a reform could ever be sponsored at home.[73]

Instead, intervention devolved to individuals and institutions. At RCSI, it was proposed that a Students' Health Service be started specifically to examine for TB. The intention was to send undergraduates to Sir Patrick Dun's Hospital for X-rays; prior to this, early diagnosis was an onerous affair, reliant on the detection of symptoms that Sir John Moore (1845–1947, Prof of Medicine 1889–1916) had listed in the previous century (a red line along the gums, myotatic irritability of the pectoral muscles, apical tenderness, 'cogwheel' inspiration[74]).

In the event, the X-ray plan was suspended until 'after the war' – which, given that this was 1942, was a somewhat arbitrary projection. In the era, few among the staff and student body of RCSI would have been untouched by the disease somehow. In 1942 alone, 4,347 TB deaths were recorded in Ireland. To take a single case, one student who began his studies in 1943 attributed his attraction to medicine to two origins: his own childhood experience of jaundice, and the death of his sister, from TB, aged 19: 'We had doctors and nurses in the house, she had a lot of treatment at home, [but] at that stage there was very little cure for tuberculosis'.[75] The student was W.A.L. ('Bill') MacGowan (Lic. 1948, FRCSI 1952) – future Professor of Surgery (1967–80) and Registrar (1980–90).

One of the most prominent anti-TB activists was Margaret (Pearl) Dunlevy (1909–2002, Lic. 1932). After graduation, she worked in Britain for a period, returning to Ireland as Assistant County Medical Officer in her native Donegal; in 1938, she relocated to Dublin as Assistant Medical Officer of Health, where she was instrumental in establishing Dublin

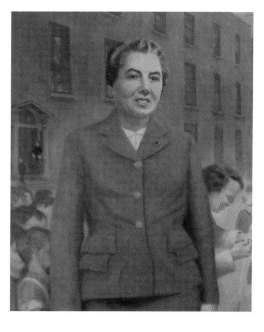

Margaret (Pearl) Dunlevy by Benita Stoney, 2019.

Corporation's primary TB clinic. Traditionally, the Irish medical establishment had followed the UK for TB treatment, but Dunlevy was one of those who looked to Scandinavia, as a result of which Dublin became the first city in these islands to institute a widespread BCG vaccination programme. According to Deeny,

> Dunlevy built up from nothing the highly efficient, beautifully organised Dublin scheme, which ran like clockwork, was availed of widely, produced no unfavourable incidents, reduced childhood tuberculosis to vanishing point, and lowered dramatically the awful incidence of tuberculosis meningitis in babies in Dublin. All this was carried out during the very difficult post-war conditions in the city.[76]

Indeed, post-war conditions were such that, as Dunlevy herself observed, medical staff were paid less for the testing of patients than vets were for the testing of cattle.[77]

It is not clear that the promised post-war radiography of RCSI students ever came to pass. In any case, by the end of the decade, the advent of drug therapies was already effectively consigning epidemic tuberculosis to history. By 1953, Dunlevy and the Dean of the Medical School, Prof Matthew Harris O'Connor (1895–1963, Prof of Pathology 1943–63), were administering BCG vaccinations to the annual intake of students.[78]

Once TB was largely vanquished, Dunlevy shifted her attention to other infectious diseases, publishing widely on childhood epidemiology, vaccination and public health. Amongst her many honours and honorifics, she was the first female President of the Biological Society (1951–52). In 2019, a portrait of Dunlevy was commissioned as part of RCSI's Women on Walls project. The artist, Benita Stoney, depicts Dunlevy – dressed in the tweed of her native Donegal – at work in the midst of those urban children whose lives she transformed.

RCSI'S FIRST - AND LAST - DENTAL PRESIDENT, EDWARD LEO SHERIDAN (1881-1949, LIC. DENT. 1902, FRCSI 1908, PRCSI 1944-46)

Between the wars, dentistry struggled for recognition at RCSI. Following Henry Gregg Sherlock's (1850–1924) tenure as Professor of Dental Surgery (1910–24), no replacement was appointed (for forty years the Dental School was staffed by Lecturers, until a general overhaul in 1965). But the mid-century status of the profession was raised considerably with the election of Edward Leo Sheridan to the office of President of RCSI.

A Council-member since 1922, Sheridan had previously been elected President of the Irish Dental Association in 1926. Moreover – and controversially – he was appointed as Chairman of the Dental Board of the United Kingdom in 1940. This provoked objections in the House of Commons, where he was denounced as 'a Sinn Fein Irish Catholic living in Dublin', but Sheridan's charm and ability ensured his success in the role.[79] At a meeting of the Irish Dental Association in 1945 – held in RCSI – one commentator noted that, whereas dentists were formerly 'regarded by many as a mere technician, with, perhaps a sadistic bent',[80] this attitude had changed a good deal lately, thanks to Sheridan.

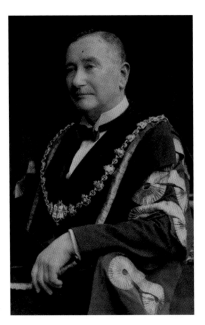

Edward Leo Sheridan, PRCSI 1944-46.

At this time, there were four dental schools in the Free State – RCSI, UCD, TCD and UCC – while all practical training was done in Dublin and at the Cork Dental School (the latter had been founded by Israel Scher (1887–1954, Lic. Dent. 1909)). Like their medical confrères, Irish dentists were educated for export – in the mid-1950s it was calculated that some 85 per cent would emigrate.[81] Generally speaking, the Irish populace's need for dental treatment was considered 'extremely high', but the demand for it was 'extremely low'.[82] To redress the former, the fluoridation of public drinking water commenced in 1964.

Since 1987, a biennial Leo Sheridan Medal (with an accompanying Lecture) has been awarded by the Faculty of Dentistry (established 1963).

'A MEDICAL UNITED NATIONS': THE INTERNATIONALISATION OF RCSI

Political independence notwithstanding, Irish medical education remained inextricably linked to developments in Britain, the latest of which was the publication of the Goodenough Report (1944). This document recommended a 'drastic overhaul' of undergraduate teaching in order to serve the embryonic NHS. Amongst its many desiderata – greater emphases on social medicine, paediatrics and psychiatry; an increase in the admission of women; the appointment of full-time teachers – the most important was the stipulation that, after passing his or her qualifying exam and before being admitted to the Medical Register, students should be required to complete a twelve-month internship in a hospital, so that they would be 'properly equipped for practice as family doctors'.[83]

When this compulsory postgraduate year was formalised by the British Medical Act (1950), Irish legislation swiftly followed (1951) to keep the local profession in step – but owing to the complicated Irish hospital scene, two years would elapse before the act came into force, a period characterised by the President of the Irish Medical Council, Richard Atkinson Stoney (1877–1966, FRCSI 1906, PRCSI 1930–32) as one of 'splitting headaches'.[84] For incoming students, it meant that the period from enrolment to independent practice was now seven years.

The prospect of such a long road did not diminish the number of applicants. In fact, 1946 saw twice the usual number of applicants for the 100 places – a recent restriction – that RCSI could offer. Many of these hopefuls were from outside Ireland: Britain, the USA and Canada, but also, as local newspapers reported with wonder, 'South and West Africa, New Zealand, British Guiana, China, Burma, and one girl has applied from Nepal, India, home of the famous Gurkha!'[85] There were German and Polish applicants too. Other Irish medical schools experienced similar rises in applications, but RCSI's non-denominational ethos would have held a particular attraction.

RCSI had been welcoming students from far and wide for more than a hundred years at this point, but these were largely scions of the colonial class.[86] Before and after the First World War, RCSI could boast of a number of notable trailblazers, such as the Bengal-born Hassan Suhrawardy (1884–1946, FRCSI 1914; he was knighted in 1932 but renounced his British honours shortly before his death) and, from Nigeria, Elizabeth Abimbola Awoliyi (née Akerele, 1910–1971, Lic. 1936), who was not only the first West African woman to gain the RCSI Licence, but the first woman in Nigeria to practise as a (Western-trained) physician.

Facing page:
'The Medical
Student as he
appears...', by
G.K. Maharaj
in *Mistura*
(Summer 1955).

But it was after 1945 that RCSI developed its reputation for internationalism. While Dublin's foreign students attended all of the city's third-level schools – and came together annually for a 'Carnival of Nations' showcase of traditional songs, dances and costumes – RCSI's comparatively small student population meant that, in the popular consciousness, 123 St Stephen's Green was particularly associated with foreign students. Indeed, by 1954, with some thirty-six nations represented, RCSI was looked on locally as 'a medical U.N.O.'.[87]

From the start, this international reputation was fostered internally by both staff and students. The lecturer who assisted students with accommodation, Gilbert Marshall Irvine (Prof of Anatomy 1959–69), cheerily told the *Irish Times* that he had never heard of 'any displays of racial prejudice against visiting students in any restaurant or public place'. Moreover, at the first sign of any discrimination 'the student body as a whole would be up in arms'.[88] Proving that point, in 1953, RCSI students withdrew noisily from the Irish Medical Students' Association when foreigners were debarred from the presidency of the organisation.

The accompanying letter of protest ran: 'It is a well-known fact that there is a large influx of non-Eire students at our medical college... and the discrimination so flagrant as this is inimical to our non-Gaelic speaking guests while on academic sojourn here.' This was not just prejudice, they said, it was blatant hypocrisy: 'Our medical and other graduates continually knock at the doorsteps of the countries whence these non-Eire students come...'[89] (In general, however, the IMSA was a force for good, bringing together medical students who might otherwise have had little contact with one another until their intern year.)

RCSI's internationalism also had a certain extracurricular, consciousness-raising influence: RCSI students were regularly numbered in protests against colonial interference in Egypt ('56) and Algeria ('58), and against apartheid in South Africa ('60); in 1962, they took part in the Aldermaston marches, in opposition to nuclear weapons. By that date, of RCSI's student population of some 700, approximately 90 per cent came from outside Ireland.[90]

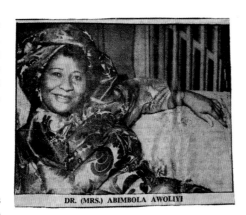

Nigerian
trailblazer,
Elizabeth
Abimbola
Awoliyi, née
Akerele.

Akelere's
signature in
the Roll of
Licentiates
(1936).

DR. (MRS.) ABIMBOLA AWOLIYI

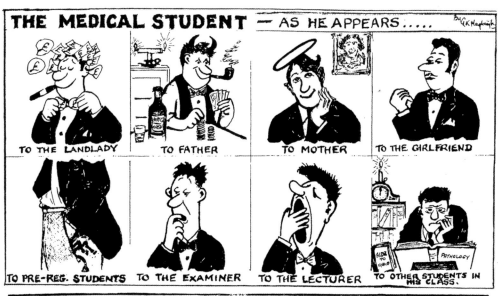

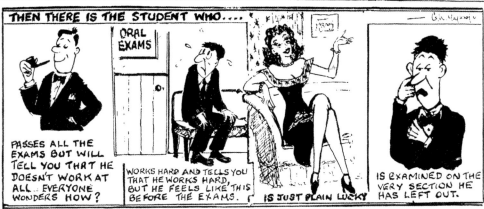

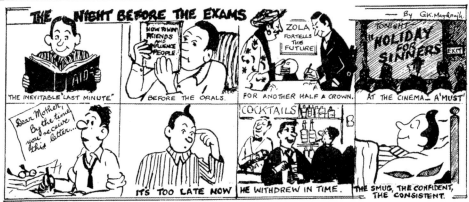

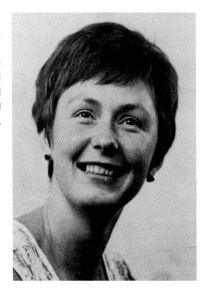

Moira O'Brien, Prize-winning student, influential teacher and researcher, and Distinguished Graduate.

If Dublin in the 1950s was a relatively inexpensive place to live, medical education itself was by no means cheap – and the cost was rising all the time: in 1947, RCSI fees per term rose from £16 to £20. 'An extreme state of hard uppishness' was how Stacey Biswas Day (Lic. 1955) described his life as an undergraduate.[91] Some students were supported in part or whole by ex-service grants, such as Kitchener Scholarships or similar equivalents.

From 1936, the Francis Nolans Prize provided free tuition to the sons (an amendment remembered to add *daughters* too) of Irish medical graduates (another amendment remembered *dental* colleagues).[92] The student who entered via this route in 1950 was Moira McMahon, aged 16 (coming first in her Preliminary Examination 'by a large margin'[93]). Winning multiple medals, she progressed to the post of Demonstrator in Anatomy and Physiology while still a student. Subsequently, as Moira O'Brien (Lic. 1956), she was a Lecturer and Reader in the School of Anatomy (1959–84), during which time she also ran a clinic for students. Her profound influence in the fields of sports medicine – in 2003 she was a Founding Fellow of the RCSI/RCPI Faculty of Sports Medicine – and osteoporosis research are widely acknowledged.

Since 2018, an annual RCSI Sports Scholarship has been awarded in O'Brien's name, and in 2020 she received the Distinguished Graduate Award.

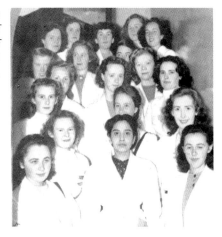

From *Surgeon's Log: Annals of the Schools of Surgery, RCSI* (1949).

In conversation with the present author, O'Brien vividly recalled her first day at RCSI, how she entered by the side door on York Street, how proper dress was *de rigueur* (skirts for the women, ties for men, policed by the Superintendent of the Schools, T.K. Digby), and how there were twenty female students in her year, all of whom sat together in the front row of the lecture theatre. The male students – including Polish ex-RAF officers perhaps twice her age – sat terraced behind.

TROUBLE WITH THE AMERICAN MEDICAL ASSOCIATION

At the end of their studies, four-fifths of the class, native and foreigner alike, would leave Ireland for work. (In fact, the great number of RCSI Licentiates working in Britain gave rise in 1953 to a London branch of the Association of Graduates.) Of the two named above, O'Brien went to Manchester and Day went to the United States. Ever since the war, the US was a popular destination for newly qualified medics worldwide, but in 1950 the American Medical Association (AMA) suddenly and unceremoniously stoppered this pressure valve for Irish doctors.[94]

They produced a list of approved overseas medical schools which were deemed comparable with their own – and none of the schools of the Irish Republic made the grade (Queen's in Belfast did). Amongst Irish medical educators, this provoked consternation; for the fledgling Republic, it was a source of embarrassment. As it happens, the AMA delegates who visited Ireland had not even bothered to inspect RCSI, blithely assuming it was an examining body only, like RCPI.[95] A flurry of medico-political lobbying ensued, from the Irish diplomatic mission to William Doolin's friendly drop-in chat with the US Ambassador in Dublin.[96]

Another AMA inspection was scheduled for September 1953. This time, RCSI was to be considered for inspection, only to be told that, owing to 'the shortness of the time available', inspectors would not make it as far as St Stephen's Green; following RCSI complaints ('because of the publicity given to the matter, it was feared that non-visitation of this school would be misinterpreted in a manner injurious to the reputation and honour of the school'[97]), additional time was found in the inspectors' timetable. But once more, after the visit, none of the southern schools made the AMA list.

Where there had been embarrassment and consternation before, there was now deep annoyance: one headline ran, 'America Keeps Ban on Doctors – Angers Eire';[98] another blustered, 'So our medical schools don't please America!'[99] All the schools were chagrined, but RCSI chose to issue a point-by-point rebuttal of the AMA findings: 'The first criticism of the visitors... [was the] inordinate proportion of the yearly budget which was provided by the students' fees – 98%.' This, they said, 'was not the fault of the College... and it is one that they would very much like to see amended'.[100] (Elsewhere, figures confirm that, of the £322,274 provided by the State to third-level institutions in 1949, RCSI received £1,500, while the lion's share, almost half, went to the much larger NUI; in 1950, RCSI's 'grant-in-aid' was raised by a handsome £3,000, but this was still nugatory compared to, say, UCD's £104,000 increase; in 1953, when UCD received £233,224 and Trinity pocketed £100,250, RCSI's grant-in-aid remained at £4,500.[101] In fairness, few would argue that *any* of the universities and colleges were adequately funded for their numbers.)

The next AMA criticism – a lack of equipment – was denied ('not true of the essential equipment'), but with a caveat ('might be so of the less important'). In any case, this was a dearth RCSI would be 'glad to remedy if more funds were at its disposal'. Likewise, the AMA critique that RCSI merely followed the curriculum of the other Dublin schools was easily dismissed: RCSI's curriculum was 'recommended by the Medical Registration Council and was in all essentials the same as that recommended by the General Medical Council'. Putting the boot in, the anonymous RCSI spokesperson said that if the required American model 'means spending time on endless note-taking and the performance *ad nauseam* of unnecessary tests and examinations, the College authorities prefer the Irish to the American way'.[102]

In some respects, this was all a repetition of the pre-war Rockefeller episode: the impecunious Irish State was not in a position to implement the Flexner-inflected model the AMA desired; or, as the *Journal of the Irish Medical Association* nimbly put it, 'Customs, social standards, and milieu vary from country to country. It would be absurd to consider that a uniform standard of education could be laid down for an entire world.'[103] The AMA recognised the essential truth of this as the decade wore on; realising that it was a tall order to inspect the 566 or so medical schools around the globe, and recognising that individual US states were continuing to grant licences to individuals, the troublesome list was abandoned.

Instead, the intern and residency system became the primary route for medical emigrants to the US, and from the late 1950s AMA accreditation was issued on an individual rather than an institutional basis, via the ECFMG exam.[104] This did not, however, mean that 'the Irish way' had scored any great victory. As the dust settled, Prof Leonard Abrahamson told the Biological Society that, while it was 'clear and incontrovertible' that Irish medical graduates could hold their own ('and, in many cases, more than hold their own') on any hospital corridor, there was also room for improvement – in particular, he said, 'the setting up of a post-graduate school should merit very close consideration in the near future'.[105] A similar note was sounded by the General Medical Council, whose accreditation of Irish schools never lapsed through the AMA fiasco – a fact that Irish defenders pointed to – but whose 1954 inspection report doubled down on the 'unstructured relationship'[106] between the schools and the hospitals.

Separately, however, as a body for higher, surgical accreditation, RCSI was in excellent standing: from 1951, reciprocity had been achieved in the Primary Fellowship examinations amongst all of the Royal Colleges, and seven years later, in 1958, RCSI became a founder member of the Stockholm-based International Federation of Surgical Colleges.

my teacher, and thrust my head fully under the water tap, allowing the water to flow over me for several minutes, after which very much like a wet terrier that has scrambled from a stream, I shook the water from my head, and left the examining ward.[111]

A pillar of the Irish Jewish community, Abrahamson was a founding member of the Jewish Representative Council and chairman of the Jewish Refugee Aid Committee (both established in 1938), and in recognition of his work a forest in Israel was named in his honour in 1951. Likewise, the Abrahamson Memorial Lecture at RCSI was endowed by the Dublin Jewish Community. As PRCPI (1949–51), he was a leading light in the IMA.[112] He died in 1961 of a coronary thrombosis – one of his specialties.

POSTGRADUATE AMBITIONS: THE FACULTIES OF ANAESTHETISTS (1959) AND RADIOLOGY (1961)

Abrahamson's post-AMA wish for a postgraduate strand in Irish medicine was an aspiration shared by many. In the late 1940s, William Doolin had devoted a great deal of time and energy to this dream, only for it to fail for lack of student interest: only two signed up. (Unusually – and perhaps tellingly – the Council commiserated, recording that 'this poor support was regrettable after all the trouble taken by Mr Doolin in its organisation'.[113]) But if the students were not there, neither were the funds to furnish facilities (when the Boxwell Memorial laboratory had opened in 1946, it was paid for in part by subscriptions from his past pupils and friends).

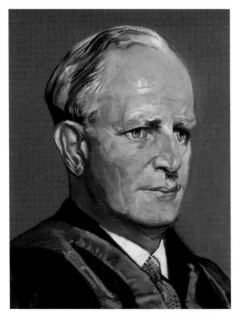

Thomas James Gilmartin, first Dean of the Faculty of Anaesthetists, by Seán Keating.

Added to that, any postgraduate courses would require, ominously, the 'co-operation of the hospitals'.[114] Doolin was probably ahead of his time; a decade later, there were distinct signs of budding postgraduate life in Dublin as a whole and at RCSI in particular: a Faculty of Anaesthetists was founded in 1959, with Thomas James Gilmartin (1905–1986, Lic. 1929) as first Dean. Gilmartin traced the rise of his discipline back to 1942, when the Conjoint Diploma in

Anaesthetics had been introduced ('the first explicit recognition by any academic body in this country of the anaesthetists' implicit status in the hierarchical structure of the specialities of medicine'[115]).

Before the advent of the Faculty, anaesthetists laboured under a host of deficiencies compared with their surgical colleagues: training was ill-defined, qualifications indifferently recognised, they had no corporate voice, no university professorships, little clout on hospital boards and were obliged to confine their work to mornings to suit the surgeons; in addition, they were paid by the operating surgeon, rather than the patient.[116] As well as addressing these issues, the Faculty introduced examinations, and then courses for such examinations.

The continuation of the RCSI/RCPI Diploma, however, sat ill with the Faculty – amongst other chafings related to finance and oversight. In 1965, Gilmartin was appointed Associate Professor of Anaesthesia at RCSI, the first such professorship in Ireland (which, admittedly, did not come with a Department or any facilities for teaching or research[117]). Credited with introducing both thiopentone (1934) and curare (1945) to the country, Gilmartin was made an Honorary Fellow of RCSI in 1974. From 1985, the Faculty of Anaesthetists – latterly, since 1998, an independent College of Anaesthesiologists – has hosted an annual Gilmartin Lecture.[118]

A Faculty of Radiologists followed soon after in 1961, spearheaded by its first Dean, Desmond J. Riordan (1909–1968, Lic. 1933, FRCSI 1935). Born out of the Radiological Society of Ireland (1932), the Faculty's stated aims were: 'to advance the science, art and practice of radiology and of allied sciences'; and 'to promote education, study and research in radiology'.[119] Although the focus was on postgraduate training, the Faculty's first lectures were in fact to undergraduates. Exams for Primary Fellowship – in radiation physics, pathology, surgery, radiological anatomy and medicine, and Final Fellowships in Diagnostic Radiology and Radiotherapy – had to wait until May 1966.[120]

Increasingly, then, RCSI's future seemed to lie in postgraduate education. When PRCSI Nigel Kinnear took office in 1961, he spoke of the desirability of 'an institute of post-graduate medical studies' with 'his college anxious to unite with the other medical colleges in forming such an institution'.[121] Others had similar ideas: as far back as 1950, the government had toyed with the idea of confining undergraduate teaching to the two universities, with RCSI becoming a uniquely postgraduate school.[122] Funds and facilities for higher research remained a want, but the period in question (1958–62) saw RCSI receiving its first corporate donations, from the likes of Ethicon, Johnson & Johnson, Pfizer, Ciba and Glaxo Laboratories, in some cases for specific research fellowships.[123]

The first annual Robert Adams Postgraduate Lecture was given in March 1962. A year later, the first issue of the *Journal of the Royal College of Surgeons in Ireland* appeared, edited by T.G. Wilson. 'At present the trend in the College is directed mainly towards the development of postgraduate education,' Wilson wrote in his first editorial: 'With this end in view, the College has purchased the six adjoining houses in York Street which will provide much-needed space for laboratories, lecture theatres, Faculty offices, and other facilities.' Demolition, he added, was already begun, while building, he hoped, would not be too long delayed.

RCSI had long had its eye on these properties, certainly as far back as 1944 ('Mr Stokes emphasized his opinion that the York Street houses would be a desirable acquisition'[124]), if not before. Council-member Thomas Adrian Bouchier-Hayes (1907–1960, FRCSI 1934) reiterated the point in the 1950s, lamenting the lack of funds to do anything about it. At this time, the intention was to provide student accommodation on the site: 'since this would remove the only criticism of any weight that can be made about the schools'.[125] (Property on Leeson Park was also considered for the same purpose, an altogether grander prospect than York Street's tenements, but this came to nothing.) Soon enough, however, funds were found, and the house nearest the College, no. 33 York Street, was acquired in 1953.

TOM GARRY'S GRIND AT 33 YORK STREET

For the best part of fifty years, no. 33 York Street was perhaps the single most important address in the unofficial history of Irish medical education. This was where Tom Garry (1884–1963) held his famous anatomy 'grind', attended by students of all of the medical schools. Garry also lived here, in conditions inversely proportionate to the excellence of his teaching. As one past pupil recalled,

> We sat around an old dissecting table, under which he kept buckets of lungs, kidneys, intestines, brains and other anatomical specimens – all floating disgustingly in formalin. The rest of the furniture of this 'room' consisted of boxes of various bones, and more piles of books.[126]

Grinding was a system of private tutoring that had sprung up in the mid-to-late nineteenth century, when so much medical teaching was off-hand and *ad hoc*. The practice largely died out in the mid-twentieth century with the appointment of clinical tutors (from 1956, all three Dublin medical schools had staff *in situ* in the various teaching hospitals[127]), but Garry's grind continued to thrive for the simple reason that he was better than everyone else. As Peter McLean (1934–2010, Lic. 1958, FRCSI 1962, PRCSI 1998–2000) recalled:

Most students of Anatomy would look back on Tom as one of the great teachers. I think they would find it hard to pinpoint what qualities he possessed that made him such an outstanding teacher. Certainly some would be impressed with his eccentricity. Some would remember him for his ability to make an uninteresting subject like Anatomy interesting. This no doubt was related to his entire devotion to the subject. Everybody would certainly feel that he had the ability of expression and used the graphic qualities he possessed to the full. Although a gentle man he still had

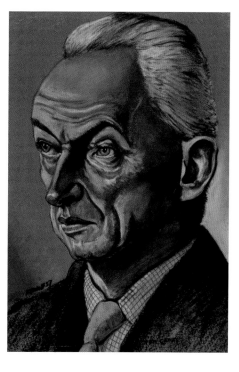

Tom Garry by Harry Kernoff, 1957.

a formidable appearance and instilled a certain amount of reverence in his students. He used the classics liberally and we always felt that he was a particularly well-educated, intelligent person and consequently expected his teaching to be of the highest standard. That he knew so much and still never qualified as a doctor created great curiosity and a certain amount of awe in the students...

Legends sprang up concerning Garry's lack of formal qualifications, usually to the effect that he disagreed with an examiner and refused to back down.[128] In any case, it was not a path he recommended to others ('get through and get out,' he advised).[129] For all his brilliance, Garry was also a difficult, disappointed man. In 1957, a fire in his rooms in No. 33 destroyed much of his life's work – the manuscripts and notebooks he had compiled over decades. Three years later, when Garry – now 76 – applied for the post of Lecturer in Anatomy, the duty to deliver the painful reply fell to Registrar Norman Rae:

The Council has instructed me to thank you for your application... I am to say that they have a great regard for you as an anatomist and appreciate all the work you have done in this connection for the schools. The post of Lecturer is intended for a younger man...[130]

Garry had long enjoyed privileges normally reserved for Council-members, but change was coming. In 1961, to facilitate the development envisioned in Wilson's editorial, Garry received a notice to quit No. 33. He wrote back to say that he would do his best to comply speedily, but to dispose of his vast collection of books, models and specimens 'in an appropriate way within a short space of time is well nigh outside the pale of possibility'.[131] But quit he did: in June 1963, he died in the room where he had lived and taught. A plaque in his memory, and a portrait by Harry Kernoff RHA, both hang in the Department of Anatomy.

INCISIONS AND UPPERCUTS: ARNOLD KIRKPATRICK ('A.K.') HENRY (1886-1962, FRCSI 1914, PROF OF ANATOMY 1947-59)

Garry's grind was an extension of his official RCSI work as Tutor and Prosector in the Anatomy Department, first under the professorship of Evatt, latterly under A.K. Henry. During the First World War, Henry had served as a surgeon in the Serbian, British and French armies; he was made a chevalier of the *Légion d'honneur* in 1918. Subsequently he was Evatt's assistant, leaving in 1925 to take a professorship at the University of Cairo; after a spell in Hammersmith at the newly established Postgraduate Medical School, he returned to his native Dublin and RCSI.

In 1927, he published *Exposure of the Long Bones*, revised first as *Extensile Exposure Applied to Limb Surgery* (1945) and again as the acknowledged classic, *Extensile Exposure* (1957), dedicated to Dr Dorothy Milne, his close collaborator, surgical assistant and, not least, wife. Even to the lay reader, Henry's personality is evident on every page, where his conversational, descriptive style vividly outstrips the more orthodox *Basle Nomina Anatomica*: 'when the thalamus is sick no surgery can cure — except the guillotine'.[132]

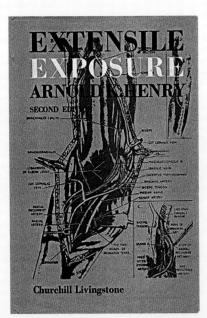

A.K. Henry's classic text.

Henry's concern for student welfare manifested itself in his push for an in-house cafeteria (a service subsequently slowed by post-war rationing[133]); located in the basement, it was named in honour of Henry shortly after this retirement.[134] Henry's other pet project was RCSI's Boxing Club, for which he secured new equipment and doubled the undergrad membership. For training, a ring was erected between the pillars of the Anatomy Room (as well as table tennis, fencing took place here too); the College Hall was used for intervarsity bouts. (Amongst those who represented RCSI in the early 1950s was Ben Briscoe, the future Lord Mayor of Dublin (1988–89); this was all the more impressive as Briscoe was never actually a registered RCSI student, unlike his siblings Joan, Brian and Joe.[135]) In 1956, Henry embraced new technology for teaching, giving the first anatomy lecture in Ireland or Britain to be relayed by television to a neighbouring room: 'the camera is placed above the operation table...'[136]

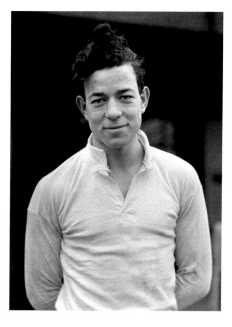

Grand Slam winner Karl Mullen. © PA Images / Alamy Stock Photo.

POST-WAR SPORTS AND A TRAGIC ACCIDENT

Outside Henry's squared circle, the sporting luminaries of the post-war years were: the rugby player Karl Mullen (Lic. 1949), who won twenty-five international caps and also captained Ireland's first Grand Slam win in 1948; and the hockey player, Anita Doherty (Lic. 1951), winner of twenty-nine international caps, as well as member of the 1950 Triple Crown-winning side.[137] The Basketball Club was another success, thanks largely to its North American players; its Canadian Captain, Al Mutchnik (Lic. 1953), established an intervarsity league, the Embassy Cup, sponsored by the US Ambassador.[138] The Rowing Club was launched, albeit after a slow start ('We had an enthusiastic club, but no boats...'[139]).

Before his retirement, Evatt instituted the Inter-University Dramatic Festival, hosted (and won) in its first year (1947) by RCSI.[140] One of RCSI's standout performers was a South African student, Emile Stone. Tragically, in 1952, Stone was one of twenty-three passengers who was killed when their Dakota

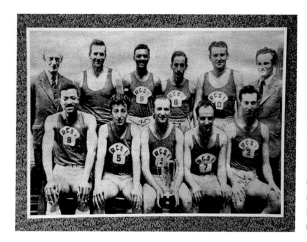

RCSI's basketball team, 1951, featuring Prof A.K. Henry (back row, left) and Alfred Mutchnik (front row, centre).

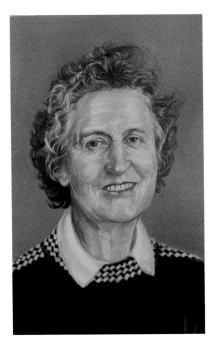

Prof Ethna Gaffney by Vera Klute, 2017.

plane crashed in North Wales (after sixteen years in operation, this was Aer Lingus' first fatal accident). The Emile Stone Memorial Cup was presented at the annual Drama Club awards for many years.[141]

Another victim of the crash was a 40-year-old doctor, James Gaffney; three years later his wife, Dr Ethna Gaffney (1920–2011), was appointed, first, Lecturer in Chemistry and Physics, then from November 1961, Professor of Chemistry and Head of the Department of Chemistry and Physics, making her at a stroke both the first female professor at RCSI and the first female Head of Department.[142] A teaching laboratory was named in her honour in 2018.[143]

NEW DECADE, NEW FACES

As the 1960s began, RCSI was saying its goodbyes to the last of the generation born in the previous century. In the span of a few months, the Council stood in successive silences for Abrahamson, for Henry and for Doolin, of whom the Minutes declare: 'There will not be his like again.'[144]

Meanwhile, every autumn term the School was reborn. In 1961, W.J.E. Jessop wrote a survey article on 'The Medical Schools in the Republic of Ireland'.[145]

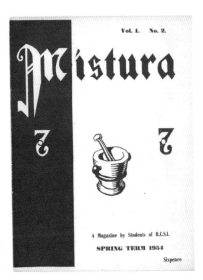

Vol. 1.   No. 2.

Mistura

A Magazine by Students of R.C.S.I.

SPRING TERM 1954

Sixpence

The student magazine, *Mistura* (1954).

A snapshot of a subject in perpetual motion, the article first makes general observations ('The courses of instruction which medical students are required to take follow the same general pattern in all the schools'), then proceeds to individual institutional sketches. RCSI, he reports, employs 'about 35 teachers formally appointed by the College and about a further 80 "recognised teachers" who are consultants in the hospitals attended by students of the College... About 85 students are admitted each year, a high percentage of whom are from overseas countries...' The general hospitals attended by RCSI students are listed as St Laurence's Hospital (that is, the collective of the Richmond Whitworth and Hardwicke Hospitals), Jervis Street Hospital, the Meath Hospital, the Adelaide Hospital, the Royal City of Dublin Hospital and Mercer's Hospital.[146]

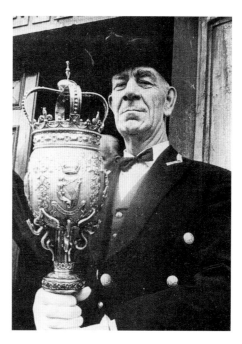

Head Porter Felix Cooper, 1971.

Teaching and examining apart, from 1962 two new members of staff in particular would influence the incoming students' RCSI experiences. The first, arriving in February, was front-of-house: this was the new Head Porter and Mace-bearer, Felix Cooper (taking over from David Maxwell). Cooper was a former boxer who, as a Guard for thirty years, had driven police escorts for five British ambassadors. Apparently superstitious, he suggested that students who used the main entrance on St Stephen's Green before their exams were doomed to fail (or perhaps he simply did not want the hassle of checking that they had closed the door behind them).

Cooper also chased locals kids away from the doorway – including one named Frank Donegan, who lived around the corner on York Street; in 1982, Donegan joined RCSI as a porter, eventually coming to fill Cooper's shoes as Head Porter from 2013.

The second notable arrival, appointed in March, was a little more behind-the-scenes: this was the new Registrar, Dr Harry O'Flanagan. RCSI's years of adversity were by no means all in the past, but the architect of its resistance – and, indeed, its eventual hard-won recovery – was now in place. ■

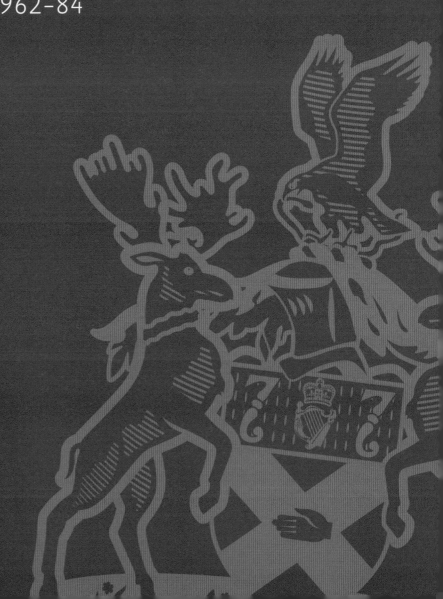

Chapter 7:
Renaissance, 1962–84

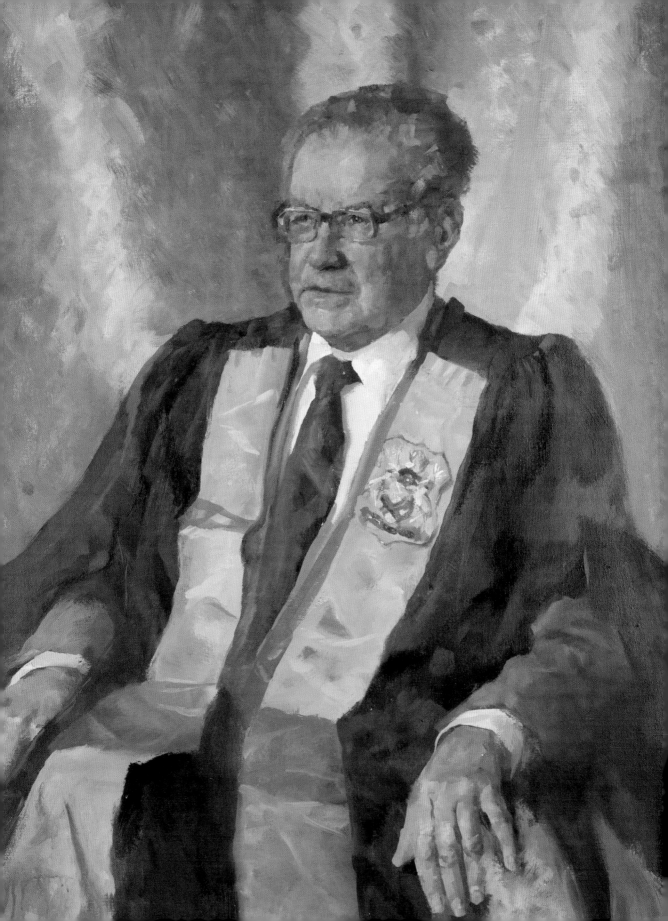

Chapter 7:
Renaissance, 1962-84

THE ASHES OF DRESDEN

On Tuesday, 13 February 1945, Dr Harry O'Flanagan (1917–2000,[1] Lic. 1939, Registrar 1962–80, Hon FRCSI 1981) sat with bomber crews in a Nissen hut at RAF Kirmington, halfway between Scunthorpe and Grimsby in the north of England. He was in his late twenties, the sole medical officer for the 2,000-strong station. Earlier that day, he and the crews had observed the ratio of bombs to petrol being loaded on to the aircraft and surmised that the coming night's target would be a distant one, at the upper limit of navigational range.

But there was general surprise in the hut when the destination was revealed: Dresden. Close to the Russian front, it was not a military city, nor did it have the usual munitions factories or railways yards. Indeed, when Bomber Command received the order, they did not even have maps of the area. Why Dresden, then? Almost fifty years later, when O'Flanagan wrote a short memoir of his experience, he had no interest in apologia or euphemism: 'This was to be a night of civilian slaughter.'[2]

Following the briefing, he moved amongst the crews as they checked their notes and emptied their pockets of any identifying objects or papers. He handed out

Previous page: Harry O'Flanagan, Registrar of RCSI, by James Le Jeune.

caffeine tablets for the nine-hour, 2,000 km journey ('Drowsiness was a real problem, particularly for the air gunner isolated in their cold turrets in the tail and midway above the fuselage'). There was little chat. Later, while O'Flanagan attempted to sleep, a first wave of 244 Lancasters dropped incendiaries and barometrically fused blast bombs; the latter exploded in the air, creating a

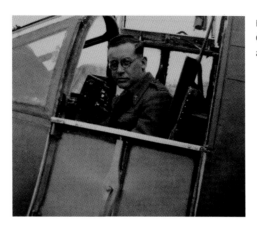

Harry O'Flanagan on active service.

firestorm. Once the city was ablaze, the second wave of twice as many bombers had a wide, bright target for their 2,000 tons of high explosives.

Back at Kirmington the next morning — Ash Wednesday, as it happened — the mood was sombre. There was none of the usual post-mission banter and repartee. The night's effort, O'Flanagan wrote, 'highly successful in operational terms, became shrouded in revulsion and disgust'. Over time, the casualties were counted: some 25,000 killed, 35,000 declared missing, close to half a million rendered homeless — and there were the numberless maimed, too. The statistics, observed O'Flanagan, 'were horrendous... I doubt if any of us who were involved in the events of that dreadful February night have not carried, and will not do so for all time, a sense of shame and guilt.'

FULL CIRCLE: LICENTIATE TO REGISTRAR

By the time O'Flanagan took up his post as Registrar of RCSI in April 1962 — the Council formally welcomed him on the same day they stood in remembrance of William Doolin — he was an experienced medical administrator. Before his Kirmington stint he had worked in the Public Health Service in Wales, where the poverty he witnessed in the Rhondda Valley, particularly of children, marked him not unlike the Dresden experience; in the latter stages of the war he was in Egypt, again with the RAF.

In peacetime he returned to his native Dublin (though he grew up in Roscrea) to join the nascent Department of Health as a Medical Inspector. Part of his role included responsibility for infectious diseases, such as the 1956 poliomyelitis epidemic in Cork (when the county qualified for the All-Ireland Finals in hurling and football that year, both matches were postponed at the request of the Dublin health authorities, lest travelling fans spread the disease); O'Flanagan was central to the subsequent national vaccination programme. His flair for administration was recognised in the Department and he went on to represent the Minister on many international bodies related to public health, including the WHO.

As Registrar of RCSI, O'Flanagan was in some respects coming full circle, having been a student in the School some thirty years earlier. At that time, Alfred Miller's tenure as Registrar still owed much to its original role of 'Clerk and Housekeeper'; his successor, Professor Rae, began the process of modernising the position, but day to day the role largely consisted of fighting a rearguard action to keep the lights on through decades of adversity. O'Flanagan was thus RCSI's first medically qualified Registrar. His bilingualism in the languages of medicine and politics proved a combination that did not merely suit the institution, but essentially saved it from extinction.

'MANIFEST DESTINY' ON YORK STREET

As O'Flanagan began, he took an inventory of RCSI's not-so-vital signs: the College's total income was £66,500, there were almost no capital funds to draw on, the State grant-in-aid sat plateaued at £4,500, and any small annual surplus scraped together was taxed at the business rate. As to the School, it required near-complete replacement of instruments and other teaching aids, and there were a mere ten professorships, of which only three were full-time positions. (In addition, dragging down the entire School's reputation, the 'chronic' student was, as it were, alive and well.) On the plus side, the Council owned the College, the School buildings behind it and five adjacent houses in York Street. The Bird Avenue playing fields, meanwhile, were leased.[3] Of all of these elements, the redress of two in particular – RCSI's tax status and the further acquisition of York Street property – would transform RCSI's fortunes.

The thirteen houses on the northern side of York Street were, by mid-century, in advanced states of dilapidation. The one nearest to RCSI, no. 33 – Garry's domain – had been bought in 1953, while the next four, up to and including no. 37, were acquired just ahead of O'Flanagan's arrival. As assets, they were of dubious value. In spite of their condemnable decrepitude, they were occupied, and the Corporation was loath to declare them unfit for habitation because of the city-wide shortage of housing.

In the event, a series of tragedies forced the issue: a tenement collapsed in Bolton Street in June 1963, killing two residents and injuring seven others; then, less than a week later, there was a similar incident in Fenian Street, where two tenements collapsed and two children perished.[4] (Fifty years after Cameron had inspected the Church Street disaster, conditions had not much changed for Dublin's poorest inhabitants.) Days later again, the roof of no. 36 York Street – owned by RCSI – fell in. Fortunately, the residents were evacuated in time and no life was lost. On the advice of solicitors, RCSI went to the District Court as a common informer against itself, seeking a closure order as the houses were unfit for habitation. The Corporation's representative was unwilling to attend until he was subpoenaed; only then were the houses declared unfit. The tenants were rehoused and demolition began.[5]

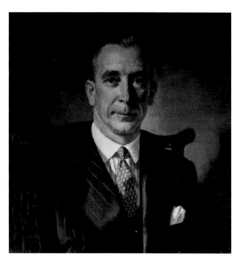

Terence Millin, PRCSI 1963-66, by Arthur Pan.

TERENCE MILLIN AND MILLIN HOUSE

No. 38 was, by contrast, in decent repair, as it had been maintained as a working-men's club, the Conservative, since the 1880s. After two years of negotiating – RCSI initially offered £3,000, the Club wanted four times that figure[6] – an anonymous donation from a grateful patient of the London-based surgeon Terence Millin (1903–1980, FRCSI 1928, PRCSI 1963–66) allowed RCSI to pay £8,000 for the building and cover the cost of refurbishing it as a student club (total: £12,110).[7] The donor's one stipulation was that the house should be named in Millin's honour.

A Council-member since 1960, Millin never practised in Ireland, so his election as RCSI President in 1963 was unprecedented in that regard. As a young surgeon in London, he had inherited a thriving Harley Street practice when his mentor, the urologist Edward Canny Ryall (1865–1934, FRCSI 1900), died suddenly; Millin's own hard work ensured his reputation thereafter (the rumour – alas, untrue – circulated that he claimed tax relief on two chauffeurs on the grounds that one driver could never keep up with his schedule).

On 1 December 1945, Millin woke up to find that he had become famous overnight. This was owed to an article he published in *The Lancet*, 'Retropubic prostatectomy – a new extravesical technique'. His own claims in it were not especially modest ('Although this report

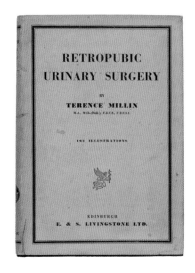

RETROPUBIC
URINARY SURGERY

BY
TERENCE MILLIN
M.A., M.B.(Dub.) F.R.C.S., F.R.C.S.I.

162 ILLUSTRATIONS

EDINBURGH
E. & S. LIVINGSTONE LTD.

The book (1947) that followed Millin's famous *Lancet* article.

is based on a relatively small series of 20 cases, the procedure represents in my view, a great advance in the treatment of prostatic obstruction'), but the journal's editor went full fanfare, making comparison to Archimedes' 'eureka' moment in the bath. Millin was soon operating around the world, often counting grateful potentates among his wealthy patients.

As Britain's top rate of tax climbed (even the Beatles were soon complaining on 'Taxman'), Millin scaled back to part-time London surgeon, part-time gentleman farmer in Co. Cork. His retirement from the operating room in 1963 allowed him to devote his considerable energies – and legendary personal charm – to all things RCSI, particularly as Chairman (from 1967) of the Finance Committee; his name 'opened doors everywhere'.[8] RCSI's annual Millin Meeting – and keynote Millin Lecture – are named in his honour.

THE GIFT OF CHARITABLE STATUS

Over the years, various plans were touted for the York Street acquisitions, from student accommodation to office space to postgraduate facilities. This last option was still the official line as late as December 1964, when the Prime Minister of Mauritius, Dr Seewoosagur Ramgoolam, presented a £10,000 cheque 'in recognition of the work the college has done for Mauritian students'. (At that time, there were approximately fifty such students at RCSI, several of them close relatives of the PM.) But coinciding with O'Flanagan's arrival, more ambitious plans were taking shape, and in 1963 a survey of the site was undertaken to ascertain its potential for School buildings. This begged the question, how would such potential development be paid for?

The answer was to change RCSI's legal – and, crucially, taxation – status to that of a charitable body. This was a coup to which the Council had aspired since the 1950s, when the Royal College of Surgeons of England won an appeal in the House of Lords against the Inland Revenue, following which all the UK Colleges gained charitable status. RCSI considered taking a similar challenge to the High Court, but there was no certainty of a positive ruling and the possible costs were eye-watering. Instead, the Council asked O'Flanagan to make di-

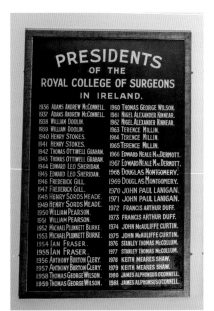

The Presidents of RCSI, 1936-1981.

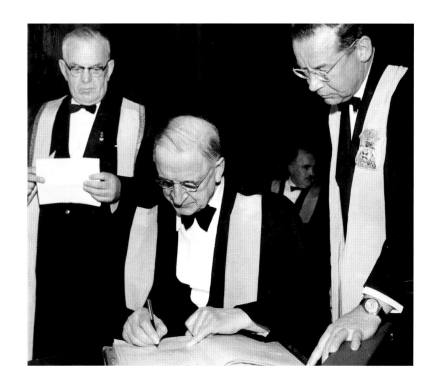

President de Valera receives Honorary Fellowship, 1964.

rect contact with the Minister for Finance, James Ryan. A medical doctor himself, Ryan was sympathetic to the proposal. He referred O'Flanagan to the Revenue Commissioners, who in turn explained that the most significant obstacle lay in RCSI's own Charter.

On the one hand, RCSI was engaged in teaching and research, which was charitable; on the other, the College could exercise disciplinary control of its Fellows, which was inimical to charitable status. Immediately, the legal wheels were set in motion to excise the latter powers from the Charter (helpfully, Revenue indicated the exact words and phrases that needed to go), and on 17 February 1965 the Royal College of Surgeons (Charter Amendment) Act was signed into law by President de Valera. No doubt he was happy to do so, having been made an Honorary Fellow the year before.[9]

At a stroke, what had been an annual albatross – in some years, RCSI's tax bill had more or less consumed its state grant – now looked like a financial phoenix: henceforth, RCSI was free to solicit and accept covenanted gifts.

THE 'GOOD OFFICES' OF ROBERT BRISCOE

As the 1960s advanced, further pieces of the York Street puzzle fell into place. Following a public hearing in 1963, Dublin Corporation acquired by compulsory

'THE ABE': LEONARD ABRAHAMSON (1896-1961, PROF OF MATERIA MEDICA 1926-34, PROF OF MEDICINE 1934-61)

Abrahamson's comments on the AMA fiasco carried more weight than most. In all medical matters, his reputation preceded him (as, indeed, did the aroma of his favoured Partagás cigars from Fox's of Grafton Street).[107] Born under Tsarist rule in Semiatich (now Poland) in 1896, from whence pogroms caused his family to flee, Abrahamson's long career meant he could see the virtue of combining the old with the new. From the 1920s, he was a recognised expert in electrocardiography, but at the same time he urged students to 'Look to the face' – as one recalled:

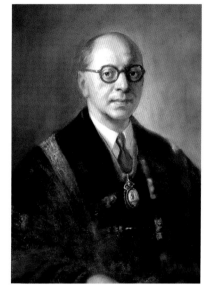

Leonard Abrahamson, RCSI professor and President of RCPI (1949-52), by Roderic O'Connor. Courtesy of RCPI.

> He was of a generation when laboratory back-up was minimal and clinical expertise was paramount... the facies of Parkinson's, myxoedema, the Dresden chin skin of aortic regurgitation, capillary pulsation on the forehead, tabetic facies, pellagra face, and sadly the Hippocratic facies of cachexia; one saw them all working with the old Abe.[108]

Another student spoke of Abrahamson as 'a legendary clinician and teacher... an extraordinary individual [who] epitomized the best in Irish medicine by his human clinical approach and the clarity of his teaching style'.[109] According to others, Abrahamson arrived at the lecture theatre at four seconds to the hour – this allowed time to walk from the door to the podium – and would then speak without notes for forty-five minutes ('at a moderated speed that facilitated note-taking'[110]). That said, as an examiner he could be terrifying; Stacey Day recalled one such clinical interrogation:

> ... never before or since have I been so grilled. Indeed there were moments when I could have retreated to the patient's bedclothes myself. I have absolutely no idea to this day as to how long precisely the examination endured. I do remember, and will never forget, that when the Abe dismissed me I was so confused that I was literally giddy, and with great effort made my way to the nearest sink, in full view of

purchase order (CPO) the remainder of the site bounded by York Street, Mercer Street and Glover's Alley (RCSI had to argue that Millin House should be exempt). A year later, certain changes in the powers of the Planning Authority and the City Manager evolved, by which the City Manager could dispose of land acquired by CPO in the best interests of the city (and not necessarily for any reasons set out in the original CPO). In October, the former PRCSI T.G. Wilson invited the former Lord Mayor of Dublin Robert Briscoe (1894–1969) to discuss these developments.

Briscoe was well-disposed towards RCSI — not because his sons and daughter had passed through (though that surely did not hurt), but because he believed RCSI's many foreign students provided a cash injection to the city. At a follow-up meeting, Wilson, Briscoe and O'Flanagan met with the City Manager, T.C. O'Mahony, to ask for the land. O'Mahony needed to convince his fellow councillors, so Briscoe agreed to lobby on behalf of RCSI. 'We must never forget Mr. Briscoe's good offices in obtaining this site for the College,' O'Flanagan later wrote. 'Without his help it would almost certainly have slipped away.'[10]

In 1966, the Corporation voted to transfer the site to RCSI at the price they had compulsorily acquired it; the sole condition they attached was that the land must be used for RCSI purposes only and could not be sold to another interest without its consent.[11] Finally, in 1969, RCSI acquired a redbrick house tucked away in Glover's Alley. This was part of a mineral water company that had been located here for many years; various trade names came and went, but its latest owner — to whom RCSI paid £8,000 — was Taylor Keith, of red lemonade fame.[12] Thus the area bounded by York Street to the south, Glover's Alley to the north and Mercer Street to the west now became an island of RCSI property. Meanwhile, in a related development out in Windy Arbour, RCSI finally became the owner of the Bird Avenue playing fields that had previously been leased.[13]

THE STUDENT EXPERIENCE –
OR, 'WILL IT RAIN LIKE THIS THE WHOLE TIME?'

September 22, 1965. Coming to Ireland. The Aer Lingus 707 dipped low on the short flight from Shannon to Dublin. The landscape below a crazy quilt of greens: some patches almost chartreuse, others greyish and strewn with rocks... Dublin Airport, a piece of cake after the pandemonium of JFK... changing money into a strange new currency with five pound notes and ten shilling notes and half crowns.

Thus begins the wonderfully vivid, impressionistic memoir of the late 1960s student experience penned by an American, Robert C. Goodwin (Lic. 1971):

A first look at the country that will be home for the next six years. *Will it rain like this the whole time?*

Settling into Dublin – *is there any way to make sense of this city?* The streets changed their names and directions every two blocks, the banks closed for lunch, and the telephone system was like something designed by Laurel and Hardy. And the rain continued...

A first look at Surgeons. Scars of bullets... The grand entrance, like the portico of a Victorian museum. Cooper, in a navy blue uniform trimmed with gold, and brass buttons the size of ha'pennies... Classmates from Goa and Guyana and Malawi and Mauritius... from more than thirty countries, converging for six years on this rain-swept edge of Europe.

Pre-reg. Wooden pews in cavernous halls. Professor Gaffney lecturing in black robes, Mrs Kenny lecturing in a maternity dress, Dr. Gallen taking attendance. *You – where's your tie?* Professor Widdess pouring millet seeds into ancient skulls... The labs... some recompense in the heat of forty Bunsen burners. The *je-ne-sais-quoi* of vapours of HCl and ammonium hydroxide wafting through the morning air. In biology, drawings of amoebae and spirogyra. Remember the dogfish?

Exams. None of your multiple guesses, or stabs at true or false. Entirely essays – 'Give an account of...', 'Compare and contrast...'

First year. Anatomy and physiology and biochem; white coats and dissecting kits and *Grant's* and *Gray's*... The vastness of the dissecting room, with a ceiling as high as a nineteenth century railway station. Dr. Rooney was all facts and nervous energy, pointing and pacing and probing. Moira O'Brien alternated threats and encouragement like a riverboat gambler dealing out aces and deuces. Geroid Lynch – brash friendly, taking the whole thing (including himself) with several grains of salt... Professor Irvine, descending the spiral staircase from Olympus. And then there was Anne Legge... Professor Moore, his manner crisp as Kane's was muted...

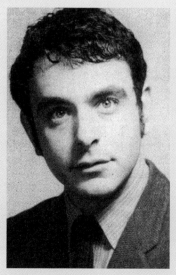

'We never left...' Robert Goodwin, 1971.

Meanwhile, something was happening. Coming from all over the world, we grew to know each other. Together we put on Revues, attended lectures at the Bi, played in the Purefoy, chatted in the canteen and (over endless pints) in the pubs... We were becoming a class, with our own legends and cast of characters. More than that, we were becoming Irishised. Steve Bohan [Lic. 1972] put it best – 'This place makes you unfit to live anywhere else.'

Spring 1968 – the Halves... ten days of exams on all the preclinical studies to date. Culling old notes review sessions, last-minute lectures, cramming into the night... We huddled in small groups. 'How did it go?', 'What did he ask?', 'Jaysus, I didn't have a bloody clue!' Frank Kane's singular way of giving bad tidings: 'You see the leaves... come back when they're brown.'[14]

And after the Halves we began at the hospitals... and slowly, imperceptibly, we learned enough to become competent. A funny thing, this matter of a medical education. You can't pinpoint what you learn at a particular time, but at the end of the process you have a body of knowledge, an accumulation of facts and experience, that you didn't start out with. The teaching was disjointed, but, like everything else, it had an Irish logic of its own. And they taught us very well.

More hospitals: the Gothic leviathan of St. Brendan's, paediatrics at Our Lady's and Temple Street. Ob/Gyn at the Rotunda or the spanking new Coombe. Alan Browne's introductory lecture: 'For some of you, delivering your first baby will be the highlight of your professional career, and you'll send the child birthday cards all your life. Others of you will be sufficiently traumatized to get out of clinical medicine altogether and take up research.' Paediatrics was mainly fun, sometimes terribly sad, and very tough. Professor Kavanagh ran a tight ship at Temple Street, and repeatedly failed more people than anyone except Bewley. There was one big difference, though. If Kavanagh failed you, you didn't graduate with your class...

Which brings us to Finals. May 1971, a solid month of them... Waiting for the results, this time the longest wait of all... Then the word came out, and Jaysus! we really were doctors... we had gone the distance... Relief and pride and a sense of completion... and no responsibilities yet. The beepers, the acute abdomens coming in at 3 a.m., the frantic days and sleepless nights would come later. For two weeks we had it all, no strings.

June 16, 1971: a cool summer afternoon, and a clear bright sky hung over the city... Bloomsday. Also Conferring. Marching two-by-two in our black gowns with light blue trim... Harry O'Flanagan reading off our names... the Graduation Ball at the Intercontinental. Our last hurrah. At some point it seemed to dawn on people that this was the end. An unsettling recognition. No one wanted to leave. We promised each other we'd write, and finally headed out into the Dublin dawn... we scattered across the world, to America, to Zambia, to Mauritius and Malawi, back to the thirty-odd nations from whence we came... Many of us vowed or threatened to come back. In a sense we never left.[15]

In Goodwin's time, South African students – barred by apartheid laws from studying at home – represented the largest cohort of foreign Licentiates, followed by significant numbers from the UK, Mauritius, Norway, Nigeria and Malaysia:

Australia (1)	Italy (2)	Sierra Leone (8)
Belgium (2)	Jamaica (6)	Singapore (3)
Canada (4)	Jordan (1)	South Africa (167)
Channel Islands (1)	Kenya (24)	Sri Lanka (16)
Ethiopia (1)	Malawi (3)	Sudan (1)
Ghana (12)	Malaysia (50)	Tanganyika (2)
Grenada (4)	Malta (1)	Tanzania (6)
Guyana (20)	Mauritius (65)	Trinidad (48)
Holland (1)	Nepal (1)	Uganda (14)
Hong Kong (5)	Nigeria (53)	UK (159)
India (7)	Norway (57)	USA (17)
Ireland (125)	Pakistan (2)	Zambia (5)
Israel (1)	Rhodesia (6)	Zanzibar (5)[16]

Uncounted here are those students who 'studied' at RCSI for many years but did not, in the end, collect any qualifications. (In the era, the rate of a student's progress was not strictly policed; one could sit and re-sit exams until a passing grade was obtained, and for some, perhaps on generous grants, there was little rush to launch oneself into professional life.) Such cases were naturally a minority, but

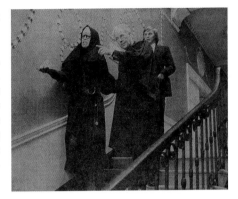

Superintendent of Schools, Seamus Gallen, escorts a gatecrasher, Sven Bjork (disguised as a nun), from the 1973 conferring ceremony. From the *Irish Press*.

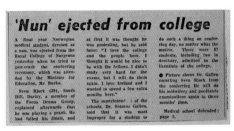

'Nun' ejected from college

A final year Norwegian medical student, dressed as a nun, was ejected from the Royal College of Surgeons yesterday when he tried to gate-crash the conferring ceremony, which was attended by the Minister for Education, Mr. Burke.

Sven Bjork (29), South Hill, Dartry, a member of the Focus Drama Group, explained afterwards that he was playing a prank. He had failed his finals, and at first it was thought he was protesting, but he said later: "I love the college and the people here. I thought it would be nice to be with the fellows. I didn't study very hard for the exams, but I will do them again. I love Ireland and I wanted to spend a few extra months here."

The superintendent of schools, Dr. Seamus Gallen, said that it was most improper for a student to do such a thing on conferring day, no matter what the motive. There were 87 students, including two in dentistry, admitted to the licentiate of the college.

● Picture shows Dr. Gallen escorting Sven Bjork from the conferring He will do his midwifery and paediatric examinations again in three months' time.

Medical school defended: page 5.

for a time RCSI's reputation was not always of the first order — especially as far as rival institutions were concerned.

Irish parents, especially doctors, also looked askance at RCSI's student profile — not because they had any apprehension about standards, but because they feared their sons and daughters were being usurped from a medical career.[17] As a result, in the mid-1960s, RCSI adopted a so-called 'rule of thirds': one third of admissions would be Irish, one third from 'developing' countries, and one third from 'developed' countries.

EXTRACURRICULAR LIFE

In the continued absence of in-house accommodation, many students lived in digs around the city. Year after year the same landladies — and, in general, they were land*ladies* — welcomed RCSI students. On occasion, however, there were culture clashes. At the annual student revue in Millin House in 1965, a sketch called 'Room at the Top' depicted an Indian student meeting his Irish landlady for the first time — with comic results. Off-stage, similar interactions could be fraught (and in the wake of the Green Tureen incident, a notorious 1963 murder case involving a South African student, there were a number of racially motivated attacks in the streets).

An independent body, the Dublin Overseas Students Advisory Bureau, was established to defend the interests of the 1,000-plus newcomers to the city (estimated numbers were 363 at Trinity, 332 at UCD, the remaining 400-plus at RCSI). In 1964, the bureau distributed a questionnaire (200 copies to RCSI, 150 to both TCD and UCD) asking if a 'colour bar' existed in Dublin, and if it was easy or difficult to make contact with Irish people. Unfortunately, fewer than twenty-five responses were received — but at least the questions were being asked.[18]

Outside of the classroom and the clinic, RCSI students' favoured haunts were Robert Roberts' Café on Grafton Street (closed 1970), the Four Provinces, which

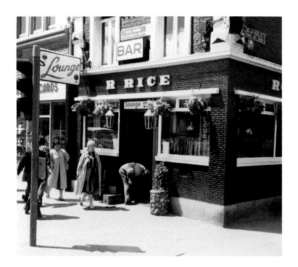
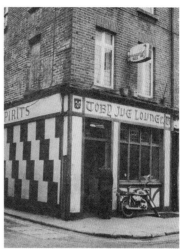

Haunts of yesteryear.

became Rice's (demolished in 1986 to make way for the Stephen's Green Shopping Centre), the Toby Jug (last orders, 1982) and Peter's Pub. ('Pass or fail,' remembered Goodwin, 'there were always the pubs'.) All the student societies held their own 'hops'. The snooker table in the Albert Hall seemed to be in uninterrupted use until 1979, when the room was converted to the Albert Lecture Theatre.

The Green Cinema, practically next door to RCSI, offered students an escape from their lecturers (and vice versa). Movie-star glamour came even closer in 1963, when scenes for *Of Human Bondage* (1964), starring Kim Novak and Laurence Harvey, were filmed in the Anatomy Room. The College happily received £100 for the day's interruption, but the students were less impressed to discover that all the extras – hired before the locations had been decided, and now pocketing an easy £3 – were Trinity interlopers. (Later, the Anatomy Room would also provide a location for *Circle of Friends* (1995), while the York Street foyer played a Garda station in *Ordinary Decent Criminal* (2000).)

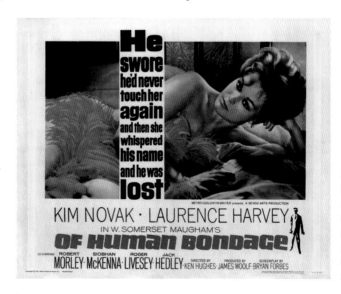

Somerset Maugham's *Of Human Bondage* (1964), also starring RCSI's Anatomy Room. © Metro-Goldwyn-Mayer.

ACADEMIC DEVELOPMENTS

As the healing art sprouted new branches, RCSI established new chairs to keep up. A Department of Clinical Microbiology was founded in 1965, and three years later Ellen Moorhouse (Lic. 1952) was appointed as inaugural Professor, a position she held until her retirement in 1995. (Her portrait, by Vera Klute, was unveiled in 2017, while the Ellen Moorhouse Laboratory at the RCSI Department of Clinical Microbiology at Beaumont Hospital was named in her honour in 2022.) Also in 1965, John Moore[19] and John McKenna were appointed inaugural Professors of Psychiatry and Psychology, respectively.

As far back as 1962, with support from the WHO, RCSI provided a course in Tropical Medicine.[20] By the end of the decade, this had evolved into a professorship held by New York-based Kevin M. Cahill (Hon FRCSI 2016). As a pre-requisite for taking the post, Cahill stipulated that his course be made part of the regular curriculum, 'on the principle that tropical medicine in the 1970s was relevant for all students from all lands'.[21] As the decade ended, Robert Douglas Thornes was appointed the first Professor of the new Department of Experimental Medicine (1969).

Some years earlier, in 1961, the Inspector of Taxes demanded income tax on Thornes' meagre stipend as a postgraduate researcher. Thornes' response was to take a case to the Circuit Court – which he won. The ruling represented a sea change in official attitudes to research funding: ever since, many thousands of Irish students have benefitted from this tax free status.[22] In 1963, Thornes was invited by Colman Kevin Byrnes (1909–1965, Lic. 1934, FRCSI 1940, Prof of Surgery 1961–65) to set up a fibrinolytic laboratory at the Richmond Hospital; it opened in 1970, named in memory of the late Prof Byrnes.

In the decade that followed, Thornes' work here was regularly rewarded with the lion's share of annual research grants from the Irish Cancer Society (headline writers got very excited when 'Irish researcher's tests show rat poison can prolong life of cancer sufferer';[23] this referred to Thornes' trials of warfarin, a drug that originally had been developed for pest control). Unusual for the era, the new chair Thornes' occupied from 1969 was co-funded by a Dutch pharmaceutical company, Organon, and Thornes was expected to devote half of his time to Organon projects.[24]

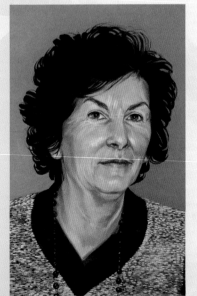

Prof Ellen Moorhouse by Vera Klute, 2017.

Into the early 1970s, there were two more first-time appointments: Brendan O'Donnell – (who was also Dublin's Chief Medical Officer) – in Social and Preventive Medicine, and Patrick J. Bofin – (who was the Dublin City Coroner) – in Forensic Medicine and Toxicology (both 1972). At the time of his appointment, Bofin noted that the most recent textbook on forensics in Ireland was William Dease's *Remarks on Medical Jurisprudence; intended for the General Information of Juries and Young Surgeons* – published in 1793.[25]

New faces were presenting older subjects too, in Medicine (Alan Thompson), Surgery (W.A.L. MacGowan), Anatomy (Brendan Patrick Rooney) and Physiology (Richard T.W.L. Conroy). On the day that Tom Garry died, the Professor of Pathology, Matthew Harris O'Connor (father of the writer Ulick O'Connor) came to work, supervised the commencement of the Primary Fellowship exam, deemed everything in order, and went home and died.[26]

O'Connor was succeeded by his assistant, Peter Dermot Joseph Holland (Lic. 1945), who held the chair until his retirement in 1980, the year he was elected PRCPI. 'The physician knows everything,' Holland once said, 'but does nothing; the surgeon knows nothing, but does everything; while the pathologist knows everything – too late.'[27] O'Connor's other assistant for many years was Dr John Hackett Pollock (1887–1964), a founder-member of the Gate Theatre; he was also a prolific novelist, poet and critic, writing under the pen-name 'An Philibín' (The Plover).

THE MEDICAL SCHOOL OF THE RCSI: A COST-BENEFIT STUDY

All this expansion and change generated drifts of paperwork like never before. PAYE had arrived in Ireland in 1960, and within a few years RCSI's auditors felt the need to hire an extra bookkeeper to keep up. From 1963, for the first time, Council Minutes were typewritten, while O'Flanagan was given permission to purchase an exotic contraption, 'a Thermofax copying machine'.[28] But the great irony is that while RCSI was, on the inside, limbering up, powerful external bodies were expecting the medical school to wipe its blackboards and close the doors.

In the four decades since independence, higher education in Ireland had been largely left to its own devices. By contrast, the next twenty years saw the sector intensely scrutinised, beginning in 1960 with the Commission on Higher Education. The Commission promised a Report, provoking some trepidation at RCSI in light of the UK's recent Willink Committee findings (1957), which recommended a reduction in the number of medical students. Another ominous trend across the water was the move to allow private medical schools – those unconnected to a university – to 'wither and die'.[29] This would have been noted with interest in the Department of Education, who were anxious to cut costs anywhere they could find them, no matter how small.

Civil service reports take their time to bloom – and so at RCSI, life went on: students studied and pooled their pennies for snooker or the bookmaker. Annie O'Mahony's tuck shop did a roaring trade. Fees ticked up almost annually. To mark the golden jubilee of the Rising, the flower-bedecked façade of 123 St Stephen's Green was resplendently floodlit. (A plan for portraits of Markievicz and Mallin was halted at the last minute when the chosen artist showed alarming samples of his work...[30]) Mother Mary Martin (1892–1975, Hon FRCSI 1966), Foundress and Superior of the Medical Missionaries of Mary, became the first female Honorary Fellow. The College Cultural Club – aka 'C-Cubed' – put on a student revue in December 1966 that dropped the curtain on Millin House; shortly afterwards, to clear the ground for a new project, the wrecking ball swung in. On Wednesdays at lunchtime, Kathleen M. Bishop oversaw recitals in the Library ('for those,' she said, 'whose musical tastes veer more towards Bach, Brahms and Beethoven rather than the Beatles, Barbra Streisand and Herb Alpert...'[31]).

Finally, after seven years, the Commission published its report. Amidst its 400,000 words the bottom line for RCSI was that 'the broad view would be that the College would regard its primary duty as being the provision of training at postgraduate level, and that, if it had to make a choice, it would prefer to develop purely as a postgraduate institution'.[32] This ominous verdict was in fact based on the comments of the RCSI Council's own representatives, potentially hoisting themselves with their own petard. But the report pushed no further, merely concluding that 'there is not a prima facie case for the closing of any of the five existing medical schools'.[33] It is likely that RCSI's reprieve here was owed in large part to the Commission's chairman, Cearbhall Ó Dalaigh, who admired the School's liberal ethos and international outlook.

The slow appearance of the Commission's report meant that other developments overtook it, notably the 1967 proposal by the new Minister for Education, Donogh O'Malley, to merge Trinity and UCD. O'Malley died suddenly the following year, and his successor, Brian Lenihan, revised the proposal: Dublin should have one university, with Trinity and UCD comprising its pair of constituent colleges. The two universities swiftly entered negotiations with each other to come up with a plan they liked better. In the meantime, the new Higher Education Authority (HEA, 1968) began preparing a sweeping set of recommendations. Where would RCSI land at the end of this? The signs were not good: despite vigorous representations to a suite of ministers, RCSI was repeatedly refused a seat at the HEA's table.

A pounds-shillings-and-pence proof of RCSI's outlier status appeared in the form of a cost-benefit study of the School by a talented young economist, Charles Mulvey.[34] (These cost-benefit studies were popular in the era – Irish Shipping, Aer Lingus and Bord na Móna had recently been given similar treatments.) The State's concern, as Mulvey saw it, was that RCSI was in receipt of public money but was catering primarily for non-Irish students. Surely this was an unnecessary drain on the country? Mulvey's analysis was based on a thought experiment: if the School closed in the morning, would the country be better or worse off? Sixty pages lat-

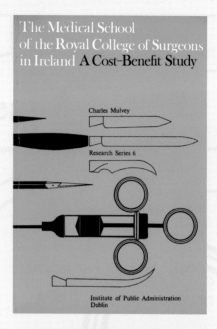

The Medical School of the Royal College of Surgeons in Ireland **A Cost-Benefit Study**

Charles Mulvey

Research Series 6

Institute of Public Administration Dublin

Charles Mulvey's economic report on the Medical School, 1971.

er, his data-driven conclusion matched what Robert Briscoe had previously intuited: 'The social contribution of the medical school of the RCSI to the product of the economy is greater than the social cost of the resources uti-lised in its production.'[35] Or, in other words, the nation as a whole benefitted from RCSI's existence.

Along the way, Mulvey had put his finger on a distinction that few outsiders grasped:

> the medical school of the RCSI is primarily engaged in providing a med-ical education for non-Irish students whereas the other medical schools in the Republic are primarily engaged in providing a medical education for students from the Republic of Ireland. In this respect the medical school of the RCSI is performing a substantially different function from the other medical schools in the country.[36]

But what of the State funding all these non-Irish students? (In 1965, the *Sunday Press* joked about a 'Viking invasion' when twenty-two Norwegian students en-rolled.[37]) Again, Mulvey was careful to make distinctions. The School, he said, makes 'a negligible demand on the state for financial support' – unlike the other medical schools, which were 'all in receipt of substantial aid'.[38] (Elsewhere, in 1967, O'Flanagan had calculated that RCSI's grant-in-aid amounted to £30 per student, whereas at Trinity it was £170, irrespective of the student's origin.[39])

Making up the shortfall in funding, the School was financed in the main by student fees. These fees were charged on a sliding scale: Irish students, subvented by the grant, paid the least (and which was only a little higher than in other schools); students from the 'developed world', whose presence attested to international standards, paid the most (necessarily competitively priced vis-à-vis their home country); while those from the 'developing world' paid an in-between figure. 'This,' observed Mulvey, 'is in keeping with the traditional commitment of the medical school of the RCSI to provide a service to the underdeveloped countries by training doctors for them at a subsidised rate.'[40] If this last comment sounds less than impartial, Mulvey himself later admitted that while he arrived merely to gather data and crunch numbers, he left with 'considerable respect' for the institution.[41]

'COLD SHIVERS': *THE HEA REPORT ON UNIVERSITY REORGANISATION*

Mulvey's cost-benefit report came out in 1971, but despite its positive findings a new nadir was ahead. When the HEA produced its Report (1972), much of the substantial document was taken up with steering a compromise between the government's single-university plan and the alternative TCD/NUI solution. Specifically in relation to medicine, the government proposed a single faculty at Trinity; the universities' preference, on the other hand, was for pre-med subjects to continue at both institutions, while clinical medicine would devolve to a 'joint University Clinical School'. In both conceptions, however, the existence of RCSI was largely steamrollered. Sounding something of a death knell, the Report found itself

> ... driven to the conclusion that any State subsidy to the College beyond its present annual token grant would not be warranted. In view of the College's long and honourable record in medical education we have arrived at this view with regret and only because we are convinced that the best interests of Irish medical education and research would be served by the integration of the College's undergraduate School, including the existing staff thereof, in Dublin's university medical complex.[42]

This sent 'cold shivers'[43] through RCSI. It also provoked anger: a response was drawn up, highlighting RCSI's lack of representation as well as the fact that there was but a single medical doctor on the board. (The first draft was so robustly worded that Nigel Kinnear wondered if it bordered on 'offensive'; others felt that 'the submission was not offensive but that it expressed the strongly felt opinions of the staff and graduates'.[44]) The new Professor of Anatomy, Brendan Patrick Rooney, put his opinion in blunt terms to the press: the report was 'uninformed' and 'badly-researched'; he also foresaw an ominous chain of events: 'If the college closed, with it would go international recognition of postgraduate degrees from this country. The postgraduate work in the college could not survive, if the undergraduate school closed down.'[45]

In the event, the response did not have much effect because it did not need to. As the universities' feet grew colder at the prospect of merger, they stalled for time, and by degrees the Report lost its momentum. Certain changes did follow – notably in relation to dentistry, pharmacy and veterinary medicine – but in the main it was the Report itself, rather than any one institution, that was left on the shelf.

THE APPEAL TO FELLOWS AND LICENTIATES

The entire episode confirmed what was already well-suspected at RCSI: its future was in its own hands. To this end, an independent survival plan had been in action for several years, one that was unbeholden to the kindness of bureaucrats. It hinged on the fact that RCSI's newly minted charitable status allowed it to accept covenanted gifts. This became the basis of a concerted Development Appeal. 'Our appeal is based on a seven-year plan of contribution under deed of convenant,' explained the College *Journal*:

> Those who are not familiar with this type of gift may like to know its advantages. If a benefaction is given under an approved deed of covenant, income tax already paid by the donor at the standard rate of tax on the sum convenanted is refunded by the Revenue Authorities to the College. Thus, in the Republic of Ireland, with income tax at 7s. in the pound, a net sum of £100 donated yearly for seven years will yield over £1,075 gross to the College. In the United Kingdom, with a standard rate of tax at 8s. 3d. in the pound, the same sum would yield over £1,150 gross. The advantages of this method are obvious.[46]

Planning for the appeal began in the summer of 1967, under the advice of professional fundraisers Hooker Craigmyle & Co. (these fiscal alchemists were given a room in the Department of Clinical Pharmacology). The ambition was, in time, to approach industrial, commercial and philanthropic sources, but early surveys suggested that such bodies would be influenced most by the rate of response to an initial appeal directed at RCSI's own Fellows and Licentiates. In this, the signs were good: even before the appeal was launched, parents and visitors to RCSI – mainly from overseas – had already donated in excess of £100,000.

The appeal proper began with a grassroots campaign in the autumn of 1968, when O'Flanagan, Millin and representatives from the advisors toured all the major Irish towns, north and south. At meetings large, small and very small – twenty-one in eighteen locations, to be exact – they explained how RCSI was in possession of a prime site behind 123 and how new buildings could be raised there; they explained how covenants and subscriptions worked, and they asked attendees at meetings to spread the word to others. As O'Flanagan later recorded, apart from the pleasant social aspect, it was 'very uphill work'.[47]

In early 1969, they ventured to the UK – to London, Birmingham, Manchester and Liverpool – a tour not without its slapstick moments ('A disco was in progress and the sounds penetrated to the basement room allocated to the RCSI. The group was very small – about six or eight people... one had refreshed himself too liberally... between the background jive and the periodic crash as our friend slipped from his chair, the atmosphere of the meeting was tense'[48]). Belts were tight everywhere, and the winter weather did not help with attendance. At first, donations trickled in: £5 and £10 per annum, then some £20s and £30s; the 'uninhibited' pledged £50. 'One learned much about human nature,' O'Flanagan said. 'Those who one expected to give much, gave little, and vice versa.'

But it was all welcome, and no one underestimated how relatively small sums might represent serious outlays for people in delicate financial situations. In 1970, O'Flanagan, Alan Thompson and the new PRCSI Douglas Montgomery brought the appeal to South Africa. 'I think those who saw us off reckoned it was a most foolhardy effort,' recollected O'Flanagan. In fact, it was an overwhelming success:

> We concentrated on Johannesburg, Capetown and Durban. Everywhere we were most hospitably treated by the Asian community. Indirectly, we were told that the Government welcomed our visit and that we should feel free to go where we wished without hindrance, in the Republic. We certainly saw for ourselves both sides of the coin, from Soweto and the slums of Durban to the prestigious areas of the cities...

One highlight was a dinner – multi-racial, O'Flanagan carefully noted – at the President Hotel in Johannesburg, when £25,000 was pledged.[49] In attendance was the local superstar surgeon, Christiaan Barnard. A short time earlier, in November 1968, within a year of his famous heart transplant operation, Barnard had visited RCSI in Dublin to give a lecture. (He was the guest of the *Irish Medical Times* that night, not RCSI, and indeed the event was picketed by anti-Apartheid groups.) Less celebrated, then or since, was Barnard's anaesthetist for the pio-

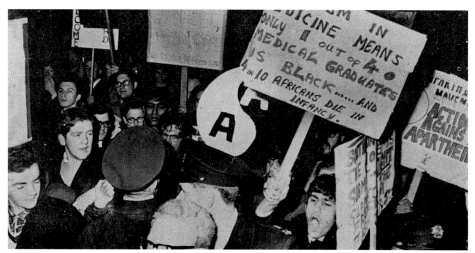

Anti-Apartheid protests on the occasion of Christiaan Barnard's visit, 1968.

neering operation, Joseph Ozinsky (1927–2017), who had trained at RCSI (Dip. Anaes. 1955) and was a Fellow of the Faculty of Anaesthetists (1961). For his contribution to medical history, RCSI had congratulated him in a rather low-key fashion: they sent him a College tie.[50]

From Johannesburg the team flew to Capetown, then drove to Durban ('the warm Indian Ocean outside our hotel, but no time for swimming'), where their host was Mohamed Essack (Lic. 1957).[51] The last stop was Lagos, Nigeria, where there was yet another outpouring of RCSI graduates' hospitality ('All the party increased greatly in girth'). There would be many future fundraising trips – the Colles-Graves Foundation (1970) was established in New York to facilitate North American donors – but O'Flanagan maintained it was the initial Irish and South African tours that taught them the most about the business of charity. It was later estimated that one in five South African doctors of Indian origin qualified from RCSI.[52]

TOWERING AMBITION AND PENNY-PINCHING

The Building Fund grew steadily, the rising tally noted at every Council Meeting: in late 1968, it was £8,381; a mere three months later, in January 1969, it had risen to £38,956; in February, it stood at £48,883. Shortly thereafter, the architects' model for the development was released to the papers.[53] The most striking element of the design was a thirteen-storey student accommodation tower on the corner of York Street and Mercer Street (at the time, the tallest building in the city was the sixteen-storey Liberty Hall, completed in 1965). Almost immediately, the opinion within RCSI was that this design was 'quite impractical'[54] (to say nothing of the pie-in-the sky price tag of £2.5 million), but matters grew

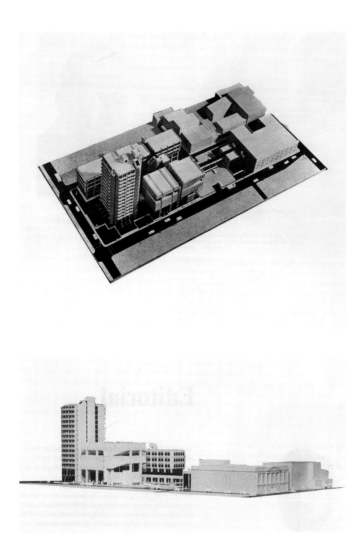

Unexecuted proposal for York Street development, 1969.

complicated when the architect, Michael Kane — brother of Prof Frank Kane (Physiology) — died after a short illness. Kane had been working with a London firm on the project, who now attempted to sue RCSI for its fees. Practically on the threshold of the High Court in London, the firm withdrew the case and paid the legal expenses.

This came as a great relief for RCSI, because even as pledges rolled in, liquid finance remained tight. At one extreme, an overdraft facility of £125,000 had recently been negotiated; at the other, attendance at the Charter Day Dinner for 1971 cost diners £5 a head (in between, the purchase of a hogshead of 1967 Château La Lagune for £295 was evidently unavoidable). The government grant decreased in 1972, from £20,000 to £18,000, while in accordance with national agreements, wages increased (up 35*s* for men, 27*s* for women in 1968–70); concomitantly, fees rose: the per annum tiers in 1974/75 were £400, £650 and £900. If the tiered structure set RCSI apart, the fact of rising fees did not: in the period, all Irish third-level institutes increased their charges.

Away from the York Street project, a separate development plan was also threatening to go awry: portions of the Bird Avenue grounds were put on the market and, in anticipation of a quick sale, some land in Tallaght was purchased for £22,875 – but then the valuation of Bird Avenue proved faulty and the sale collapsed, leaving the undeveloped Tallaght site looking very like a white elephant. Council-member J.G. Maher (FRCSI 1954) pointed out the irony that while RCSI aspired to build a massive city-centre extension at vast expense, it did not have the funds to level a playing field.[55]

Elsewhere, the Finance Committee sought to make savings: the *Journal* – increasingly handsomely produced as the years went by – began to look like an unnecessary expense. It was saved by becoming a 'conjoint' venture in 1971, with the new title *Journal of the Irish Colleges of Physicians and Surgeons* ('With this issue the *Journal* enters on a new phase – it shares it pages with its sister College and becomes the official organ of both'[56]). When its editor, Prof Widdess, retired in 1973, Eoin O'Brien (Lic. 1963) took over.

THE COLLES BICENTENARY

A different expense loomed in the early 1970s: the bicentenary of the birth of Abraham Colles. Behind the scenes, there was much frenetic activity to work out how best to mark the occasion, and how not to break the bank in the process. (RCSI's suggestion, to the Minister for Posts and Telegraphs, of a commemorative Colles stamp did not, alas, stick.) In the end, a three-day surgical conference was settled on ('the meeting should go ahead in as dignified and comprehensive form as possible even if a certain loss was incurred by the College'). As it happened, 300-plus guests enjoyed the very successful Colles Bicentenary in May 1973, complete with a champagne reception (happily, the loss on the event 'would not be anything like as great as was originally estimated'[57]).

Rather more grimly, certain topics the conference addressed – shock, metabolic response to trauma, the management of injured viscera and limb salvage – were timely in the context of the recent flare-up of violence north of the border. Indeed, in the aftermath of Bloody Sunday (30 January 1972), Prof Conroy (Physiology) led some 500 staff, students and technicians from RCSI to the British embassy to protest the killings. 'We are an international college representing students from Ireland and almost the entire world,' Conroy told the assembled crowd. 'We hope that this is the first international response and condemnation of the appalling happenings in Derry over the weekend.'[58] Bearing placards with the names of their many homelands, the RCSI protestors marched to and from the embassy in silence.

THE FACULTY OF NURSING, MARY FRANCES CROWLEY
AND THE IRISH RED CROSS HOSPITAL AT SAINT-LÔ

In 1974, following several years of hopeful discussions, RCSI started an important new chapter with the inauguration of a Faculty of Nursing, the first of its kind in Ireland or Britain. The first Dean (1974–79) was Mary Frances Crowley (1906–1990).

One of the remarkable episodes of Crowley's life and career was the period she spent as Matron of the Irish Red Cross Hospital at Saint-Lô in northern France. Arriving at Dieppe on Christmas Eve, 1945, she was met by her translator-driver-quartermaster, a Dubliner by the name of Samuel Beckett. (The future Nobel Laureate proved a talented translator and quartermaster, but his skills behind the wheel would win no prizes.) Their destination was, in Beckett's first impression,

> just a heap of rubble, la Capitale des Ruines as they call it in France. Of 2,600 buildings, 2,000 completely wiped out, 400 badly damaged and 200 'only' slightly. It all happened in the night of the 5th to 6th June. It has been raining hard the last few days and the place is a sea of mud...[59]

Amongst the other volunteers at Saint-Lô were Dr James Gaffney, who would perish in the North Wales air disaster; the serving RCSI Vice-President, Frederick Gill (1895–1960, FRCSI 1921, PRCSI 1946–48); and Beckett's friend since his schooldays, Alan Thompson, the future Professor of Medicine. The *hôpital irlandais* closed on 31 December 1946, having treated 1,427 patients. In 1948, Crowley and other members of the hospital management were awarded the silver Medal of French Gratitude (*La Reconnaissance française*) at the French legation in Dublin.

Back home after the Saint-Lô experience, Crowley became a leading figure at the Dublin Metropolitan School of Nursing; when it closed in 1969, she approached RCSI to provide a successor post-registration training body. The College was interested, but the heavy financial lifting devolved to the nurses themselves: eighteen original Foundation Members – Crowley amongst them – each contributed £100 towards a Foundation Fund; further donations came from the Irish Nurses' Organisation (£100), the Irish Matrons' Association (£500) and the Ethicon Suture Company (£250). By the end of the decade, the Faculty was in a

Facing page:
Mary Frances
Crowley
by William
Nathans, 2019.

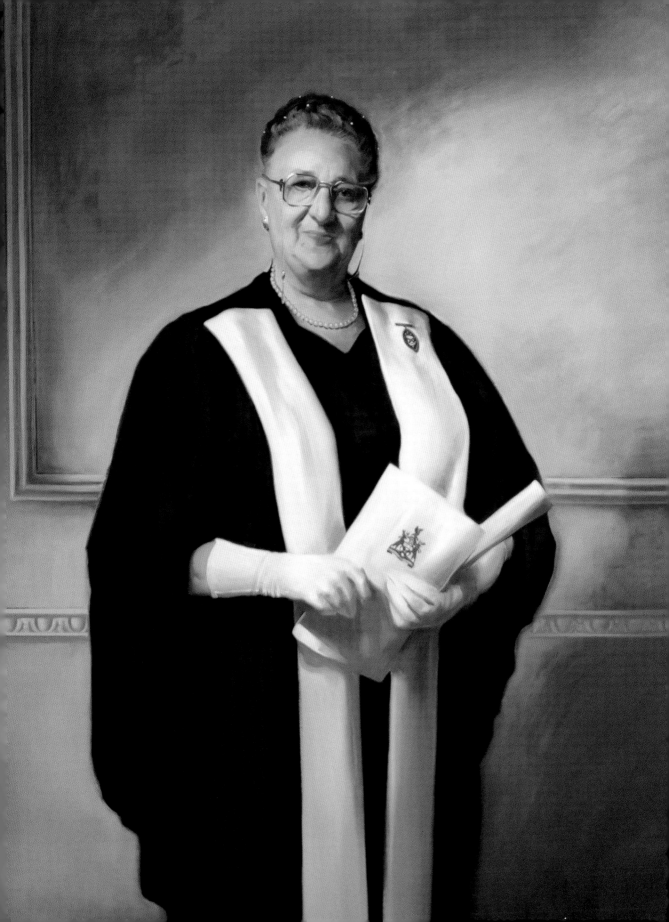

position to donate £25,000 to the RCSI Building Fund.

On the occasion of the inauguration of the new Faculty (which, owing to exams at RCSI, in fact took place at RCPI), Dean Crowley observed that the quality of any healthcare service depended on the quality of the nursing service: 'This means that nurses must be educated on a parallel with the medical profession, taking their place on the health team with full responsibility and assurance of expert service.'[60] A gifted administrator, Crowley took an interest in every aspect of the Faculty, even designing the Dean's medal and black-and-white gown.

Crowley also travelled the country to encourage nurses to further their qualifications; within a few years, Nursing had grown to become RCSI's largest faculty. By 1979, over 1,000 nurses were taking courses, while a Fellowship was offered from 1982. The Faculty's annual Mary Frances Crowley Award honours her memory, and in 2019 Crowley's portrait, by William Nathans, was commissioned as part of the Women on Walls project.[61]

THE START OF THE FACULTY OF DENTISTRY AND THE END OF THE DENTAL SCHOOL

Predating the Faculty of Nursing was the Faculty of Dentistry (founded in 1963) with Rodney Dockrell as inaugural Dean. This was a high point for the profession – at least at the postgraduate level – as exams, and later courses, led to the award of FFDRCSI. There was good news too at the undergraduate level – that is, in the School of Dentistry – when five new full-time appointments were made in 1965.[62] However, that momentum turned out to be relatively short-lived.

A year later, strike action occurred at the Dental Hospital, where the three dental schools in Dublin – RCSI, TCD and UCD – shared the same clinical facilities but had no control over them; conversely, the Dental Hospital had the facilities but no power to control student intake, resulting in overcrowding. Nor were the lengths of undergraduate courses identical in the different schools: RCSI students worked harder than their coevals elsewhere as they were obliged to follow the same preclinical course as medical students (one benefit of this was that Dental Licentiates had the option to 'top up' to a medical qualification later on).

Moves towards standardisation began in 1964, following the visitation of the General Dental Council. To alleviate overcrowding at the hospital, RCSI suspended its intake in October 1965 (Trinity was expected to do likewise but at the last minute chose not to). After the fact, this looked to some like a lack of confidence in the Dental School – despite public pronouncements to the contrary. As the new whole-time positions suggested, RCSI did not want to lose its undergraduate school, and no one knew the effect such a loss would have on the thriving post-graduate Faculty; on the other hand, student numbers were in the single digits, and the comments by Minister O'Malley as well as the Ó Dalaigh Commission's Report indicated that, as far as officialdom was concerned, the future of Dublin dental education belonged to Trinity.

In early 1976, RCSI discovered that meetings were taking place between TCD, UCD and the HEA; following expressions of protest, RCSI was invited to the table – discouragingly located in Trinity – in June. In essence, everything was already decided (indeed, this was part of a greater rationalisation strategy that allocated pharmacy to Trinity and veterinary medicine to UCD). On the day of the meeting, RCSI made do with assurances that its place in postgraduate dental education would be respected by both universities.

Then, in the quiet month of August – when most members of the School Dental Committee were away on leave – PRCSI John McAuliffe Curtin let it be known that the undergraduate School was to close. As something of a last-ditch stand, those committee-members who were present emphasised the importance of retaining the right to confer Dental Licences into the future. This was upheld – but only until 1985, when the necessary safeguard was omitted from that year's Dental Act.[63]

Those students about to commence dentistry at RCSI in the autumn of 1976 found themselves transferred to Trinity; those about to end the second professional year stayed on at RCSI.[64] Over the course of almost a century, some 1,600 dentists had been educated at RCSI. By way of memorial to this long contribution, a traditional-style dentist's chair still sits in the foyer of 123 St Stephen's Green.

THE NEW MEDICAL SCHOOL ON YORK STREET

PRCSI McAuliffe Curtin (Lic. 1940, FRCSI 1945, PRCSI 1974–76) had a happier task on 11 December 1974, when he laid the foundation stone of what was called the New Medical School. 'We shall go steadily from strength to strength,' he said on the occasion, 'fortified by the knowledge that our college is destined to hold an expanding place as a centre of surgical and medical education and research.'[65]

A new architect, Frank Foley of Buchan, Kane and Foley, had been appointed to the project in early 1971.[66] In light of the last lofty false start, Foley was given a tightly controlled brief for the already restricted site; his drawings, presented in December, were approved by Council ('practical and economical' were O'Flanagan's watchwords[67]).

Initially, Foley imagined a suite of connected buildings to be built in phases: immediately west of the old College would be an administrative block (later known as the 'Link Building'); next was the enlarged cuboid heart of the school;

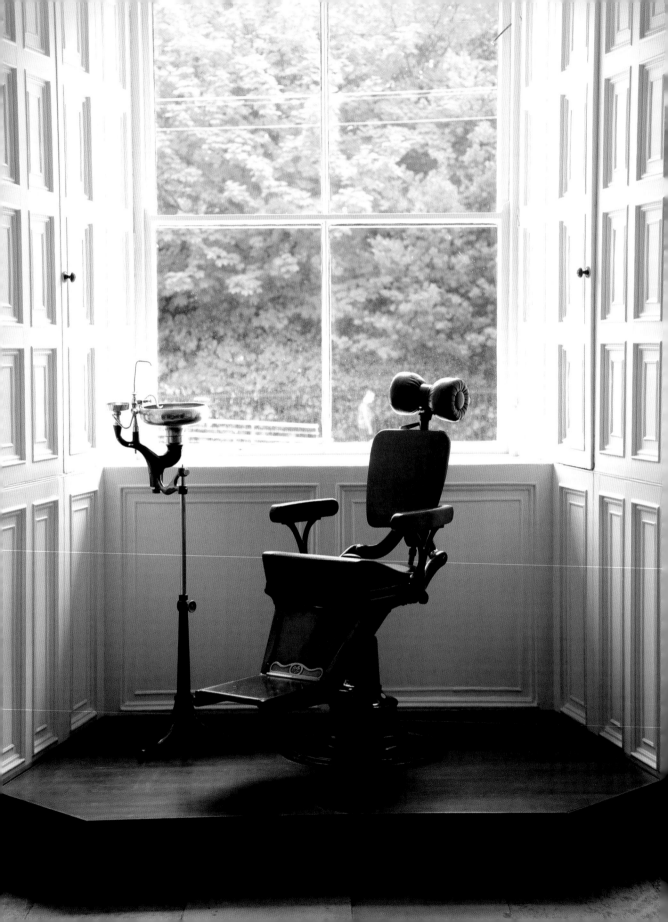

two further blocks running along Glover's Alley and Mercer Street were to frame a grassy piazza concealing an underground carpark. Dublin Corporation granted planning permission, McLaughlin and Harvey won the contract, and work began on Phase One – the central block – in September 1973, at an estimated cost of £1.3 million.[68]

Foley designed a complex structure in a deceptively simple building. Constrained by height – the project had to harmonise with the 1827 building fronting onto the Green – he conceived of three storeys over basement and sub-basement with a vast hollow core at the centre. Working with a second architect, Andrew Devane, who had trained with Frank Lloyd Wright, Foley inserted into this space an inverted cone of three lecture theatres, two seating 200, one seating 400; the steep rake of the seating was a trade-off to maximise circulation space in the concourse outside the theatres. (Later, these were named the Cheyne, the Houston and the O'Flanagan Theatres.)

Below street-level, tucked under the cone's tip, was a student space complete with a gym, a squash court and a coffee bar. Directly above the theatres is the cavernous double-height Examination Hall, accommodating 800 students comfortably (if they've studied). This space was originally lit with natural light, until later expansion put more buildings on the roof. The RCSI coat of arms high on the west wall was a gift from the Royal College of Surgeons of England in 1981 (the same year the former Examination Hall in the old building was renamed 'College Hall').

Encircling – or, strictly, ensquaring – the upper floors are classrooms, offices, laboratories and, originally, a restaurant. This uninterrupted interior is made possible by the defining feature of the exterior: the massive precast perimeter panels which in fact bear the load of the building. (The use of precast concrete tells its own story: widely utilised since the war to rebuild bombed cities – such as, say, Dresden – it also became the fashionable choice among architects for its modern, egalitarian aesthetics, particularly in higher education, UCD's then-rising Belfield campus being a local example.) Foley and his engineering consultants – Ove Arup and Partners – laboured over these panels.

A full storey high, 3.2 m wide and weighing nine tons, they were amongst the largest used to date in the country; even lifting them into place was a feat. For good or ill, massive precast concrete panels will always look like what they are, but Foley's iteration exhibits a thoughtfulness in its detail: the windows reflect the ratios of the first-floor windows of number 123, while the surface aggregate of Coolkenna quartz with a white cement binder relates well to the Georgian stone next door. Staining, the bane of concrete structures, is avoided with a vertically ribbed texture, the idea being that wet Irish weather will accentuate this detail

Facing page:
The dental
chair in the
Entrance Hall.

Frank Foley's plans for York Street, 1971.

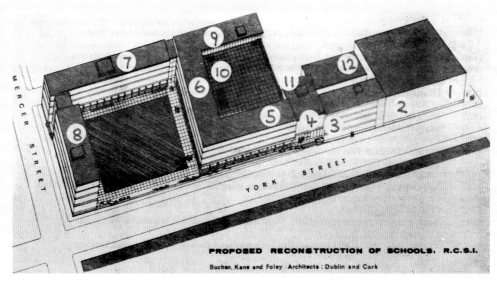

Left: The Foundation Stone is laid by PRCSI McAuliffe Curtin, December 1974. Right: Phase One, looking north-east, January 1975.

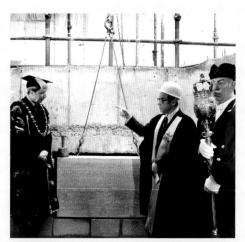
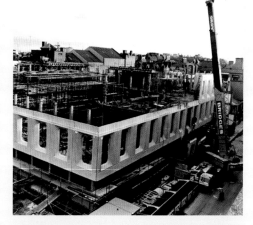

Left: Progress photographed by *Construction and Property News*, February 1975. Right: 'Aerial view', looking south-west.

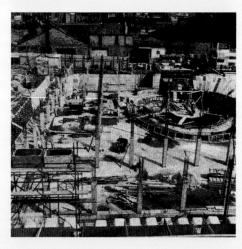
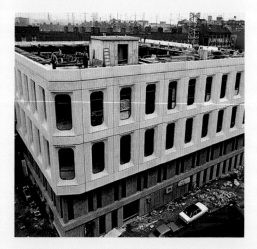

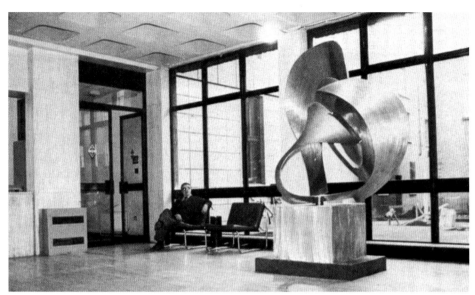

The foyer
of the New
Medical School,
with Arnold
Haukeland's
sculpture.

rather than deface it. And inside, after 165 years, RCSI had a new entrance foyer, with floors, walls and staircase surfaced in bright travertine marble tiles (the St Stephen's Green door was henceforth for formal occasions only). For the architectural journal *Plan*, the New Medical School was, in short, 'one of the most unusual buildings of 1975'.[69]

The achievement is all the more extraordinary when one considers that the Building Fund had been launched only a few years earlier, in July 1968. But by now the Fund had evolved into a smooth-running machine, guided by Senator Patrick McGrath (RCSI Court of Patrons 1980[70]): gone were the fivers and tenners in a bucket in basement rooms; instead, by the time of the topping-out ceremony (April 1975), a seat at a fundraising dinner in New York's Waldorf Astoria cost £150 per person (appropriately, the hotel's long-time resident doctor, James Jackson-Moore, was a Licentiate (1902; he died in 1966). The building was formally opened on 27 April 1976 by Cearbhall Ó Dálaigh, now President of Ireland as well as first Patron (1973) of the College and Honorary Fellow (1975).[71] He and 300 others, including the Taoiseach, Liam Cosgrave, and the Tánaiste, Brendan Corish, were welcomed on the occasion by PRCSI McAuliffe Curtin.

J.B. LYONS AND THE BORDERLANDS

While the future was being lifted into place, RCSI's past was also being written. In February 1975, a Department of the History of Medicine was established – another first of its kind for Ireland and Britain. Widdess' successor as Librarian, John

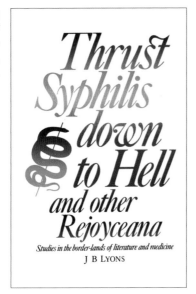

The striking cover of one of J.B. Lyons' many publications, 1988.

Benignus Lyons (1922–2007), was appointed to the Chair, a position he occupied for the next twenty-five years. Widely travelled as a ship's surgeon – he voyaged around the Mediterranean and North Africa, as well as to India, Japan and South America – Lyons practised in the UK before returning to Ireland in 1955. His clinical interests led to *A Primer of Neurology* (1974), and for many years he was president of the Irish Epilepsy Association.

By this time, Lyons had published several novels (he used the pseudonym 'Michael Fitzwilliam', derived from the hospital where he worked in Dún Laoghaire and the city-centre address of his consulting rooms), but increasingly he turned to medical biography and history. Probably his best-known work was *Brief Lives of Irish Doctors* (1978), but his two volumes of RCSI biographies – *An Assembly of Irish Surgeons* (1984) and *A Pride of Professors* (1999) – bring to vivid life personalities only hinted at in the broader brushstrokes of Cameron and Widdess. He was also an authority on the dropout medical student James Joyce.[72]

Lyons' pre-eminence in his domain was invoked in a *Festshcrift* for his 80th birthday, *Borderlands: Essays on Literature and Medicine in Honour of J.B. Lyons* (2002), edited by Davis Coakley and Mary O'Doherty (from 1985, O'Doherty, provided invaluable research support to Lyons – and, indeed, to the entire RCSI community). As a regular contributor to the hypnopompic borderland that is RTÉ Radio's *Sunday Miscellany*, Lyons probably did more than anyone else to sprinkle RCSI history into the dreamlife of the nation.

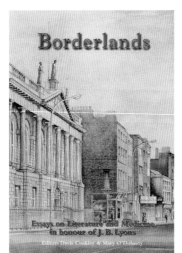

A scholarly tribute to Lyons from Davis Coakley and Mary O'Doherty, 2002.

THE QUESTION OF UNIVERSITY DEGREES

Not everything about RCSI's long history was a boon, however.[73] One particular problem concerned the nomenclature of the qualification that RCSI conferred. The long-standing 'Letters Testimonial' – or Licence – had served perfectly well for RCSI's first hundred years: LRCSI was qualification enough to see one's name entered on the Medical Register, as per the 1858 Medical Act. When the act was amended in 1886 and a triple qualification was required – in medicine, surgery and midwifery – RCSI joined with RCPI to issue a Conjoint Licence. For the next eighty-five years, those who passed their final exams assembled at 123 St Stephen's Green in the morning to receive two RCSI diplomas (surgery and midwifery), and then in the afternoon reconvened in Kildare Street to receive two more diplomas (medicine and midwifery). Shoe-leather was saved from 1973 when the Conjoint conferring ceremony was hosted in either College in alternate years.[74]

If such pageantry had its charm on the day, by the 1960s, in an increasingly international medical world, aspects of the old ways were throwing up obstacles. Put simply, licences were not degrees, and without a primary degree one could not obtain a higher degree – MD (that is, 'doctorate in medicine') or PhD – without which, in turn, one was effectively barred from an academic career. Another aspect of the same problem was acutely felt by RCSI Licentiates in the United States, where their contemporaries exited medical school with the degree of MD (in this case the same letters simply denoted 'medical doctor').

Even in the UK (where many art and technical colleges were lately raised to degree-awarding status), a conjoint licence was starting to look dubious by virtue of the fact that one could register for it a few months before obtaining one's MB – meaning, as the Todd Report put it, it smacked of 'a form of insurance against failure to get a degree'.[75] With good cause, then, aggrieved students and Licentiates complained to RCSI of 'permanent disadvantage' and a 'ceiling' on their ambitions.[76] And it was not only students who were disadvantaged: RCSI itself was held back by being unable to retain or attract talent to the research programmes of its various departments.

There was one obvious solution to the problem: RCSI could start to grant its own degrees. This option was closely considered from at least 1968 until well into the next decade.[77] Legal opinion was sought and a close reading of the Charters revealed clauses which suggested that the College reserved this right (the lines in question come from the Supplemental Charter of 1844: '[it is] lawful to and for the Council, or a majority of such Members thereof as shall assemble... to make and publish and also to alter, change, or annul, from time to time, such Bye-laws, Rules, Ordinances, and Constitutions as to them may seem requisite for the regulation, good government, and advantage of the said body and Licentiates of the said College...'). Moving gingerly, by 1971 RCSI had drafted new bye-laws outlining how its Licentiates would be awarded the primary degrees of Bachelor in Medicine (MB) or – the Dental School was then still in existence – Bachelor in Dental Surgery (BDS). The proposals were duly sent to the Minister for Education for the necessary government ratification.[78] Trinity and UCD were also apprised of the move.[79]

Anyone hoping for a quick rubber-stamping was to be disappointed. Time passed – a year, another, a third, a *fourth* – and no decision was forthcoming. (The HEA Report of 1972 was surely a factor in the delay: why offer degree-awarding status to an institution hitherto treated with, at best, benign neglect? For its part, Trinity had also written to the Minister setting out its opposition to the proposal.) For the RCSI community, disappointment turned to frustration. The College repeatedly urged the Department to approve the bye-laws, while the Graduates' Association urged the College to press ahead and grant degrees 'by Ordinance';[80] six hundred students also signed a petition to similar effect.[81] (No doubt they were reacting to alarming newspaper comments – inaccurate, as it turned out – suggesting that when Ireland joined the EEC (1973), the medical profession would be limited to those with university degrees.[82]) PRCSI McAuliffe Curtin took the matter up personally with the government, and finally, in late 1975, the Minister made his decision: 'only a University could award a degree'.[83]

Having broken this bad news, the only sop the Minister offered was to suggest that RCSI should approach the universities directly about working towards some degree-awarding agreement. A small 'task force' was duly set up and initial, informal meetings took place in June and July; more formal discussions followed in December 1976. Chaired by the new PRCSI, Stanley McCollum (FRCSI 1944, PRCSI 1976–78), RCSI's 'Basic Principles' were as follows:

1. It would continue to appoint its teaching staff.
2. There would be minimal university control over the individual departments.
3. It would select its students, accepting matriculation as the minimum standard of entry.
4. The Licentiateship of the Colleges would be maintained.

Perhaps surprisingly, neither university baulked at any of these conditions. Instead, they each made proposals that would allow RCSI students to earn degrees. Trinity's proposal was on the model of oversight and accreditation that it had already worked out with the Dublin Vocational Education Authority. The UCD alternative offered RCSI the status of a 'recognised college' of the National University of Ireland (NUI). (The year before, 1975, saw Carysfort College, Blackrock, St Patrick's College, Drumcondra and Mary Immaculate College, Limerick all attain this 'recognised college' status; Maynooth College, meanwhile, had been a pioneer in this regard since 1910.)

McCollum and his negotiators (amongst whom were VPRCSI Keith Meares Shaw, PPRCSIs McAuliffe Curtin and Frank Duff and, representing the academic side, O'Flanagan and W.A.L. MacGowan[84]) brought their findings back to Council, whereupon the 'heart searching' began.[85] Many thought an arrangement with Trinity was a shoo-in (McCollum himself was at that time Trinity's Regius Professor of Surgery), but at a Special Meeting of Council in January 1977, it was agreed that the status of 'recognised College' under the NUI aegis was 'the more clear-cut and defined system of relationship'.[86] (As one commentator subsequently put it, 'to many of that Council, the rejection of TCD must have conflicted strongly with their own traditional inclinations'.[87]) The Senate of the NUI gave their approval in the summertime, and so it was the graduating Class of 1978 who first took home the new haul of postnominals: LRCSI, LRCPI, MB, BCh, BAO (NUI). In addition, arrangements were made whereby *all* RCSI graduates, *past* and *present*, were henceforth eligible for postgraduate degrees (MCh, MAO, PhD), provided they fulfilled the necessary conditions.[88]

All involved in the negotiations were conscious of the historical coincidence – or irony – that, six-score years before, it was RCSI that awarded its qualification to students of the NUI's forerunner, the Catholic University Medical School in Cecilia Street. Without that Licence, the Cecilia Street students would have had no access to the all-important Medical Register. The wheel, as it were, had turned full circle. Or, as NUI Chancellor T.K. Whitaker put it in his address on that Friday in June 1978: 'The kind foster-father of the second half of the nineteenth century has placed himself under the spreading wing of his former foster-child.'[89] There was no ceiling now – semantic or otherwise – to the ambitions of RCSI students.

THE END OF THE O'FLANAGAN ERA

And while figurative ceilings were being lifted off, there was still literal building work to be done. That same year – 1978 – a contract was signed for Phase Two, connecting the St Stephen's Green edifice to the New Medical School. The contractors were the same as for the previous phase, McLaughlin and Harvey (who were not told, when tendering, that no one else had been invited to compete). The architect was again Frank Foley. Three storeys without a basement, the new 'Link Building' was not likely to elicit much excitement – though the collective Council pulse was raised when the cost went from an anticipated £150,000–£200,000 to the final £350,000-plus (principally because the floor area was increased from 9,000 to 12,000 square feet).

The pre-existing buildings on the site – in fact, parts of the School dating to 1810 – were demolished; the east–west passage between the new construction

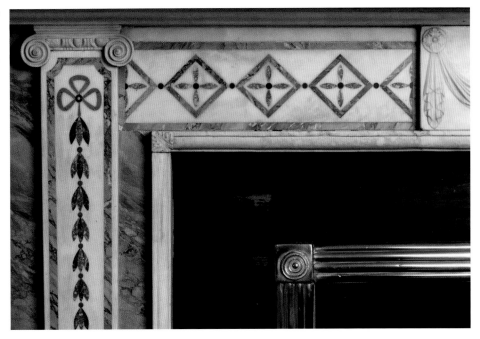

Detail of the Adam fireplace in the President's Room.

and the Anatomy Room (once an outdoor alley) was re-roofed and re-floored; the York Street entrance familiar to generations was closed up; and plans for tiered theatres and laboratories were let go in favour of administrative offices and seminar rooms (the postgraduate Faculties in particular benefited from this badly needed space). Outside, facing York Street, Georgian-proportioned windows are set amid granite slabs; at street level, these slabs are bevelled in vague imitation of the same effect on the 1827 podium around the corner. Above, bands of concrete mark off the floors.

During the same period, Foley had more interesting projects inside the older building: the students' hang-out, the old Albert Hall, was converted to the elegantly tiered Albert Theatre, with its 1861 ceiling preserved. Foley was asked to include the Colles Room in his renovations, and in 1980 a ceiling (*c.*1750) from a house in South Frederick Street slated for demolition was gifted to RCSI and rehung (at a cost of £11,000) in this room.[90] Similarly, a Robert Adam fireplace presented by the paediatrician Patrick MacClancy (Lic. 1941; the MacClancy Medal in Neo-Natal Medicine is named in his honour) was installed the following year.[91] Foley also supervised the cleaning of the 1827 façade and the renovation of the stone balustrade running above the cornice on St Stephen's Green and York Street (cost: £100,000).

The 'Link Building' was the last major infrastructural project of Harry O'Flanagan's tenure as Registrar. It was completed in 1979, at which time the Building

Fund had raised £1.3 million towards an overall target of £2.65 million.[92] The other planned building phases, which would have created a grassy piazza over a subterranean carpark, never came to pass, but O'Flanagan enjoyed some good luck with certain other, mired ventures. Away from St Stephen's Green, for example, the long-standing riddle of how to develop Bird Avenue and/or the Tallaght land resolved itself. The latter – last seen as a financial white elephant – became subject to a Compulsory Purchase Order in 1975.

By way of compensation, Dublin County Council offered a different site on the far-off north side, at Castleknock. RCSI resisted, launching an appeal. Then the County Council offered £8,000 per acre (October 1979), totalling £120,000.[93] Given that the site had cost less than £24,000 in the first place, this offer was snapped up. ('The President complimented the Registrar,' noted the Council Minutes.[94]) This put the focus back on Bird Avenue. Through the 1970s, various plans had come and gone: when planning permission was secured for 115 houses, developers came knocking, and various types of deals (such as land swaps and partnerships, impossible because of RCSI's charity status) were proposed.

Another idea was, with the new NUI degrees, maybe RCSI could share the facilities at Belfield? No thanks, said UCD – and in the end, very little happened. Then, by 1977, RCSI was suddenly interested in the prospect of playing fields on Dublin's north side, owing to a separate development: the traditional city-centre teaching hospitals of the Charitable Infirmary, Jervis Street, and St Laurence's Hospital – aka 'the Richmond' – were scheduled for amalgamation and transfer to a green-field site at Beaumont. Moreover, by this time RCSI's finances were effectively transformed – thanks to graduates' generosity – and there was no longer any great pressure to off-load the Bird Avenue site. The one amenity that was still sorely missed by RCSI was student accommodation, and to that end plans were made early in the new decade to develop a 'hostel with sports pavilion' on the site (estimated cost: £1.8 million).[95]

Within the RCSI community, some, by this stage, were asking the question: was there too much emphasis on building in O'Flanagan's time? To what extent did the needs of teaching and, in particular, research suffer as a result? O'Flanagan himself considered this criticism 'a valid view'. However, he said, 'it was decided to concentrate our finances on wiping out the debt on the building and equipment'.[96] Few would argue – especially in the lean 1980s ahead – that this decision was not vindicated. That said, as his tenure wound down, the days of the Building Fund's dominance over all other concerns were numbered (in February 1979, the Council adopted the Finance Committee's proposal that monies borrowed from pension and research funds, as well as rainy day caution money, in order to finance building, 'should be repaid... at the earliest possible time'[97]).

Having retired in 1980, O'Flanagan – already with an annual RCSI Lecture named in his honour, as well as many other international awards and tributes – was conferred with the College's highest award, Honorary Fellowship, in 1981. (As it happened, the ceremony was a sombre affair, coming the night after the Stardust disco fire; a minute's silence was held for the victims.[98]) O'Flanagan continued to serve Irish medicine, notably as president of Irish Medical Council. A giant of twentieth-century Irish medicine, he died at the end of his century's final academic year, in August 2000. His portrait, by James Le Jeune RHA, hangs in RCSI. For a time – as was said of Colles before him – he *was* the College.

MORE AMERICAN FRIENDS

Someone who ought to have been conferred with Honorary Fellowship alongside O'Flanagan was the American neurosurgeon, Loyal Davis (1896–1982). He had accepted the invitation, but as the occasion drew closer he was unable to travel, first because of his wife's ill-heath, then because of his own (he had contracted pneumonia at the inauguration of his son-in-law, Ronald Reagan, as US President). Council duly decided that if the surgeon could not come to Dublin, Dublin would go to the surgeon, and in July 1981 Honorary Fellowship was conferred on Davis at a ceremony at the Irish embassy in Washington DC. (In a way, this was of a piece with the recent tradition – spearheaded by PRCSI McCollum – of the Council convening in Belfast, Cork and Galway.)

Fourteen representatives of RCSI travelled to the American capital, including

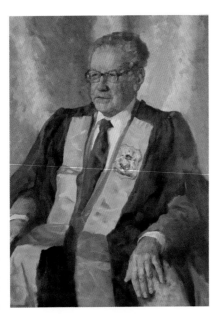

Harry O'Flanagan, Registrar, by James Le Jeune.

PRCSI James Alphonsus O'Connell (FRCSI 1941, PRCSI 1980–82) and O'Flanagan's successor, William MacGowan. On the day, President Reagan kept a low profile, not wanting to steal any thunder. In a short speech, he said: 'You have honoured one of the most distinguished citizens of our country. And we're not at all bothered that your charter comes from George III, shortly after he had an argument with us...'[99]

In truth, international politics were uppermost in many minds, if not necessarily those of the RCSI emissaries; in the background were the ongoing H-Block hunger strikes, and there was much tension as to whether Reagan would weigh in with a comment. Curiously, with the RCSI occasion providing access to the President, the Irish government in fact made a behind-the-scenes request for US intervention.[100] In the event, no comment was forthcoming, and all enjoyed a dinner at Decatur House, where a Marine Corps quartet played Mozart and Moore's *Melodies*. Davis died the following year, but in June 1984, when President Reagan visited Ireland, Nancy Reagan came to RCSI to unveil a portrait of her father.[101]

THE BEGINNINGS OF THE BEAUMONT HOSPITAL SAGA

As with the higher-education sector, scrutiny turned to healthcare and the hospital system in the late 1960s. The key document in this regard was the Fitzgerald Report (1968),[102] which characterised the inherited hospital sector as 'outmoded and a hindrance to good medicine'.[103] Political inertia failed to follow through on many of the report's carefully considered findings, but a major development on the north side of Dublin can be traced to this analysis.

In 1978, O'Flanagan and McAuliffe Curtin were amongst the RCSI personnel on hand to watch Minister for Health Charles Haughey turn the first sod on what would become Beaumont Hospital. Conceived of as a replacement for RCSI's traditional teaching hospitals at Jervis Street and the Richmond, RCSI kept a close eye on Beaumont's progress for much of the decade it took to build – with good reason. Early on, it was discovered that the HEA did not propose to accept responsibility for the provision of clinical teaching facilities; in short, if RCSI want-

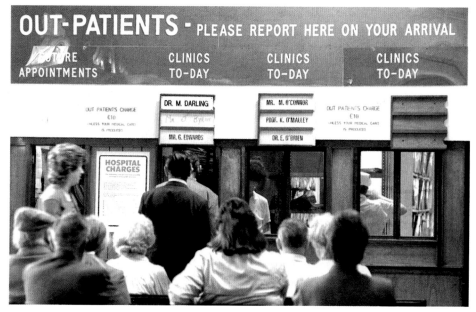

From *The Charitable Infirmary, Jervis Street, 1718–1987: A Farewell Tribute* by Eoin O'Brien (ed.), 1987. © Creative Commons.

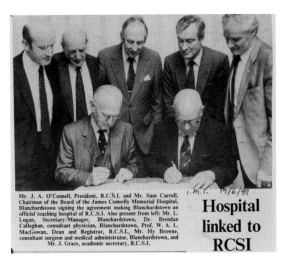

Mr. J. A. O'Connell, President, R.C.S.I. and Mr. Sam Carroll, Chairman of the Board of the James Connolly Memorial Hospital, Blanchardstown signing the agreement making Blanchardstown an official teaching hospital of R.C.S.I. Also present from left: Mr. L. Logan, Secretary/Manager, Blanchardstown, Dr. Brendan Callaghan, consultant physician, Blanchardstown, Prof. W. A. L. MacGowan, Dean and Registrar, R.C.S.I., Mr. Hy Browne, consultant surgeon and medical administrator, Blanchardstown, and Mr. J. Grace, academic secretary, R.C.S.I.

**Hospital
linked to
RCSI**

ed them, RCSI could build them.[104] It even fell to RCSI to provide the hospital's architect with a schedule of such facilities. There were fears too that there would be fewer beds in the new hospital than there were in the old ones.[105]

It was not until November 1982 that a formal teaching agreement with the hospital was concluded – by which time RCSI was already heavily invested: the estimated budget for teaching facilities had doubled from £500,000 in 1979 to £1 million in 1983. Later again, it transpired that there was no adequate provision for accommodation for doctors, nurses or students.[106] (Another bump concerned the hospital's name: Eoin O'Brien's strong advocacy to name the hospital after Dominic Corrigan – in which he was supported by RCSI and the various hospital boards – ultimately came to naught.[107])

During these years, RCSI was also securing teaching agreements with other hospitals, starting with James Connolly Memorial Hospital in Blanchardstown, with which there had been an unofficial agreement since 1973, formalised in 1981; four provincial hospitals were added later that year in time for October rotations: Our Lady of Lourdes, Drogheda; Louth County Hospital in Dundalk; Our Lady's in Navan; and St Luke's in Kilkenny. These were not cost-free ventures: inevitably, some refurbishment of local teaching facilities generally followed. Blanchardstown alone was spruced up to the tune of £17,000.

How to pay for it all? RCSI had lately turned a corner – in 1976/77, the College brought in £845,463 but spent £953,693; in 1977/78 income (£953,690) at last – and just about – exceeded expenditure (£914,129).[108] The ship had been righted, but that counted for little in the face of a prolonged recessionary tide. Closing his first *Annual Report* (1981), the new Registrar, W.A.L. MacGowan, spoke of 'the ominous inflation now affecting the country as a whole'.[109] Already, however, moves were being made to secure RCSI's future by looking to the east.

PROF W.A.L. MACGOWAN AND RCSI'S EASTERN CONNECTIONS

MacGowan had taken up his duties in the autumn of 1980, but he had had a long history with RCSI before that. He had enrolled during 'the Emergency' ('It was in the middle of the war... practically all Irish students in the year, very few overseas or anything like that. They couldn't get to Ireland anyway'[110]), qualifying in 1948 with first-class honours and the Council's gold medal for special merit; he became a Fellow in 1952. After stints in Ireland and Britain, he worked at the University of Khartoum in Sudan, beginning a long, productive relationship with that country. (In Sudan about this time, approximately 300 qualified doctors and 600 medical assistants were handling some 34 million out-patient visits; by

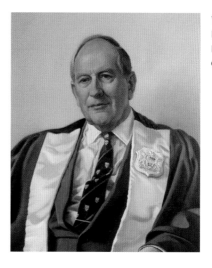

W.A.L. MacGowan, Registrar, by Carey Clarke.

the time Ahmed Abdel Aziz Yacoub – MacGowan's trainee and friend – was conferred with Honorary Fellowship of RCSI (1980), it was projected that soon more than half of Sudanese surgeons would have been trained in Dublin.[111] For his contribution to Sudanese healthcare, MacGowan was awarded the Order of the Two Niles in 1993.) Returned to Dublin, MacGowan performed one of Ireland's earliest kidney transplants at the Richmond. He was appointed Professor of Surgery at RCSI in 1967, shaping the department into a 'modern, progressive scientific unit'.[112]

By the time MacGowan was appointed Dean of the Medical Faculty (1974), eastern enquiries were under way. It had all begun the year before, when RCSI was invited to London to call on the ambassadors of Egypt, Kuwait, Bahrain, Saudi Arabia and Libya to discuss medical education. The travelling delegation comprised the Vice President (McAuliffe Curtin), the Registrar (O'Flanagan) and MacGowan. Relations with Kuwait were the first to take off: O'Flanagan visited the university in 1974, and again in 1976 for the foundation of the Medical Faculty; the following year an agreement was signed, and the Dean of Postgraduate Studies, Gearóid Lynch (Lic. 1955, FRCSI 1959), went out to organise a Primary Fellowship course.

Visiting RCSI staff came to teach and the Primary Fellowship exam was conducted there in 1978 (the examiners were from a number of Irish medical schools). This was the first time that a College examination was held outside Ireland, setting an exciting precedent for all involved. Provision was also made whereby Kuwaiti trainees could enrol in training courses in Dublin. As candidate numbers increased annually, relations were strengthened by Kuwait's donations towards RCSI research and building funds (£250,000 in 1978, £100,000 in 1983). In 1982, Dr Na'il Ahmed Al-Nageeb of the Kuwaiti Ministry of Health was conferred with Honorary Fellowship in Dublin.[113]

Similar progress took place in Saudi Arabia. In 1979, MacGowan was seconded to Dammam's King Faisal University, and the first RCSI Primary Fellowship course was held there in the winter of 1980. Thirty-three candidates took the exam the following January; when it ran for the second time a year later, the numbers had more than doubled.[114] Into the 1980s, an increasing number of Irish staff travelled out (in an interview in the *Irish Medical Times*, MacGowan described his time in Dammam as 'the most rewarding and exciting experience of his career'; he also warned, 'Watch who you go driving with!', as road traffic accidents were the commonest cause of hospital admissions[115]). A major milestone was reached in January 1985 when, for the first time outside Ireland, the Final Fellowship exams were conducted in Dammam. The first Saudi Honorary Fellow was the individual responsible for bringing MacGowan to the country, Dr Tawfik Mohammad Al-Tamini (1982) of King Faisal University.

In neighbouring Qatar, an agreement was signed in 1977 – in conjunction with RCPI – whereby consultant-level expertise would be provided in Doha, while Qatari students, nurses and para-medical staff would be educated or trained in Dublin.[116] A short time later, officials in the nearby island nation of Bahrain approached RCSI with a view to an agreement on the Qatari model.[117] An agreement of co-operation followed in September 1980, providing postgraduate surgical training as well as assistance with a proposed 'Pan Arab medical school'.[118] To attract further consultants, the Bahraini authorities took a full-page advertisement in the *Journal*: 'a very pleasant island to live on for Europeans without many of the irritating restrictions of its neighbours... about the size of Co. Dublin... originally a British protected state... became independent in 1971... well equipped but currently understaffed... the terms are very attractive by Irish standards'). In 1984, a further five-year agreement was signed with the Bahrain Defence Forces Hospital. The first Bahraini Honorary Fellow was the Emir since 1961, Sheikh Isa Bin Salman Al Khalifa (1995).

By contrast with all of the above, relations with Libya did not take off in the same way. As early as 1976, RCSI staff – notably Gearóid Lynch and Bill MacGowan – were at Garyounis University in Benghazi, contributing to the education of the first doctors to graduate from a Libyan medical school.[119] The students were enthusiastic, but facilities were basic and relations with the authorities 'unsatisfactory'[120] (in short, the university failed to pay RCSI for its services while advertising the prestigious connection[121]). The saga dragged out until RCSI cut ties in 1980. Then the following year Albert Reynolds, Minister for Transport, made a new effort to establish an Irish–Libyan exchange, inducing RCSI to get involved again. Warily, RCSI agreed to 'co-operate with any efforts... in the national interest'[122] – but nothing, as far as RCSI was concerned, came of this.

SUCCESS AND SUCCESSION: TWO FUTURE REGISTRARS, KEVIN O'MALLEY AND MICHAEL HORGAN

At the time of O'Flanagan's retirement, there had been lively speculation in the medical press as to his successor, as this would indicate RCSI's future priorities.[123] MacGowan himself later speculated that it was his experiences in the Middle East and Africa that made him the successful applicant in a contested field.[124] Described as a 'formidable figure', who brooked little interference with the implementation of his ideas – in his tenure, a few 'upheavals' with RCSI Presidents would occur – it was also noted that, in MacGowan, the College had 'no better servant'.[125]

The 'surprisingly smooth'[126] transition from the O'Flanagan era was due in no small part to the administrative team O'Flanagan had built up, notable figures being Joseph Grace, who started in 1973 as Academic Secretary – a role designed to take some weight from O'Flanagan's shoulders – and Michael Horgan (Hon FRCSI 2009), whose arrival in 1976, as Administrative Assistant, began three decades at RCSI that would eventually see him appointed Registrar/CEO in 2004. From the start, Horgan's affinity with the student body manifested itself in invitations to address the graduating class in their yearbook.

In 1976, another future Registrar/CEO joined RCSI. This was the new Professor of Clinical Pharmacology, Kevin O'Malley (Hon FRCSI 2004, PRCSI-MU Bahrain 2004–09), who brought with him ideas developed during postgraduate stints in Atlanta and Dundee. Indeed, O'Malley's career at RCSI may be seen as the necessary corrective – and then some – to the research deficiency O'Flanagan had admitted was the price of his infrastructural focus. Or, to quote Eoin O'Brien, who shared O'Malley's reformist zeal: 'The body-building phase is over and an era of intellectual development is now mandatory.'[127]

Even before O'Malley's appointment as Dean of the Medical Faculty (he succeeded Alan Browne in 1983), this progressive push was in evidence, whether at the level of scholarly citation – as incoming editor of the College *Journal* in 1979, he was the one to adopt the new Vancouver style[128] – or steering investment in expensive computational hardware.[129] (As a nation, Ireland had one of the lowest levels of medical research funding of any country in the EEC.) Addressing the Biological Society in November 1981, O'Malley made the point that medical research was not only 'an essential activity in a vibrant and progressive medical school', but also one that 'contributes significantly to patient care'.[130] Reflecting his particular interests, he pointed at strides made by pharmaceuticals: 95 per cent of all drugs in common use, he said, were entirely unknown thirty years before. That said, he did not expect panaceas: 'most drugs are used to control disease – few cure. There are therefore great challenges ahead.'

SECOND-WAVE FEMINISM AT RCSI

The Biological Society to which O'Malley addressed these remarks was in rude health, having celebrated its fiftieth session in 1980. Repeatedly over the years, the Society aired issues in advance of the media and medical mainstreams. 'LSD and its psychedelic effects' could be the subject one night, or 'the Biological Clock' another, led by Prof Richard Conroy (whose eminence on the subject of human circadian rhythms earned him invitations to address the European Space Research Organisation and other globetrotting bodies).[131]

Another night, the topic was homosexuality — then essentially criminal — when Prof Thomas Lynch (Psychiatry) argued that words like 'treatment', 'reform' or 'patients' were 'objectionable'.[132] In advance of Pope John Paul II's visit to Ireland in 1979, the Society held a tinderbox debate on family planning, with speakers including the future President of Ireland, Mary Robinson (Hon FRCSI 1994). (Two years later, following an assassination attempt, the Pope was treated by Prof Kevin Cahill (Tropical Medicine).)

Often it was students who brought the freshest perspectives, such as the occasion when Caroline de Costa (Lic. 1973) delivered her paper 'Motherhood without Marriage' in 1971.[133] De Costa was one of seventeen women in her class, along with 103 men, and her vivid memoir, *The Women's Doc* (2021), records barriers faced — and faced down — by female students in the era. ('No trousers on women in here young lady!' she was told on her first day. 'You'll have to go home and change. Come back in a decent skirt!' Within a year, the literal rise of the miniskirt made trousers suddenly acceptable.) De Costa also recalls in glowing terms Dr Anne Legge (Anatomy), a founding member of the Irish Family Planning Association, whose clinics were clandestine at the time and subject to Garda raids. De Costa was an activist herself, travelling on the famous 'Contraceptive Train' with her friend Nell McCafferty in 1971:

> In Belfast we bought condoms in large numbers, as well as clothes that were much cheaper there than in Dublin... We also wanted the Pill, but lacked prescriptions — so we bought aspirin tablets instead, figuring that Irish customs officers wouldn't know the difference. (They didn't. Some of them also apparently didn't know what a condom looked like; they thought they were searching for items the size of an erect penis.)[134]

In society in general, change is rarely linear — nor was it within RCSI. In 1976, PRCSI Frank Duff made a prescient case for facilitating mature students to study medicine (he proposed a quota system: 40 per cent of places for students with top grades, 40 per cent for those with average grades but who demonstrated motivation, and 20 per cent for the older cohort) – but on the same occasion he wondered if women were taking up too many places. 'In the long term,' he reasoned, 'it was more difficult for women to put the same energy and man hours into their practice as did their male counterparts...'[135] His bias here was roasted by a correspondent to the *Irish Times* letters page.[136] Not quite ten years later, in 1985, the same correspondent, Gemma Hussey – by then Minister for Education – again called out RCSI for discriminatory practice when she refused to attend a dinner to which women who were not Fellows were not normally invited. 'That is one tradition in Ireland we can do without,' she told the press.[137]

In 1982, there was a grand total of twenty-one Irish women surgeons, including – conferred with her Fellowship that year – Eilis McGovern.[138] Twenty-eight years later, in 2010, McGovern would be the first woman elected PRCSI (2010–12), making her the first female President of any of the Royal Colleges. (McGovern's status as lead surgeon at a new cardiac unit opened at St James' Hospital in 1999 earns her a fleeting mention in Barry O'Donnell's mammoth directory, *Irish Surgeons and Surgery in the Twentieth Century* (2008); for all that work's depth and significance, its dedication to 'the wives of all the Irish surgeons of the twentieth century' tells its own story.[139]) To To complete the picture, at undergraduate level, approximately one fifth of RCSI students were women; by the time of the Hussey dinner embarrassment, this had risen to one third. Gender parity was not reached until the early 2000s, after which the balance increasingly tipped in favour of women; a decade later, this figure had risen to 50 per cent.[140]

THE ADMISSIONS QUESTION

PRCSI Duff had (stumblingly) put his finger on a very contentious issue: how were medical students to be selected in the first place? And did top academic achievers necessarily make top practitioners, or was there room for other criteria? These questions needed to be set in the greater context too: how many medical students did a country need? How many could it afford to educate? Indeed, in the late 1970s and early 1980s, the Irish government set about reducing the numbers of medical students, making competition for entry more intense. At the turn of the decade, some 2,000 school-leavers applied through the Central Admissions Office (CAO) for 340 places at the four medical schools of Trinity, UCD, UCC and UCG.[141]

As the economist Mulvey had recognised a decade before, RCSI was a place apart – in its particular case, one that eschewed a strict points-based process. (RCSI's ongoing freedom to select its own students had been a key point in negoti-

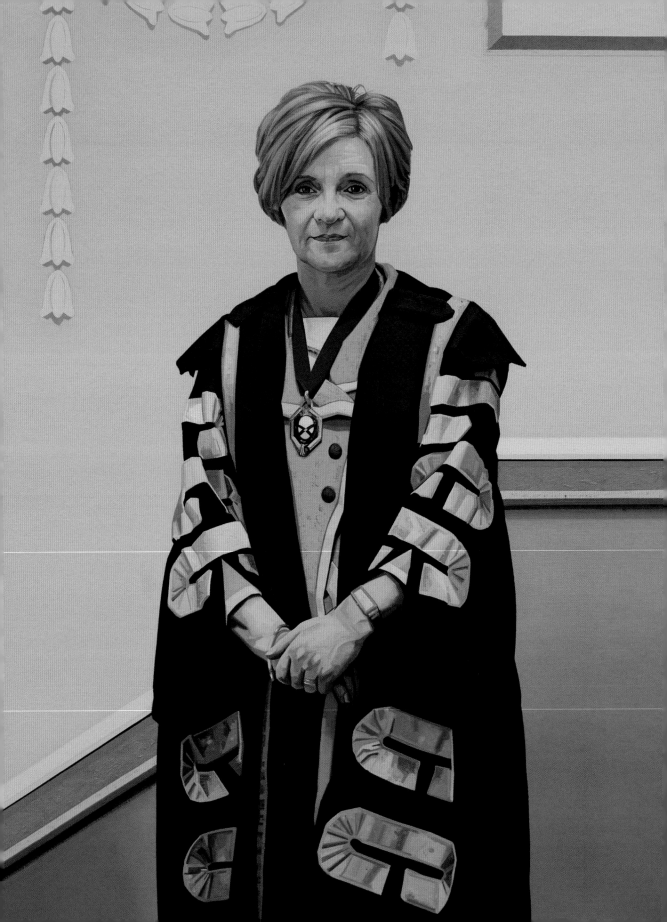

ations with both NUI and TCD regarding degree status.) Although RCSI accepted some applicants based on their Leaving Certificate results, its 130 places were not part of the CAO. Instead, by tradition, RCSI ran its own entrance examinations, on the results of which certain prizes were disbursed; later, formal interviews were also added to the process.[142] For the academic year beginning in autumn 1980, the HEA suggested that RCSI should reduce its number of Irish students to a trickle – that is, twenty-five. This was strenuously resisted, not least as such a reduction would effectively destroy the School's carefully curated 'rule of thirds'.[143] (UCC likewise disregarded the HEA's similarly reductive prescription.)

Being essentially self-financing, RCSI was in a position to ignore the HEA recommendations. But staying self-reliant was no easy matter, especially when the Irish punt was spiralling downwards in value. For students – that is, for their parents and sponsors – this meant rising fees: in 1975, incoming Irish students paid £450 per annum, those from the developing world paid £700, and those from the developed world paid £1,000. Five years later, in 1980, the respective figures had soared to £1,185, £5,645 and £6,995 (that year, as the punt continued to tumble, consideration was given to charging overseas students in sterling).

For Irish pockets, RCSI was at the painful vanguard with its prices – but within a few years the other schools were catching up; one 1983 report noted that fees for 'the State-subsidised medical schools are now nearly as high as those of the RCSI, which receives a miniscule grant from the State'.[144] (To put figures on this, RCSI's grant of £18,000 had not changed in a decade; UCD's medical faculty, meanwhile, received £3,000,000 in 1983.[145]) During this period, snipes at RCSI's admissions system were not uncommon in the Irish medical press, the grievance being that the College did not participate on a level playing field, that 'connections' put a thumb on the scales. It fell to Academic Secretary Joseph Grace to defend RCSI's practice:

> It is generally acknowledged that there is no perfect system of medical student selection – this College has evolved over many years a fair and reasonable system which produces a good standard of student and doctor. The College considers that its present system bears comparison with that in use elsewhere – in that it retains an element of evaluation and is not solely dependent on a computer print-out.[146]

In any case, with annual applications in the era cresting more than a thousand, RCSI could afford to – and could not afford *not* to – select its students with care.

Facing page: Eilis McGovern, PRCSI 2010-12, by James Hanley.

FIXTURES, FITTINGS AND FACES: THE 1980S BLEND OF OLD AND NEW

Any incoming students who made their way down York Street in the early 1980s met a mix of the old and the new. On the south side of the street were the remaining tenement houses as well a three-storey Salvation Army hostel;[147] on the opposite side, the whole street was now RCSI, itself a mix of old and new. Some of the old was showing its vintage: the stone work at the corner with St Stephen's Green was in poor repair, owing to the iron cramps that pinned granite blocks together having rusted ('Not alone was this unsightly but it was a possible hazard to pedestrians';[148] the fix would cost £150,000 and take several years). Inside, there were other changes: the Anatomy Room was refurbished with a new tiled floor and stainless-steel dissection tables; surgical scrub facilities were added too (total cost: £100,000[149]).

In the 1810 building, the hall and staircase were redecorated, while the Board Room received an extensive overhaul, notably with the addition of a new carpet from V'Soske Joyce of Oughterard, Co. Galway. (This bespoke carpet was much admired by guests, including Nancy Reagan, who reputedly ordered a similar model for the White House; the Board Room's ceiling is reflected in the carpet's decoration.) Out front, the façade was cleaned and new railings added either side of the door. All of this sprucing up was in anticipation of the upcoming Bicentenary year, 1984.

The new students did not see change, because they themselves were the change: they were greeted by the new Head Porter, Terry Slattery, who first took up the ceremonial mace in 1981 and made the role entirely his own. (The bedel's flat, in which his unfortunate predecessor had been imprisoned in 1916, was gone now too, replaced by a new audio-visual department.) For many years, the York Street foyer was presided over by Slattery and a large stainless-steel installation by the celebrated Norwegian artist Arnold Haukeland. This was unveiled in 1980 on Norway's national day, 17 May, by which time – apart from a resurgence in the 1990s – the heyday of Nordic students at RCSI had largely passed. As more and more students came from the Middle East, a prayer room was installed (1981). (Amongst the general populace, it was generally assumed that any Muslim people in the city were either trainee technicians at Aer Lingus or RCSI students. Catering for both groups, Dublin's first official Islamic Centre opened in Harrington Street in 1976.)

Student traffic was outbound too: from 1979, RCSI students participated in The Overseas Elective Scheme (TOES), whereby they spent extended periods working in hospitals in the developing world ('Though our contribution appears small,' wrote one participant, James Lucey (Medicine 1983), 'we believe an enormous amount of practical assistance can be given by students of the College.'[150]) The

Facing page: Head Porter Terry Slattery by James Hart Dyke.

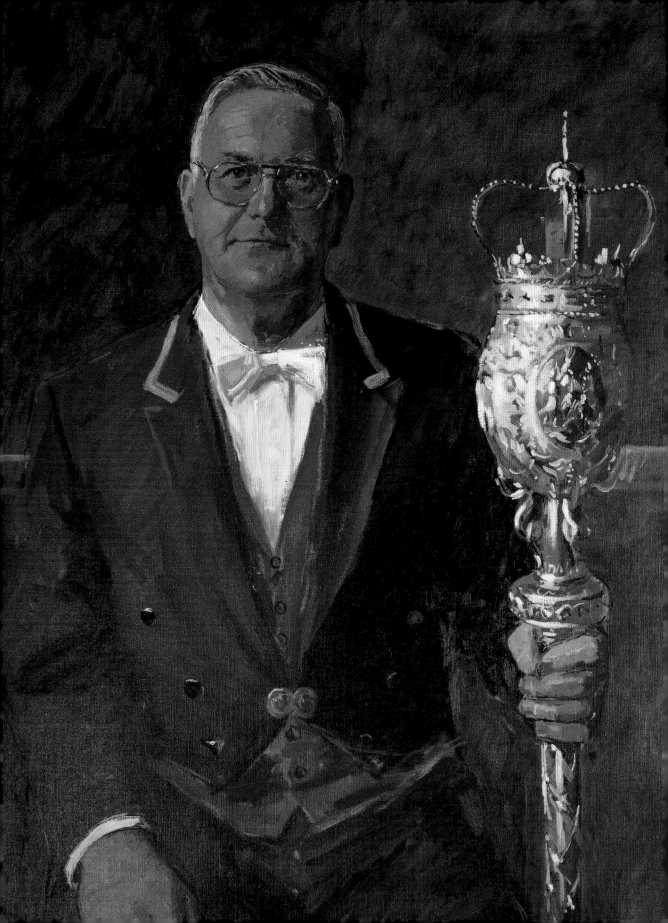

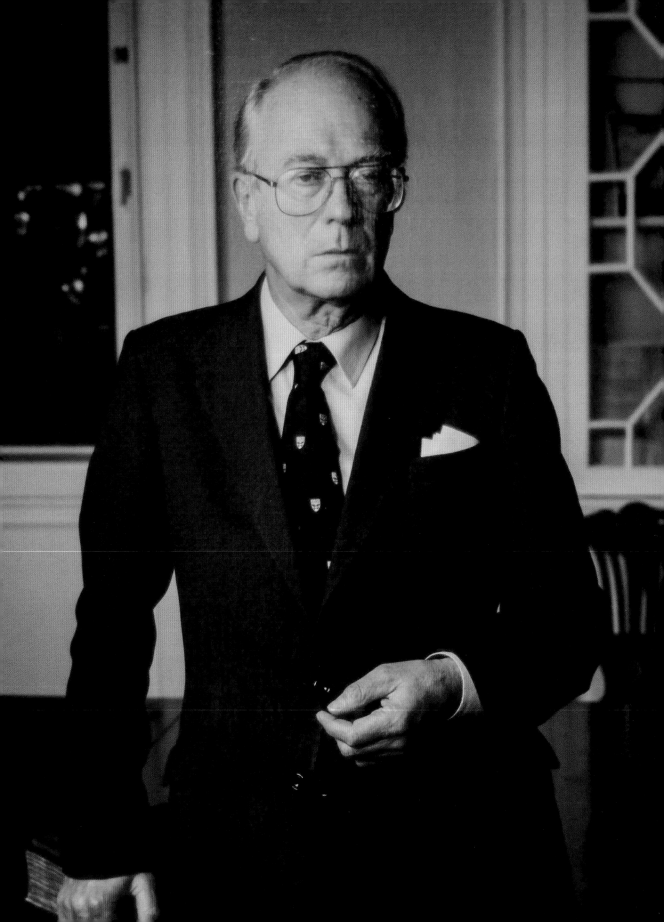

best record of RCSI's unique mix of cultures may be found in the annual Student Yearbooks. The same yearbooks pay passing tribute to the likes of Doreen Burns, the doyenne of the cafeteria, who was otherwise unlikely to feature in the more drily official records.[151]

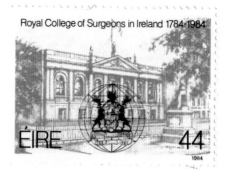

Stamp of recognition. RCSI celebrates its Bicentenary, 1784-1984.

In the Library, too, students and researchers grappled with old and new: a review of all facilities and resources was proposed in 1980, but the changes that came were piecemeal: late opening – until 9 p.m. – happened Tuesdays and Thursdays; an Apple II computer was acquired for literature reviews ('The cost of a basic search is £20.00, which covers up to 30 mins. computer time and can include up to 10 online references'[152]); a new ventilation system was installed, though it did not reach all areas: in the basement area, the Arthur Jacob collection, already suffering from dry rot (and 'the attention of rodents in the past'[153]) was steadily decomposing ('it would seem that a slow-eating fungus is attacking them'[154]). Space for readers was a problem too, and overflow seating was made available on the top floor of a house in Harcourt Street.

The need for accommodation space in general remained an issue. Bird Avenue had been slated for 'hostel' development, but a different solution arrived out of the blue, one that would solve the Library's problems too: in 1983, it was announced that the nearby Mercer's Hospital, including its adjacent nurses' quarters, was going to close, and before the end of the year, RCSI had bought it at a reported price of approximately £1 million. In many respects – not least with the Bicentenary around the corner – this acquisition had a pleasing symmetry: Mercer's was the site of RCSI's first settled location, and the hospital itself had a long association with many College Presidents, Professors and Council-members, such as Richard Butcher, William Wheeler, Leonard Abrahamson and Thomas Adrian Bouchier-Hayes (FRCSI 1934). The future development of the site was overseen by a committee, chaired by James Dermot O'Flynn (FRCSI *ad eundum* 1968, PRCSI 1992–94).

THE 1984 BICENTENARY CELEBRATIONS

Thoughts had been tending towards the Bicentenary celebrations for more than a decade – essentially, ever since the Colles Centenary had passed – but formal planning was in train from 1978, when a College Conference Centre was established; the inevitable sub-committees followed soon after.[155] House-

Facing page: Eoin O'Malley, PRCSI 1982-84.

keeping repairs and preservations were launched (not all of which, alas, were quite finished in time). The main Bicentennial elements followed the Colles event, just on a much grander scale. The year 1984 saw a suite of publications, including Lyons' *Assembly of Surgeons*, a new edition of Widdess' history, and an illustrated volume, *A Portrait of Irish Medicine*, by Eoin O'Brien, Anne Crookshank and Sir Gordon Wolstenholme; there was also a special issue of the *Journal*, which in addition to its historical essays also carried many of the contemporary letters of tribute that flooded in. 'It is with the greatest pleasure that I send my warmest congratulations and good wishes to the Royal College of Surgeons in Ireland on the occasion of its Bicentenary,' wrote the President of Ireland, Dr Patrick Hillery (Hon FRCSI 1977):

> Two hundred years of distinguished achievement have earned it well deserved respect and renown in the annals of healing. The College's contribution to the progress of medicine and surgery has been a most generous one. By their dedication and skill its alumni have brought lustre to its name everywhere.[156]

The year was also punctuated by an extensive programme of meetings, lectures and conferences, beginning with the formal Charter Day 'Symposium on Surgical Education and Training'. In September, RCSI hosted the International Surgical Scientific Conference in association with the Surgical Research Society and the Association of Surgeons of Great Britain and Ireland. The Faculties, too, convened commemorative meetings. The year's-worth of scholarship was published in two handsomely slip-cased volumes of 'proceedings'. International congratulations were generally addressed to the sitting PRCSI, Eoin O'Malley (FRCSI 1947, PRCSI 1982–84).

Few deserved the focus as much as O'Malley – 'the most influential surgeon in the Republic between 1970 and 1990'. A long-time Mater Hospital surgeon, and Professor of Surgery at UCD, O'Malley served 'on every local and national healthcare committee of consequence and was the first port of call when the Department of Health needed advice on almost anything'.[157] Trained as a general surgeon, his heart was in cardiology: he performed Ireland's first open-heart surgery (1957), and he was the first to use a heart-lung machine (1961) and the first to replace both a mitral and aortic valve (both 1965).[158] He was integral, too, to the formation of the National Surgical Training Centre (1970). At the Mater, the cardiothoracic unit he established was later named in his honour. In the Bicentenary year, he was conferred with honorary fellowships of the Royal College of Surgeons of England and the American College of Surgeons.[159]

As RCSI was honoured, via O'Malley, it too honoured others in return, conferring a record twenty-two Honorary Fellowships on surgical colleagues from Ireland, the UK, the USA, Germany, Switzerland, South Africa and Australia. The wider populace was appraised of the celebrations via an RTÉ documentary and – fulfilling a desideratum dating back to the Colles event – a stylish commemorative stamp, designed by the artist and dentist Fergal Nally (Lic. 1959, Lic. Dent. 1959, FFD 1969; the Fergal Nally Lecture was established by the Faculty of Dentistry in 2003). Appropriately for RCSI, Nally's stamp was priced for international mail.

And, as in 1884, there was of course a banquet, held on Charter Day. Four hundred guests at the black-tie event enjoyed a menu of smoked salmon, tomato and orange soup, roast fillet of beef, cheese board, desserts, coffee and *petits fours*, all complemented by dry sherries, Riesling and Château Palmer Margaux 1976. There were many distinguished guests, but the most senior was 85-year-old Dr Michael Elyan, who had received his Licence in 1921 (looking back on six decades of medicine, Elyan named antibiotics and lasers as the great innovations, while other changes impressed him less: 'In my time we dressed and looked like doctors, some of them look like tramps now...'[160]). In fact, the Charter Day dinner was the first of three banquets: the second, for the Council only, occurred in the Board Room of the Rotunda on 6 March, commemorating the location of the very first RCSI meeting on 2 March 1784. The third banquet came at year's end when, for the first time, *all* staff were invited to the Christmas party, a tradition that has endured. Lastly, a commemorative oak was planted in St Stephen's Green, close to Lord Ardilaun's statue.[161]

The closing words from this significant year go to PRCSI O'Malley, who was – characteristically – already looking ahead:

> An institution does not (or should not) grow old. It continues to exist; it may even mature, but it can and must avoid senescence. We must be careful not to be imprisoned in our history; we must be prepared to abandon any activity which is no longer useful and, if necessary, to get involved in new ventures.[162] ∎

Chapter 8:

New Ventures, 1985-2010

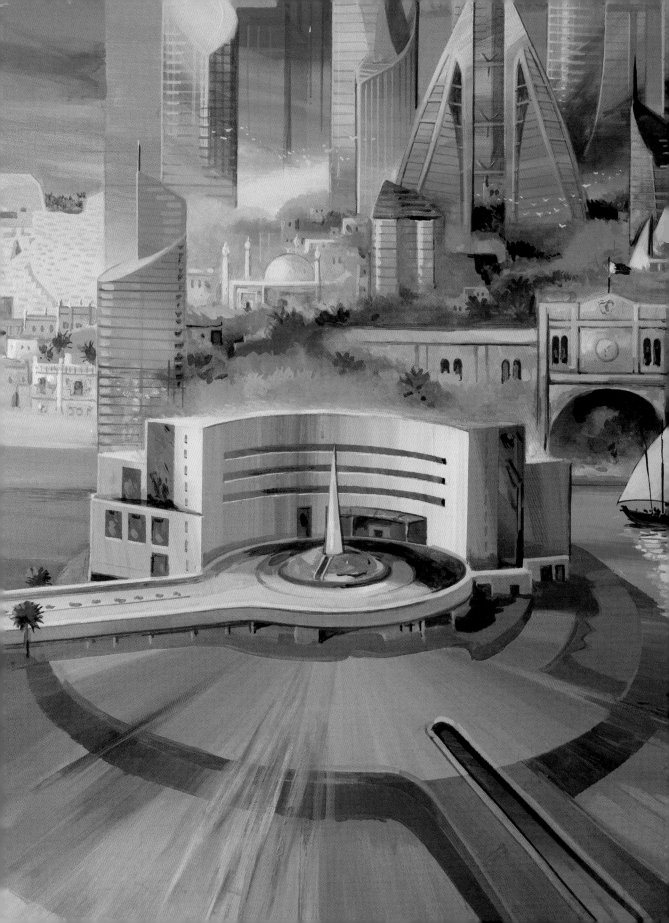

Chapter 8:
New Ventures, 1985–2010

TWO INTO ONE AT BEAUMONT

As RCSI entered its third century, two projects in particular were the outstanding priorities: the opening of a modern teaching hospital and the provision of student accommodation. Both were underway – the former at Beaumont, the latter in the precincts of the old Mercer's Hospital – and both would eventually prove successful. But neither had an untroubled time getting there.

The delivery of Beaumont Hospital was a protracted operation that covered none of its major players in glory. Begun in 1978, it was essentially finished in 1984, but did not open its doors until 29 November 1987. Blame for the delay is still debated, but certainly in the late stages it hinged on stand-offs between the government and consultants over the provision of on-site private practice. Throughout the process, RCSI was watchful, vocal and, unfortunately, largely powerless (commentary in Council Minutes and Annual Reports speak of 'anxieties', 'major disappointment' and the 'long drawn out saga'[1]).

There were concerns about the number of beds – for patients, for teaching and indeed for on-call doctors and nurses – and even after opening there was

Previous page: RCSI Bahrain (2011) by Abbas Al Mosawi. Presented to Kevin O'Malley, Founding President (2004-09).

widespread puzzlement about the campus's non-intuitive access points (this was a legacy of the cost-cutting idea to build the hospital as a carbon copy of Cork Regional Hospital – now Cork University Hospital – which had been tailored to fit its uniquely shaped site in Wilton). And yet for all that, it was a 'momentous' occasion, easily the highlight of RCSI's year. 'The transfer to Beaumont represents the merging of the two major teaching hospitals,' said Kevin O'Malley, then finishing his term as Dean of the Medical Faculty:

> and while this was not without some tension, it is true to say that we have settled in quite quickly on the new campus. We must consider ourselves most fortunate as academics to have such a first rate facility at our disposal. It provides great opportunities for academic development both educationally and for research.[2]

MILLIN HOUSE REDUX

Back in the city centre, the possibilities for the Mercer site seemed endless at the time of purchase – there would be a student hostel, yes, but maybe also a museum? Possibly a presidential suite? The Mercer's Committee, under the chairmanship of James Dermot O'Flynn, focused minds. With construction divided into phases, there would be accommodation, a new Library over three floors, and a General Practice clinic.

An initial architecture and engineering survey (July–September 1984) threw up some complications due to Dublin Corporation's ambition to run a road through part of the freehold of the Nurses' Home (that is, the southernmost section of the building along Mercer Street Lower as far as Little Longford Street). A quid pro quo agreement between RCSI and the Corporation resolved the issue. (In 2001, this corner was named in honour of the much-loved actor, Noel Purcell (1900–1985), born on the site.) The survey concluded that the building was essentially sound, but the city Fire Officer insisted that the old timber floors should be replaced by concrete.[3] Thus, having acquired the hospital at a 'very competitive price', a new and unavoidable expense presented itself. RCSI duly complied with the recommendations, the silver (or concrete) lining being that the reinforced structure would allow for an extra floor to be added on the roof.[4]

Phase 1 of the Mercer project, the transformation of the Nurses' Home into Millin House student residence – the name resurrected from the long-gone York Street location – was relatively swift. PRCSI Reginald A.E. Magee (FRCSI 1947, PRCSI 1986–88) officiated at the opening, on 30 October 1986, by which time all rooms were already occupied.[5] (The Belfast-based Magee knew the impor-

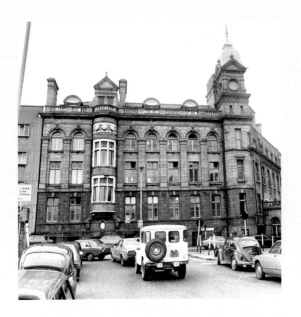

Mercer's Hospital, before the renovations.

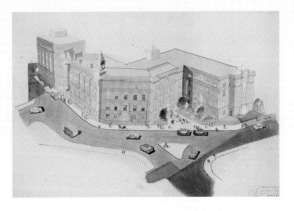

Architect's sketch for Mercer development, *c*.1988.

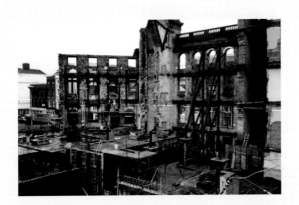

Mercer development, November 1989.

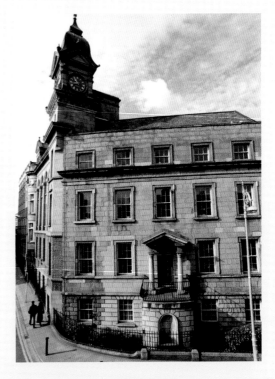

The completed Mercer building, with its first clock in the clock tower.

tance of a 'home away from home', not least as RCSI rented an apartment for him overlooking St Stephen's Green.[6] An obstetrician of international reputation, Magee was also politically active; he was elected to Stormont in 1973 as a member of the Ulster Unionist Party.)

THE MERCER LIBRARY

Phase 2 was the more complex provision of the Library and basement health centre. The utter transformation of Library services began with the appointment of Beatrice Doran, the RCSI's first professionally qualified Chief Librarian, in the spring of 1986. Among her first actions was the production of a 'comprehensive report' on Library facilities in St Stephen's Green.[7] There was long-standing affection for the space – at one point the Council expressed a hope to maintain the 'current character... in so far as it was possible'[8] – but Doran judged the 'present state of the library is totally inadequate for today's needs'.[9] Lock, stock and barrel relocation to the Mercer site was the only way forward. (Once Beaumont opened, Doran and her team were responsible for Library services there too; this was the largest hospital library in the country at that time. The first full-time professionally qualified librarian, Grainne McCabe, was appointed at Beaumont in May 1996.)

The adaptation of Mercer's 1960s Nurses' Home had been relatively simple – not so the rest of the hospital, parts of which dated to the mid-eighteenth century.[10] An Taisce – Ireland's National Trust – objected to RCSI's initial intention to demolish the building. By way of compromise, the façade was retained (adding £150,000 to the bill[11]); in addition, the clock tower was furnished with working clocks, something it never had before. Construction began in the summer of 1989; two years later, some 66,000 volumes were moved to their new home during the Easter break. (Not coming with them was Kathleen M. Bishop, Sub-Librarian, who had retired the previous December, after twenty-four years of service.)

Spread over three floors, and covering 2,500 square metres, the finish of the Mercer Library drew inspiration from contemporary American medical libraries; the entrance hall had a polished floor of pink Irish granite and dark-maroon Italian marble and oak-panelled walls, while the top floor featured purpose-built compact storage for archive materials (not just RCSI muniments, but also records salvaged from Jervis Street and the Richmond hospitals[12]). The greatest innovation, however, was the highly computerised nature of the Library service. Well ahead of the building's official opening, keen students were already at their new desks from April 1991.

A DEPARTMENT OF GENERAL PRACTICE

By this time, the General Practice at the basement level was already operating. This was at once a health centre catering for the local community and a pedagogic unit, the first Department of General Practice in an Irish medical school. Chaired by Professor William Shannon, the Department had begun life in the College's Harcourt Street premises in 1987,[13] while fourth-year students interned in some thirty practices in Dublin and Wicklow.[14] The benefits of this early introduction to patients were manifold, as RCSI lecturer Dr Peter Harrington outlined:

> Most obvious is the range of morbidity seen almost exclusively in general practice. More crucially, however, is the opportunity to see community aspects of illnesses which are otherwise seen by the student in a hospital setting. The student sees patients from presentation to resolution of illness, and sees management of illness in the community setting in which it occurs. The student is also introduced to psycho-social aspects of organic diseases. He or she can witness the effect of serious disease or disability on the family unit and the production of ill health through family dysfunction. Through domiciliary visiting the student gets the opportunity to meet the sick patient in the comfort or discomfort of his own home. How much different the rheumatoid arthritis sufferer looks sitting clothed by the fireside of her first floor flat than she did bathed and powdered in her hospital bed![15]

Coupled with expansion of the Departments of Psychology and Community Medicine and Epidemiology, this represented a new commitment to areas of training which, as the Dean of the Medical Faculty, Kevin O'Malley noted, previously 'did not have the prominence they should have in the Medical School'.[16] In some respects, the expansion of these population-based departments (as opposed to hospital-based) represent the embryonic stages of O'Malley's vision for RCSI – complemented later with the establishment of Schools of Physiotherapy and Pharmacy – as a multi-disciplinary health sciences institution with university aspirations.

The Mercer Building was officially opened on 12 September 1991 by President Mary Robinson (Hon FRCSI 1994), who noted that the occasion was 'not an opening in the usual sense, but rather the beginning of another phase in the history of Mercer's which has been part and parcel of the life of Dubliners for many generations'.[17] President Robinson was drawing on Prof Lyons' latest work, *The Quality of Mercer's: Mercer's Hospital, 1734–1991*, much of which concerns the institution's endless fundraising – including, most famously, the first ever performance of Handel's *Messiah* in 1742.

The new Library cost £4.1 million, raised largely by the College Development Fund and the generosity of graduates, Patrons and the Faculties.[18] Notable too was the 'Friends of the Library' campaign led by Doran and Dr Cliona Buckley (FFARCSI 1982, Physiology), whose events included one-woman performances by Fiona Shaw (known to one generation as a celebrated Shakespearean actress, to another as Harry Potter's aunt, and to PRCSI O'Flynn as his niece). The Department of General Practice, which also launched a research programme, received a substantial donation from the newly created Mercer's Hospital Foundation.

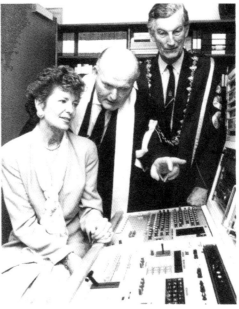

On the occasion of the official opening of the Mercer building, 12 September 1991.

THE PRESIDENT WAS SHOWN THE CLOSED CIRCUIT TELEVISION ROOM IN THE GENERAL PRACTICE UNIT WHICH IS USED FOR TRAINING MEDICAL STUDENTS TO DEAL WITH THEIR PATIENTS. PICTURED HERE WITH THE PRESIDENT, IS PROFESSOR WILLIAM SHANNON, HEAD OF THE GENERAL PRACTICE UNIT (CENTRE) AND PRESIDENT OF THE RCSI, WILLIAM P HEDERMAN.

The third and final phase of development on the site was the construction of further student accommodation, called Mercer Court. Begun in December 1992, with a seven-week archaeological dig, the residence was officially opened by Minister for Education, Niamh Bhreathnach TD, on 27 September 1993.[19] On the occasion, Bhreathnach voiced her willingness to support RCSI's long-cherished desire for the right to award degrees. A 'working party' was swiftly set up, chaired by Peter McLean, to steer strategy towards this goal. 'There are a number of routes we could take,' he later told an interviewer: one possibility was to become a constituent college of the NUI (a step beyond the current 'recognised college' status); another was to break with the NUI and establish a relationship with another university; and a third option – the most ambitious one, harmonising with O'Malley's disciplinary expansion – was to pursue wholly independent degree-awarding status.[20]

RCSI IN MALAYSIA: PENANG MEDICAL COLLEGE

Outside commentators expressed admiration that RCSI could accomplish so much without receiving substantial state funding[21] – but the truth was that the College walked a financial tightrope. The Bicentenary year, for example, was generally considered a great success, but there was also 'admonition' from the auditors for a too-heavy reliance on tuition fee income. A little later, in 1988, Joseph Grace spoke of how RCSI's financial resources were 'pulled in many directions at the one time... it is proving increasingly difficult for the College to satisfy all needs and at the same time to break even on its operation'.[22]

The Finance Committee had its work cut out in these years, as did long-serving accountant Cyril Irwin; he was later joined by Mary Alexander, who earned multiple entries in the College's roll-call of 'female firsts' as, successively, Planning and Management Accountant (1989), Financial Controller (1994) and Director of Finance (1998). The findings of a 1991 Financial Review in particular were somewhat stark. As future Registrar Michael Horgan later observed: 'The situation came to a head... when it was realised that, with hostilities building in the Persian Gulf, students from that region might be unable to get to RCSI, and those already in Ireland might be unable to access funds from their home countries... RCSI would be unable to survive more than a year or two without those fees.'[23]

For several decades now, RCSI's greatest asset was its internationalism, and so once again it looked outward to anchor its operations in diverse soils. This commitment to nurturing international connections was perhaps most visible in the form of Overseas Meetings – of which Arthur Tanner (FRCSI 1976) noted, 'There can be no future to a college that remains insular and introspective. Only by travelling abroad and witnessing first hand the problems and their solutions in other communities, can we address adequately the problems that arise in our own island.'[24]

Six of these Overseas Meetings took place in the run-up to the millennium: the first and fourth in Bahrain (1988 and 1995[25]); the second in Singapore (1989); the third in Malaysia's capital, Kuala Lumpur (1991); the fifth in Durban (1998); and the sixth back in Malaysia, this time in Penang (2000). On these occasions, RCSI Council and Fellows conducted formal and informal colloquia to exchange views and consolidate links; the conferring of Honorary Fellowships was a regular highlight.

Multiple visits to the Far East had similarly successful outcomes. Malaysian students had been coming to RCSI in Dublin since the mid-1970s; in the early 1990s, they represented the single largest overseas cohort, one quarter of the student body, many of whom were on scholarships from the Malaysian Ministry of Education. (Perhaps the most notable of these alumna is Wan Azizah Wan Ismail (Medicine 1978), Malaysia's first female leader of the opposition and first female Deputy Prime Minister.) In 1992, RCSI and a number of other international medical schools partnered with Malaysian authorities to establish Kuala Lumpur's International Medical College (IMC; from 1999, with university status, IMU), a

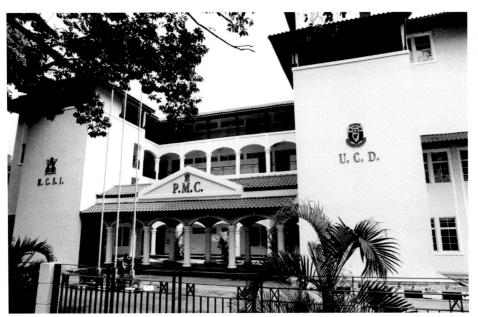

Penang Medical College, established 1996.

scheme by which students would spend their pre-clinical years at home, then undertake their clinical years in, and graduate from, a partner school such as RCSI.

In 1996, RCSI embarked upon an even more ambitious Malaysia-based venture: Penang Medical College (PMC), in the north-west of the country.[26] For this venture, RCSI was obliged to invite UCD to partner on the project, in order for PMC students to obtain the same NUI degrees awarded in Dublin; this was part of the complex, pre-existing arrangement worked out between RCSI and the NUI.

Almost immediately, the country's late-1990s financial crisis caused concern – but the RCSI's commitment to PMC was only strengthened by the official opening, in May 2000, of a Medical School building. From the start, PMC operated a reverse of the IMC model: students pursued their pre-clinical studies in Dublin, then returned home for their clinical years, where they were taught by RCSI staff as well as locally appointed consultants. Thomas Hennessy (FRCSI 1963, PRCSI 1994–96) was appointed Foundation Dean and Professor of Surgery. Named as an Irish medical university in the World Directory of Medical Schools, PMC became RUMC (RCSI-UCD Malaysia Campus) in 2018.

By the time it celebrated its twenty-fifth anniversary, in 2021, some 2,000 students had graduated from its programmes. To cater for this ever-expanding Malaysian community, RCSI had opened an alumni office in Kuala Lumpur in 1995. And a further milestone lay ahead: the launch in 2011 of a medicine programme in conjunction with Kuala Lumpur's newly established Perdana University.[27]

NELSON MANDELA'S TRIBUTE TO RCSI

Although fewer South African students now came to RCSI, the Overseas Meeting in Durban (1998) nonetheless underlined an enduring relationship. Two years before, in March 1996, a delegation travelled from Dublin to Cape Town to confer Honorary Fellowship on President Nelson Mandela, who paid this tribute:

> During the dark days of apartheid, your College provided places for many South Africans who were excluded by racist laws from the medical schools of their own country. More than 300 of the South African doctors practising medicine in our country today graduated in Dublin between 1950 and 1990. Through these doctors, you are making an inestimable contribution to the healthcare needs of our people.[28]

Many of those present in the Tuynhuys that day would have turned their thoughts to the late Dr Mohamed Essack of Durban, one of RCSI's first South African graduates and one of its greatest benefactors and supporters. There were other connections, too: the first Muslim elected to the Irish Dáil, in 1992, was Dr Moosajee Bhamjee, a South African Licentiate (1971) of RCSI. And in 1999, the College sent 2,500 soccer kits to children in a township outside Port Elizabeth. The presentation was made by Jim Sherlock, RSCI Soccer Team Manager as well as Head Porter (2001–13) in St Stephen's Green.

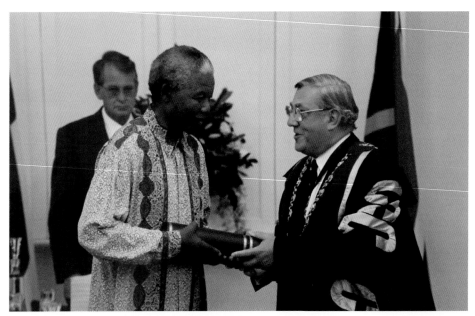

Nelson Mandela with Thomas Hennessy, PRCSI 1994-96.

RCSI RUNS A HOSPITAL IN SAUDI ARABIA

Through these years, teaching and examining continued to take place in several Gulf states, such as in Kuwait; in Jordan; and in Saudi Arabia, in Buraydah, Dammam, Jeddah and Riyadh. Two years after Crown Prince Abdulla Bin Abdulaziz al Saud came to Dublin to receive an Honorary Fellowship (1988) – PRCSI Desmond Kneafsey (Lic. 1945, FRCSI 1948, PRCSI 1988–90) made the point that the Crown Prince was only the second member of any royal family to visit the Royal College[29] – Saudi Arabia also became the location of RCSI's single most challenging overseas project of the 1990s.

Against competition from England, France, Canada and the US, RCSI won a contract from the Saudi Ministry of Defence and Aviation (MODA) to manage a 400-bed military hospital in the north-west of the country, at Tabuk. For the first time then, from July 1990, RCSI had a direct involvement in the running of a hospital, with responsibility to appoint senior staff, set standards of care and quality control, and develop education and research programmes. In turn, RCSI would receive Saudi financial support for its own research and development funds. W.A.L. MacGowan led the new project as Contract Director, having lately stepped down after a decade as Registrar. Day-to-day management of the hospital was subcontracted to Witikar Saudi Arabia Limited (WSAL).

A similar enterprise had been running in Iraq since the early 1980s, where a subsidiary of Aer Lingus, PARC, managed a hospital in Baghdad.[30] Following the Iraqi invasion of Kuwait (2 August 1990) and the outbreak of the first Gulf War, the PARC hospital was bombed. As a consequence, across the border in Tabuk there was an 'appreciable exodus' of both medical and nursing staff.[31] In the aftermath of the conflict, difficulties continued: promised consultant posts were hard to fill, local funding was cut by 37 per cent leading to shortages of supplies and delays in staff salaries (PRCSI Hennessy's 1995 Report spoke of 'a somewhat traumatic year'[32]).

Even so, there were many accomplishments and highlights: renal and corneal transplant services were established, an obstetrics and gynaecology outpatient clinic and a cardiac catheterisation clinic were opened, and several international symposia were hosted.[33] Laparoscopic surgery was introduced soon after it was pioneered at Beaumont. The Diploma in Child Health was a particularly successful programme. RCSI's contract was renewed twice – decisions not taken lightly in Dublin[34] – until the hospital was handed over to Saudi authorities in 1997. MacGowan later estimated that the Tabuk contract generated some £9 million for RCSI.[35] In a period when the College was running a deficit of about £500,000 per annum, this was both vital and hard-earned.[36]

A GROWING PROPERTY PORTFOLIO

There was widespread sadness at RCSI in May 1993, when news broke of the death of 'the most highly regarded and most universally liked person in the College'. This was John Robinson, porter and car-park attendant, known to several generations of staff and students as 'Johnny Carpark'. 'You could know the President and the Professors and the Deans,' said the Professor of Surgery, David Bouchier-Hayes (FRCSI 1969), 'but you could not get into the College of Surgeons unless you knew Johnny Robinson.'[37] If Robinson was irreplaceable, his domain was not: on this site, in 1996, RCSI – or, strictly speaking, a subsidiary holding – began construction of a 525-space multi-storey carpark.

The project was not without its critics, not least on environmental grounds, but Department of Finance tax breaks incentivised such construction (in 1990, there were four multi-storey carparks in the city centre; by 1998, there were twenty-two[38]). RCSI's contribution is aesthetically more sensitive than most, concealed behind a street-facing hotel with pedestrian-level retail units. The rationale for this development was simple, as PRCSI Hennessy put it: 'This College functions independently of Government support and must therefore behave very much as a business as well as an institute of learning.'[39] The car park was a joint venture, he explained; when a thirteen-year period elapsed, the entire income would revert to RCSI.

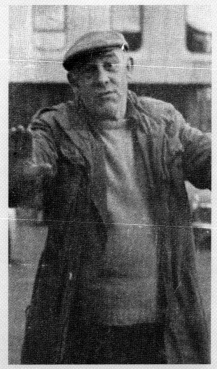

John ('Johnny Carpark') Robinson in his heyday.

In the meantime, RCSI would step further into the property development scene ('RCSI, venerable though it is, has a modern approach to property,' approved the *Irish Times*[40]). In 1987, RCSI acquired the former Carmichael School building off Aungier Street. There was a certain apt symbolism in this, given the schools' amalgamation some ninety-eight years before; but symbolism only went so far, and the same premises were offloaded in 1991. RCSI's three houses on Harcourt Street were sold in 1989, netting £1.6 million. At its best, RCSI could conjure inspiring space out of the most unlikely places, as in the metamorphosis, during the summer of 1998, of an outdoor yard behind the President's Room into the light-filled, chequerboard-floored Atrium.[41]

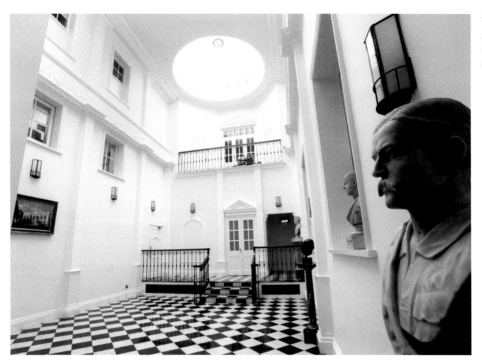

The elegant Atrium, formerly an outdoor yard.

The Mercer development dominated the next few years, but in early 1997 RCSI acquired 121/122 St Stephen's Green.[42] The Scott Tallon Walker-designed building cost £4.5 million – prompting PRCSI Hennessy to explain: 'Funding for the acquisition is borrowed and will be repaid through the earning capacity of the building, College reserves not being used.'[43] Tenants – including the Danish Embassy – remained *in situ* (for now). Around the corner, RCSI had in the mid-1980s acquired for a snip (£35,000) a small plot known as the 'Keatinge site'; playing a long game, the College patiently bought adjoining properties until it owned an island on which to build Beaux Lane House (2002).

By this time, third-level education in Ireland had moved to a free-fees model – though RCSI, being independent, did not qualify. Barry O'Brien, Director of Estate and Support Services, reiterated the College's policy: 'Any income from the office investment would be used to fund medical training.'[44] At the turn of the millennium, RCSI acquired its southside neighbour on York Street, the three-storey Salvation Army hostel (this was a site swap, whereby the hostel moved to modern facilities at the rear of Mercer Court, keeping its old name 'York House'). None of these city-centre developments would have been noticed by students, unless they read the property supplements. Other major changes, however, affected them directly – at Bird Avenue, at Dardistown and at Beaumont.

ADMISSIONS UNDER REVIEW

First things first: the students had to get in. With more applicants than places across all medical schools, the annual media-driven 'points race' frenzy generated the usual light, heat and, due to RCSI's singular interview-based process, complaints. In a 1991 interview, the Registrar, Prof O'Malley, rejected such sour grapes. As a scientist – he received a DSc based on published research from NUI this year, and was named as one of the top ten medical researchers in Europe[45] – he preferred to point to the evidence: 75 per cent of that year's intake had no obvious medical connections whatsoever; RCSI offered four full Irish scholarships and more partial ones, comprising a substantial proportion of the local student cohort; and the interview process, far from being a name-dropping opportunity, was designed in-house by the Department of Psychology as 'a serious attempt to assess the qualities' of future doctors.[46] (Elsewhere, the Professor of Psychology, Ciaran O'Boyle, pointed to the destructive nature of nepotism: 'Rather than living out their own lives,' he suggested, 'many people spend a lifetime trying to live up to parental expectations.'[47])

In fact, RCSI launched multiple initiatives to ensure prospective students had a clear-eyed vision of what a life in medicine entailed. These included free Christmas lecture series ('So you want to be a doctor?') and 'Open Days', including bus transport to Beaumont (somewhat ironically, these were so popular that there was a lottery for places). In a similar spirit of openness and outreach, RCSI launched the 'Mini-Med' programme, designed to bring the latest in medical education and research to the general public. In 1996, 450 Irish students were interviewed for forty places; the following year, when RCSI joined the CAO system, and applicant numbers rose to approximately 3,000, the interview system was retired. RCSI's separate entrance examination was held for the last time in 2000; thereafter, scholarships were awarded based on Leaving Certificate results. In 1985, the entrance fee for Irish students was £2,120;[48] in 1997, when the fee-free system started elsewhere, RCSI employed a two-tier fee structure: an EU fee (£4,600) and a non-EU fee (£16,000).[49]

There was a realisation in the late 1980s that, in a competitive global market, RCSI's reputation alone was insufficient to attract consistent numbers of overseas students.[50] A greater sense of strategy was required. The provision of campus accommodation was part of this, but so too were trips overseas by senior staff to promote RCSI, notably in the traditional markets of the Middle East, Malaysia and North America. Dividends followed: 1995 saw the highest number of applicants to date – 1,150 – from fifty-six countries. Students from Malaysia (forty-eight), USA (twenty-six), Kuwait (fourteen) and the United Arab Emirates (twelve) comprised more than half the incoming year; Irish student entrants were set at forty; there was also renewed representation from countries not seen in a while, such as India, Pakistan and Norway.[51] As these numbers suggest, the old 'rule of thirds' was giving way; some years a 1:4 ratio of Irish to overseas was not unusual, but any external pressure to reduce this further was 'resisted most strenuously'.[52]

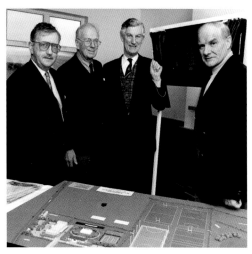

The official opening of Dardistown sports ground, December 1990. (L-R) Kevin O'Malley, Eoin O'Malley, William Hederman (PRCSI 1990-92) and Joe Grace.

MENS SANA IN CORPORE SANO: DARDISTOWN'S LEVEL PLAYING FIELD

The strong presence of Irish students was vital to protect RCSI's reputation, both at home and abroad, as an Irish school. But it was the cultural mix – showcased in events such as the annual 'International Night' – that gave RCSI its unique character, and in any given year, it was usually extracurricular activities that created lasting impressions. A Student Services Council – including, crucially, student representatives – was established in 1987. As well as advocating for student welfare – new health and counselling services were introduced – this body oversaw RCSI's vibrant sports and social life.

The 'Biological Society' remained the linchpin, where an annual highlight was the students' TOES reports (run by the Department of Tropical Medicine, this was one of the largest programmes of its type in Europe, with students on overseas electives in China, Pakistan, Vietnam, Kenya, the Solomon Islands, Uganda, South Africa, Ghana, Botswana, Zambia, Tanzania and the Gambia). By the mid-1990s, there were ten societies and twenty-six clubs, all receiving financial support. A major development in RCSI sport was the sale, in 1989, of the playing fields at Bird Avenue. This netted some £4.8 million, which at once funded the Mercer project and made possible the purchase and development of a new thirty-plus-acre sports ground at Dardistown, located south of Dublin Airport and north of Beaumont Hospital.

'Healthy bodies are synonymous with health minds,' declared PRCSI William Hederman (FRCSI 1957, PRCSI 1990–92), a keen sportsman himself, when he cut the ribbon on the grounds in December 1990:

> We regularly hear professional people saying that they have no time to
> look after their own health and their own bodies. This is a particularly

sad irony for those in the medical profession who are committed to the health and welfare of others. Through our Opening Ceremony here to-day, the Royal College of Surgeons is leading the medical profession by example and is stating loudly and clearly that sport and recreation have a lifelong, vital role to play in the hearts, bodies, minds and lives of all associated with this College.[53]

Further afield, RCSI sports teams embarked upon international tours, including Malaysia and Singapore (hockey, 1992), and the US and Canada (rugby, 1990; soccer, 1994; basketball, golf, 1996). From 1999, thanks to John V. Coyle (Lic. 1962, Distinguished Graduate Award 2002), RCSI participation in the Boston Marathon became an annual fixture. Rugby remained a key sport: from 1991, RCSI participated in an annual challenge match with Université Pierre et Marie Curie (now part of Sorbonne Université).[54] In 1995, final-year student Niall Hogan was

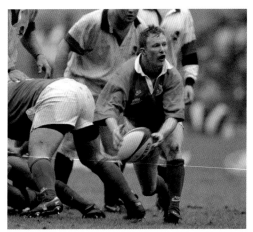

Ireland Captain and RCSI graduate, Niall Hogan, in action.

selected for the Irish national team, thereby missing his graduation ceremony (happily, a delegation from the College followed him to South Africa to present his graduation parchments). In 1991, the entire RCSI community mourned the sudden death of undergraduate Medicine student and keen sportsman Dan Kelly. An award in his memory was instituted, the Dan Kelly Gold Medal for 'all round excellence'.

CURRICULUM REFORM, DEPARTMENTAL EXPANSION AND THE NEW SCHOOL OF PHYSIOTHERAPY

In the immediate aftermath of the Bicentenary, there was talk of curriculum change, but the eventual report (1986) on the matter met with a 'mixed' reception.[55] One recommendation – early exposure of students to patients – had come to fruition via the Department of General Practice. Implementation of other elements – emphasis on genetics, immunology and infectious diseases – were more piecemeal. In 1988, the new Dean of the Medical Faculty, David Bouchier-Hayes, hoped that the humanities could be introduced in undergraduate teaching, but this did not come to pass.[56]

His successor, Hyacinth Browne (Lic. 1956, FRCSI 1969), also pushed for re-

forms: 'The curriculum is overcrowded,' he believed. 'Students are
being overloaded with facts, they're
being stifled in their development.
There's no room for any progres-
sion of free thought.'[57] One of his
aspirations was to reduce by a year
the long haul towards qualification
(this did not happen, although the
Graduate Entry Programme, introduced in 2007, offered a different
solution). In 2000, during the tenure of the next Dean, Alan Johnson
(Prof of Biochemistry, Hon FRCSI
2007), it was noted that new structures and procedures were 'consol-
idated': 'Curriculum reform contin-

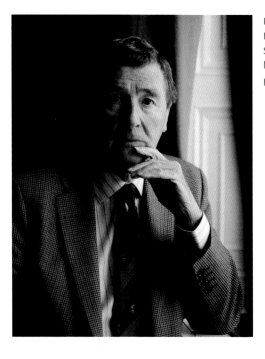

David Bouchier-
Hayes, Prof of
Surgery and
laparoscopic
pioneer.

ues at evolutionary rather than revolutionary pace.'[58] All reforms, of course, had
to conform to the guidelines of the Medical Council.

In some instances, however, those who believed in the virtue of impatience went
ahead with their own localised reforms – notably Stanley Monkhouse (Prof of
Anatomy), who reorganised teaching in his department by allotting a demonstrator for every two tables. His blue and pink student textbooks, as well as his published volumes *Cranial Nerves* (2006) and *Clinical Anatomy* (2007), further transformed the curriculum. One of his most important contributions to RCSI was his
introduction, in 1989, of the first Interfaith Service of Thanksgiving and Remembrance for those who donated their bodies for teaching and research. Relatives
and friends of the donors were invited to the service, the first of its kind held in the
Republic. A short time earlier, there had also been a Service of Remembrance for
Dr Anne Legge, long-serving Lecturer in Anatomy, who died tragically in 1987.

Between the Bicentenary and the millennium, academic expansion continued
steadily. Departments inaugurated in the period include Ophthalmology (1985),
Otolaryngology (this was a first for the Republic; 1991), Radiology (1992) and
Orthopaedic Surgery (at Cappagh Hospital; 1992).[59] Signalling further expansion
were relations with the Irish Society of Chartered Physiotherapists. This dated to
the 1980s, when the Society was a tenant in Harcourt Street; in 1994, the Society launched its programme of accreditation in the College; in 1998, RCSI was a
Founding Member of the Intercollegiate Academic Board of Sport and Exercise

Medicine – all of these strands reaching a culmination in the establishment of the School of Physiotherapy in 1999, with Prof Marie Guidon as its inaugural Head of School. This was a key move in the diversification of undergraduate courses offered by RCSI, and a major step towards the (as-yet *sotto voce*) ambition of creating a healthcare university. To accommodate the new School, Pathology and Microbiology moved to RCSI's latest major building project, the Smurfit ERC at Beaumont Hospital.

INVESTMENT IN RESEARCH AND DEVELOPMENT

In the late 1980s and early 1990s, medical research in Ireland was in a parlous state. When Kevin O'Malley spoke of the 'pathetically inadequate level of funding made available by the state,' he was referring to swingeing cutbacks imposed on the Health Research Board, whose budget fell in 1989 from £2.3 million to £1.3 million. 'Meaningful research is being carried out on a shoestring in this country...'[60] Within RCSI, excellent proposals were being turned down due to lack of funds. But a culture shift coinciding with O'Malley's tenure as Registrar turned RCSI into a research powerhouse. Early signs came in the form of an expansion of the main pharmacology laboratory (1986), which in time led to the founding of SurGen, a gene-mapping joint venture between RCSI and a French company, Genset.

As the new Prof of Clinical Pharmacology, Desmond Fitzgerald, explained: 'the beauty of the map is the huge scale of genetic investigation it facilitates, compared to cumbersome studies of familial links of disease which were invariably done

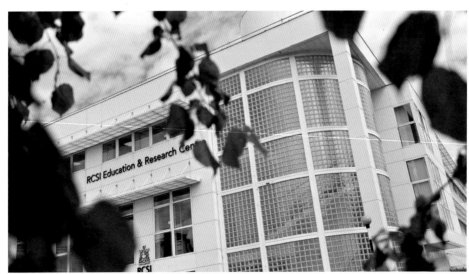

RCSI Education and Research Centre, Beaumont.

in the past'.[61] SurGen was housed in new £1.5 million facilities on the roof of the Medical School. Indeed, all departments became intensively research-active: staff publications were so numerous that by 1997 the Annual Report had to be split into two parts to accommodate the full list of references. As more academic departments relocated to Beaumont, space on the hospital campus became increasingly scarce. A new Clinical Science Building was proposed in 1994, becoming the focus of another fundraising drive within the RCSI community. Opened in September 2000, the three-storey RCSI Education and Research Centre, Smurfit Building, was financed by the HEA, alumni and donors – notably Michael Smurfit, the first Irish business-person to receive Honorary Fellowship (1997); the final cost came to £10 million.[62]

The major surgical innovation in this period was the advent of laparoscopic – that is, keyhole – cholecystectomy into Irish surgery (1990), led by Prof Bouchier-Hayes. No sooner was this introduced than training courses and best-practice guidelines were formulated. A new surgical skills simulation laboratory followed (1995), largely furnished by a £30,000 donation from Ethicon Ltd. By this time, the Report of the Science, Technology and Innovations (STI) Advisory Council had opened government eyes to the importance of STI in a modern high-tech economy.

When the ensuing Programme for Research in Third Level Institutions was launched (1998), RCSI successfully bid for inclusion, receiving a first tranche of £331,000. In the next decade, PRTLI funding would change the face of biomedical research in Ireland, with RCSI's share growing larger in each cycle. Between this programme and the flagship ERC Smurfit Building, RCSI had come of age as a modern, research-focused institution. That said, not every brilliant idea required vast sums of money and the latest technology. A project initiated by Dr Joseph Barnes (Tropical Medicine) and taken further by Dr Kevin McGuigan (arriving as Lecturer in Physics in 1991) involved the use of solar UV radiation to disinfect drinking water in low-income countries. For this project, Prof McGuigan was awarded the 2019 UNESCO Prize for International Research in the Life Sciences.

MANAGEMENT THINKING – OR, *WHO MOVED MY CHEESE?*

The challenge of these years was managing unprecedented levels of change at all levels of the institution. Unsurprisingly, then, management was a watchword of the era: as early as 1988, Prof MacGowan had identified the need to 'introduce management as a subject into the undergraduate medical course, so that our future doctors will, at least, have some exposure to the principles of management, which they can further develop in their postgraduate careers'.[63] Catering for doctors already at work, a Diploma in Healthcare Management was launched in 1992.

The course was run in collaboration with the Institute of Public Administration, with the RCSI contribution steered by Prof Bouchier-Hayes and Prof Austin Leahy (Leahy also edited the *JICPS* and its successor, *The Surgeon*, a joint publication of RCSI and RCS of Edinburgh). The success of this programme led to the establishment of Ireland's first Master of Business Administration in Health Sciences (1996), a collaboration between RCSI and UCD's Graduate School of Business and Faculty of Medicine.

Almost a decade later, RCSI's expansion into the field would see fruition in the Graduate School of Healthcare Management (2005); in the meantime, Spencer Johnson, author of two multi-million-selling business books, *The One Minute Manager* (1981) and *Who Moved My Cheese?* (1998), visited to share his insights; this was a return visit for Johnson, having qualified from RCSI in 1968. And in another sign of the times, the title 'Registrar', in use since 1832, no longer carried the weight it used to, especially for outsiders; the designation was thus expanded towards the turn of the millennium to 'Registrar and Chief Executive Officer'.[64]

RCSI's achievements did not go unnoticed by the wider Irish business community: in 2004, RCSI received the Ernst & Young Entrepreneur of the Year Special Award for an Organisation. On that occasion, many followed the lead of former Taoiseach Garret FitzGerald (Hon FRCSI 2002) in pointing to Kevin O'Malley's 'crucial role' as Registrar/CEO.

FELLOWSHIPS AND SURGICAL SPECIALTIES

In some respects, management and leadership development were hardly new at RCSI. This, essentially, was the institution's brief since 1784, at least as far as Irish surgery was concerned. But 200-plus years on, the many functions of that responsibility operated according to a Gordian knot of a system, especially when it came to postgraduate training. Prof Eoin O'Malley was famously succinct ('His most imitated characteristic was that of never using one word where none would do'[65]), but even he found the 'rather confused situation' difficult to cut through.[66] This was the end of the 1980s; the next decade was characterised by widespread if incremental reform, with minds focused by the prospect of greater European integration. Conditions for Fellowships of any of the four Royal Colleges of Surgery were also being overhauled.

When Fellowships were first introduced – 1843 in England, a year later in

Ireland, thanks to the Supplemental Charter – the accreditation designated a fully trained surgeon. Subsequently, as training expanded in duration and complexity, the Fellowship came to denote a midpoint in eventual qualification. In the aftermath of two world wars, when specialties made great leaps forward, the Royal Colleges' Fellowship fell out of step with North America and Australasia, where specialty board certificates and Fellowships were awarded at the end of specialty training. As a result, the fact that the Royal Colleges' Fellowship still designated mid-training accreditation was an anachronism and, perhaps worse, confusing to aspirant students overseas.

In 1989, intercollegiate exit examinations were introduced, after which Specialty suffixes were awarded – such as FRCS (Orth). Candidates thus had two Fellowships by examination, one in general surgery and one in a chosen specialty. The year 1991 saw the first of a new breed, the Intercollegiate Fellow,[67] while the Calman Report (1993) further changed the process, dividing training into two periods, Basic Surgical Training (BST, two years) and Specialty Training (five to six years). For candidates who entered BST after July 1996, the Fellowship of the Royal Colleges would once again represent an exit qualification and the hallmark of a fully trained surgeon.[68] (If Sir Kenneth Calman's report provoked some headaches at the Royal Colleges, no one at RCSI held it against him: he was awarded Honorary Fellowship in 1997.)

Beyond these islands and Europe, RCSI had been a founding member of the International Federation of Surgical Colleges since 1958; from 1984 to 1991, the Secretariat of this body was based at RCSI, with Prof MacGowan as Honorary Secretary.[69] Fruitful joint meetings took place with the American College of Surgeons (1988, when Joseph Murray was awarded Honorary Fellowship, two years before his Nobel Prize) and the Mayo Clinic (1996). American relations were to the fore in the wake of the 9/11 attacks: President of RCSI Thomas George Parks (FRCSI *ad eundum* 1983, PRCSI 2000–02), who was admired for his 'conciliatory' style, hosted a reception at the ACS annual meeting in New Orleans the following month; as Parks' successor, Michael R. Butler (FRCSI 1969, PRCSI 2002–04) noted, 'The support of so many Irish Fellows was greatly appreciated so soon after the tragic events'.[70] PRCSI Butler served on the Council for more than twenty years and chaired numerous important committees before his presidential tenure.

And yet, for all these advances, there was some inertia too. Despite 50 per cent of the undergraduate population being female, 92 per cent of consultants were male; the glass ceiling remained firmly in place.[71] RCSI elected its first female Council-member – future PRCSI Eilis McGovern – in 1994.

AMBASSADORS FROM THE REPUBLIC OF CONSCIENCE – AND ELSEWHERE

As specialisation – and medical education generally – became increasingly all-consuming, RCSI regularly invited guests to raise the institution's collective gaze. Many of these visitors were invited by Prof Kevin Cahill, under the auspices of the Department of International Health and Tropical Medicine's annual lecture. Speakers included the MP David Owen (1991) – himself a medical graduate – and

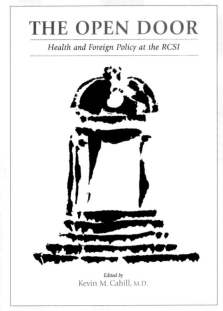

former UN Secretary-General Boutros Boutros-Ghali ('It might be appropriate in these ancient medical halls to note that, in my experience, preventing the malady of conflict may be even more difficult than preventing the diseases that afflict the mind and body of human beings',[72] 1997); Dr Oliver Sacks, author of *Awakenings* and *The Man Who Mistook His Wife for a Hat*, told his audience that 'one cannot be a physician without imagination and empathy, without an intense effort to imagine oneself in another's position'[73] (1998).

The Open Door: Health and Foreign Policy at the RCSI (1999), edited by Kevin Cahill, with cover image by Louis le Brocquy.

Amongst Irish speakers was John Hume, three years before he received his Nobel Prize, who quoted Martin Luther King:

As long as there is poverty in the world, I can never be rich even if I have a billion dollars. As long as diseases are rampant and millions of people in this world cannot expect to live more than twenty-eight or thirty years, I can never be totally healthy even if I just got a good check-up at Mayo Clinic. I can never be what I ought to be until you are what you ought to be. This is the way our world is made. No individual or nation can stand out boasting of independence. We are interdependent.[74]

There would have been those in the audience who remembered when the Troubles threatened to come to RCSI's door: in December 1985, the Academic Board had to hurriedly adjourn a meeting due to a bomb scare in the College.[75] US Senator George Mitchell and Hume's SDLP party colleague Seamus Mallon would receive Honorary Fellowships in 2002 and 2006, respectively.

Another key player in the Peace Process visited RCSI in 1998: US President Bill Clinton. The occasion was not uncontroversial – Clinton was embroiled in scandal at home and had recently authorised air strikes on Sudan and Afghanistan (also, his visit displaced a graduates' ten-year reunion) – but the new car park, bedecked in flowers, allowed his cavalcade to sweep in discreetly for lunch in the College Hall. Among the 200 guests were Gerry Adams and Seamus Heaney – the latter a regular visitor to RCSI since his 1992 A.K. Henry lecture (again, RCSI stole a march on the Swedish Academy by three years).

Heaney was awarded Honorary Fellowship of RCSI in 1998 – but even when he was absent, he could make his poetic presence felt: on one occasion when he was unable

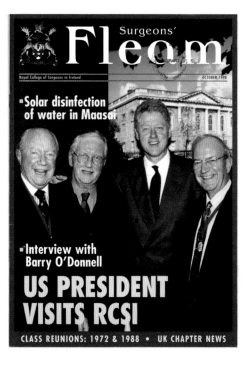

Surgeons' Fleam, with (L–R), Barry O'Donnell (PRCSI 1998-2000), Kevin O'Malley, Bill Clinton, George Parks.

to attend the Charter Day dinner, he sent his apologies in the form of a 22-line rhyming letter addressed to Louise Loughran, then Conference & Functions Officer, later Chief Communications Officer. Other eminent authors who visited – again in 1998 – were Toni Morrison (Nobel Prize for Literature 1993) and John McGahern.

Continuing the literary theme, the publisher Paul Hamlyn was made an Honorary Fellow and a member of the Court of Patrons in 1993; for many years, he had sponsored scholarships for students from Lesotho. Another Nobel Laureate, Samuel Beckett, had personal ties to RCSI figures – Dean Crowley and Prof Thompson – but he never quite represented the College. Or did he? On the occasion of Trinity's 400th anniversary, RCSI's gift to the Provost was a copy of *The Beckett Country: Samuel Beckett's Ireland* by Prof Eoin O'Brien. The book was signed not by the author, but by his friend, the subject: 'the only book Beckett signed that he did not write'.[76]

Dean Crowley died in 1990; two years later, her citation for Mother Teresa as the first Honorary Fellow of the Faculty of Nursing was read at the conferring ceremony in the courtyard of Rome's San Gregorio church. A year later, Mother Teresa came to Dublin, where she was awarded Honorary Fellowship of the College. 'She offers a remarkable inspiration to our young doctors, who are graduating today,' said PRCSI O'Flynn, 'many of whom will travel to distant countries to care

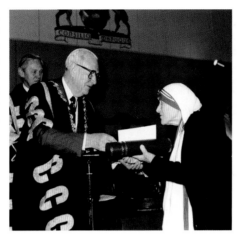

Mother Teresa
receives her
Honorary
Fellowship
(1993) from
James Dermot
O'Flynn, PRCSI
1992-94.

for the sick.'[77] (Others, such as Dr Jack Preger MBE (Lic. 1971, Distinguished Graduate Award 1995), founder of Calcutta Rescue, discerned a great gap between religious devotion and actual medical care.[78])

Through these years, RCSI continued its tradition of honouring Irish Presidents with the Honorary Fellowship: Mary Robinson was thus conferred in 1994, and Mary McAleese – who, as Prof McAleese of Queen's University, had previously delivered the 1996 Gilmartin Lecture – in 1998. Michael D. Higgins delivered the Robert Adams lecture in Galway in 1993, as a government minister; as President of Ireland, he received his Honorary Fellowship in 2016.

Y2K AND BEYOND 2000

The single greatest change in medicine and medical teaching between the Bicentenary and the year 2000 was in computerisation. RCSI's pioneering prime mover in the field was Michael Horgan, who succeeded Angela Butler (after forty-six years' service) as Assistant Registrar in 1985. The Annual Report that year noted the proud purchase of a DEC Vax 11/750, a waist-high 'minicomputer' with 8MB of memory.[79] Initially, the ambition was to allow for word processing in administration and streamlining in finance, but opportunities related to examinations and student and graduate record-keeping were quickly recognised.

Soon enough, Council recommended that 'a Computer Professional' – note the singular – 'be appointed to the Administrative Staff to take responsibility for computer/information systems in the College'.[80] A lectureship in Biostatistics and Medical Computing was also proposed, and filled by Rónán Conroy in 1987. At this time, RCSI had a single fax machine, located in the Library. Following Horgan's lead, Beatrice Doran made the Library central to RCSI's embrace of technology: state-of-the-art library management software was purchased, which connected to Beaumont Hospital Library via a leased Telecom Éireann data line; barcoded library cards for staff and students were introduced for the first time;[81] and when Mercer opened, the digital jewel in its crown was the Medical Informatics Laboratory equipped with twenty-four Macintosh LC computers. The future was the CD-ROM, particularly for Medline searches – until the future became a newfangled thing called 'the Internet': in 1993, a makeshift cable linked networks in Mercer and St Stephen's Green, superseded by a 64KB line to the HEA network. In 1996, RCSI launched its first official website, a quiet development with Gutenberg-like ramifications.[82]

From October 1995, students were being issued their own personal laptops (the Macintosh Power-Book). This was a first for any European medical school, spearheaded by Michael Horgan. By the end of

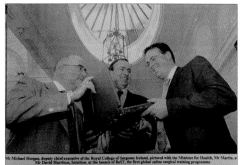

BeST (Basic electronic Surgical Training) is launched, 2000.

the academic year, 39 per cent of students had email accounts.[83] In 1999, RCSI students received the first Apple iBooks delivered to Europe. The much-feared Y2K changeover came and went without a sound. Finally, in March 2000, at the overseas meeting in Penang, a major new Training and Education project, BeST (Basic electronic Surgical Training), was launched. Again conceived by Horgan, BeST attracted worldwide press coverage as the first online training programme for surgeons. With surgical content guided by Dean of Postgraduate Studies, Oscar Traynor (FRCSI 1978), more than 100 practitioners and academics contributed to BeST's 5,000-plus webpages of modules, tutorials and interactive programmes.

AMENDMENT OF THE CHARTER AND ARTICULATION OF A 'NOBLE PURPOSE'

As a charity since 1965, RCSI's fiscal rule of thumb was to break even while using any gains to fund ongoing activities. For much of the first decade of the new millennium, RCSI was in bullish financial health, allowing for rapid expansion in all directions. The running deficit of the mid-1990s had been reversed; in the year ending September 2000, RCSI recorded a surplus of £1.6 million (this included income from the car park and in-house subsidiary companies such as SurGen). A year later, the surplus ran to £2.3 million, though day-to-day costs continued to 'present a challenge'.[84]

In 2002, Beaux Lane House opened (instantly fully let, rental income was projected to cover borrowings and interest in seventeen years), and in December RCSI purchased a second investment property, the Ardilaun Centre, on the corner of St Stephen's Green and Cuffe Street, the £75 million cost of which was financed by a long-term loan. At this point, the declared ambition was to avoid large surpluses, with expenditure closely matching income,[85] but after an initial dip, surpluses rose sharply, from €3.98 in 2006 to €16 million in 2007, the latter spike explained by the sale of a portion of the land at Dardistown. Staff numbers also increased significantly, almost doubling from 300 to 580 in the eight years from 1993 to 2001; by the end of the decade, the figure had risen further to 822.

To guide such expansion, RCSI engaged the services of the management consultants, McKinsey and Company. One result of this commission was the articulation in 2004 of what was called RCSI's Noble Purpose:

> Building on our heritage in surgery, we will enhance human health through endeavour, innovation and collaboration in education, research and service.

That surgical heritage came under pressure from within and without. Within, there was a need to modernise governance, particularly in relation to the Charter. Last modified in 1965, when the transformative charity status was secured, this was not something the College entered into lightly. Inviting the input, not to say interference, of outsiders, was inherently risky. Indeed, as soon as the bill was proposed, there were 'off stage mutterings'[86] from certain quarters of the Dáil about the College's 'royal' designation.

In extensive Seanad debates, this objection — and every aspect of the proposed changes — was debated at length, with independent Senator Joe O'Toole expressing forcefully the general consensus:

> People who cannot accommodate their history should find a different place to live. This is the name of this distinguished college. I might say this is the distinguished name of this distinguished college. In that sense we should reflect on the fact that this is where it is rooted and that is what it means. It is a good reminder of the length of our history and that we should not spend our lives flattening out the spaces in history. That is not the way we do our business; we look at it in the round and we deal with it. I hope we have matured as a nation. I certainly know that everybody in this House will have grown up and matured to the point where we do not need to blow up Nelson's Pillar once again. We can leave it sitting there and deal with it. This college has given significant and important service, both to this island and abroad, and has brought the image of Ireland, in practical and special terms, to other places. It has done us much service in that area. It behoves us to be supportive of this attempt by the college authorities to progress and also to look at ways they can make changes in the future.

Others, equally supportive, took the view that a 'royal' name was 'plainly just a common sense marketing tool'. Approved in both Houses, the Royal College of Surgeons in Ireland (Charters Amendment) Act 2003 was signed into law by President McAleese on 14 July – Bastille Day. For RCSI, perhaps the most revolutionary detail of the act's twenty pages of close-printed legalese was Section 30 (b), under the rubric of 'Additional powers of the College':

> ... to provide courses and examinations and *to award degrees* [emphasis added] in such of the following disciplines, that is to say, surgery, medicine, nursing, radiology, pharmacy, anaesthesiology, physiotherapy and dentistry, and in such further disciplines, as may be provided for by Bye-Laws made by the Council of the college.

For the remainder of the decade, this extraordinary development sat quietly on the books. In the meantime, myriad other deletions and insertions attempted to clear up inherited confusions and redundancies. (Consider, for example, the somewhat farcical spectacle of Edward Haughey accepting his Honorary Fellowship in 1998, by swearing an oath that 'I am twenty-five years of age and upwards... and that I do not now practice the business or profession of an apothecary or druggist, or indirectly sell drugs or medicine, and that I will not, so long as I shall be a Fellow of the said College, practise such business or profession.'[87] Haughey – Baron Ballyedmond – was a multi-millionaire pharmaceutical entrepreneur.) Two other notable changes allowed the College to confer Membership, as opposed to Associate Fellowship, on basic surgical trainees, and to confer Fellowship by special election, as opposed to by examination. The first recipient of the latter award was Prof S. William Gunn of the WHO Medical Society, in 2005.

COLLABORATION WITH THE COLLEGE OF SURGEONS OF EAST, CENTRAL AND SOUTHERN AFRICA

With the Charter hurdle cleared, the College continued to shift surgical training from the inherited apprenticeship model to a more active, taught, competence-based model. While statutory oversight of postgraduate training lay with the Medical Council, the Council in turn relied on the RCSI-led Irish Surgical Postgraduate Training Committee to manage the programmes. As Director of Surgical Affairs, Professor Arthur Tanner steered RCSI through the major questions of the day: the European Working Time Directive, surgical audit, manpower, human factors, investment in virtual reality simulators, to name but a few.

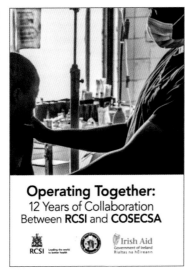

Operating Together (2019). Cover photograph by Antonio Jaén Osuna.

BeST was in worldwide use by now, and regularly edited and overhauled, augmented by a complementary online platform, SCHOOL for Surgeons. Both catered to trainees where they were, avoiding the need to travel. So too, in its own way, did the Mobile Surgical Skills Unit (on the road from 2006). Sometimes, however, travel was a pleasure, as in the Overseas Meetings – in Hong Kong (2002[88]), Dubai (2004) and – the focus of so much RCSI energy in the decade – Bahrain (2006).

Also overseas, the last pillar of the Noble Purpose – service – was exemplified by RCSI's collaboration with the College of Surgeons of East, Central and Southern Africa (COSECSA). This had its origins in the wards of Jervis Street in the 1970s, when two early-career surgical registrars – Gerald (Gerry) O'Sullivan from West Cork and Krikor Erzingatsian (Lic. 1969, FRCSI 1976) from Addis Ababa – became friends. Some thirty years later, in 2006, PRCSI O'Sullivan (2006–08) was invited by COSECSA's President Erzingatsian to attend an AGM in Malawi.

At the time, O'Sullivan brought a €10,000 donation from RCSI, but all involved knew that piecemeal funding, however welcome, would not adequately address the region's ratio of one surgeon for every 200,000 inhabitants (the Irish ratio, by way of contrast, was 1:10,000).[89] In August 2007, a memorandum of understanding was signed to develop an inter-institutional structure for surgical training and assessment. RCSI's embrace of electronic surgical training tools, coupled with Ireland's reputation as a non-colonial nation, fostered the process. Funded by the Department of Foreign Affairs' Irish Aid, the RCSI-COSECSA collaboration flourished; by 2019, more than 600 surgical trainees were enrolled in COSECSA programmes,[90] and that same year saw the publication of a history-so-far, *Operating Together: 12 Years of Collaboration between RCSI and COSECSA*.

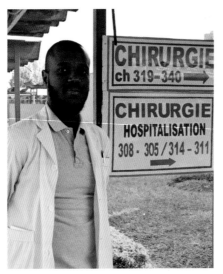

Dr Clovis Paulin Baramburiye, COSECSA trainee, Burundi.

In 2011, PPRCSI O'Sullivan was awarded Honorary Fellowship of CO-SECSA, while RCSI returned the favour to Prof Erzingatsian in 2016. On the same theme, RCSI underlined its commitment to humanitarian work by awarding Honorary Fellowships to Live Aid founder and lead Boomtown Rat, Bob Geldof, and US President Jimmy Carter (both 2007). Similarly, in March 2009, the United Nations presented its first ever award in Human Rights, Reconciliation and Humanitarianism, to Prof Kevin Cahill.

Closer to home, the College was obliged to react to national legislative developments, such as the Medical Practitioners Act 2007, obliging

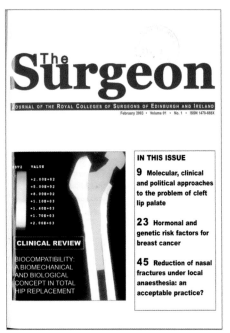

Ever-closer ties with Edinburgh: *The Surgeon*, 2003.

healthcare professionals of all types to register with their designated body to record Continuing Professional Development. For surgeons, this was via RCSI's Colles Portal. As international harmony was worked towards, the UK's introduction in 2005 of the Postgraduate Medicine Educational and Training Board (PMETB) meant that for the first time RCSI no longer had a role in the quality assurance of surgical standards or in training instruction in Northern Ireland. Conversely, RCSI enjoyed ever-closer relations with its Edinburgh counterpart. From 2003, both Colleges jointly edited a new journal, *The Surgeon* (the new title replaced the *JICPS*[91]); for Edinburgh's 500th anniversary (2005), Dublin gifted a stained-glass window to Nicolson Street (the artist, George Walsh, had recently completed a millennium project triptych of windows in the Albert Theatre (2002).

Above all, the surgical focus through these years was on an initiative known in planning as the Colles Institute. This was to consist of three elements: a National Surgical Training Centre (NSTC), a Centre for Clinical Research and Development (CCR&D) and a Centre for Innovation in Surgical Technology (CIST). The Institute was to be built on York Street, where the remaining houses – Georgian in appearance but in fact 1940s replicas – were in poor repair. In 2005, Dublin City Council sold one third of the site to RCSI for €12 million, then demolished the entire stretch. Smart, modern social housing was built on the portion retained by DCC, opening in 2009. RCSI's ambitious new contribution to the street, for which excavations – the first set – began in 2008, would take a little longer.

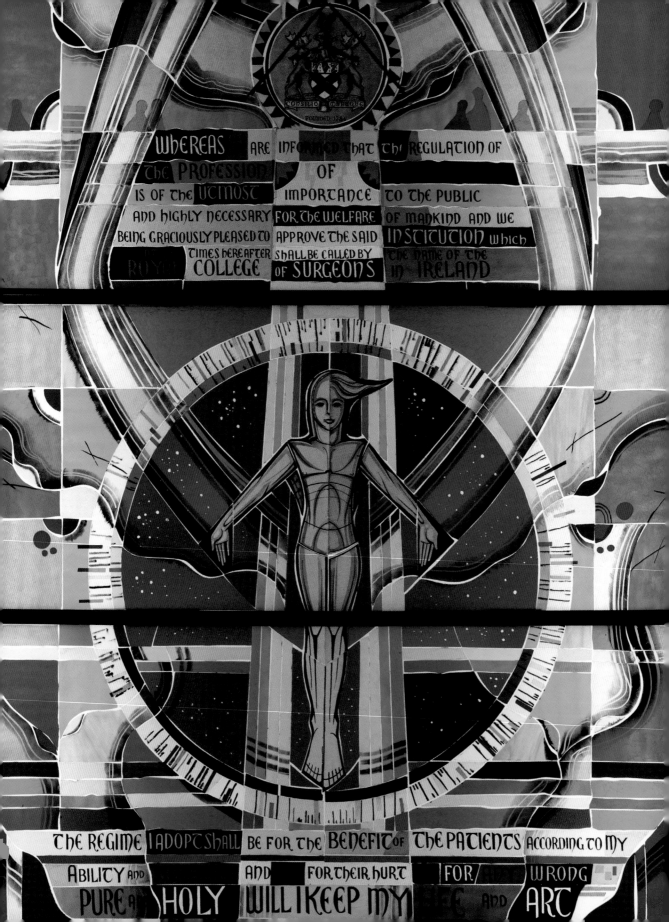

THE GRADUATE ENTRY PROGRAMME AND SANDYFORD

The world's first university was founded in Bologna in 1088, and it was in Bologna again in 1999 that European Ministers of Education issued a Declaration to work towards a more harmonious system of easily readable and comparable qualifications. The trickle-down effect of this was to produce curriculum change in RCSI. Moreover, RCSI voluntarily committed to adopting the World Federation of Medical Education Guidelines, for which a new Curriculum Board was established, chaired by Prof Cathal Kelly. A Beaumont-based vascular surgeon, Kelly was a graduate of RCSI (Medicine 1985, FRCSI 1990) and winner of a number of prestigious awards, notably the Patey Prize of the Association of Surgeons of Great Britain and Ireland. The revised curriculum's modular structure was the catalyst to introduce a four-year Graduate Entry Programme (subsequently renamed Graduate Entry Medicine to differentiate it from similar routes to other disciplines).

The first sixty entrants (half of them EU students, half from North America) commenced the GEP course – the first in the country – in September 2006.[92] Based in RCSI's latest acquisition, Reservoir House, in Sandyford, the addition of these students made RCSI the largest medical school in the State. (Sandyford is 7km from St Stephen's Green, but thanks to Dublin's reintroduction of a tramway system in 2004, students could flit from one campus to the other in the time it took to queue for a latte – Ireland's first Starbucks opened on the same Luas line in 2005.)

Clinical facilities for GEP students were at new facilities in Connolly Hospital, opened in September 2007. Prof Alan Johnson (Biochemistry) led the GEP programme, having completed his eight-year tenure as Dean of the Medical Faculty in September 2006. One of the last major innovations he oversaw was the 2005 introduction of a Virtual Learning Environment (VLE), Moodle. He was succeeded as Dean by Prof Cathal Kelly.

THE SCHOOL OF PHARMACY AND YORK HOUSE

Having started a new phase of growth with the 1999 establishment of the School of Physiotherapy, the Faculty of Medicine and Health Sciences (this was a broader designation than heretofore, introduced mid-decade) continued to expand in the new century. In 2002, RCSI established the second School of Pharmacy in Ireland (the other was at Trinity), with Prof John Kelly as its inaugural Head of School; in September, fifty-four students began their four-year programme leading to the degree of BSc (Pharmacy). Entry to the School's first postgraduate programme – MSc in Industrial Pharmaceutical Science[93] – also took place that year.

Facing page: From George Walsh's Millennium triptych (2002), in the Albert Theatre.

345

York House, York Street, on the site of the Salvation Army's hostel of the same name.

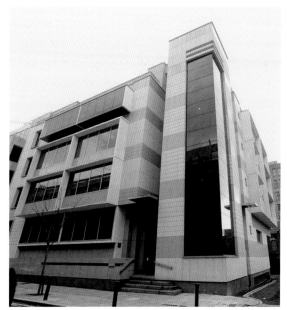

The new School benefitted immediately from close links to the College's Biopharmaceutics Research Institute. In 2004 both parties had the good fortune to move into a new, purpose-built home for pharmaceutical sciences, York House – officially opened by An Taoiseach Bertie Ahern the following June – on the site of the former Salvation Army hostel. The laboratories and office space of York House also accommodated the new Centre for Human Proteomics and the Centre for Advanced Drug Delivery. In 2009, the School won a competitive tender for the provision of the National Pharmacy Internship Programme for all student pharmacists in Ireland, for which successful interns were awarded a Master's in Pharmacy (MPharm).

THE SCHOOL OF POSTGRADUATE STUDIES AND THE INSTITUTE OF LEADERSHIP

As such fourth-level activity expanded College-wide, a School of Postgraduate Studies was established in September 2006, with Prof Kevin Nolan (Chemistry and Physics) as Foundation Head of School.[94] The School introduced structured PhD programmes, which encompassed taught modules, laboratory rotations, and university and industry placements both at home and abroad. Also under the Faculty's umbrella was the Institute of Leadership (founded in 2005 as the International School of Healthcare Management), which brought together the management and leadership training activities of various RCSI departments and units.

Directed by Prof Ciaran O'Boyle, the Institute was based at Reservoir House in Sandyford, and in Dubai Healthcare City, from where it also ran programmes in neighbouring states, notably Jordan and Bahrain. To return to the School of Physiotherapy, towards the close of the decade it introduced Ireland's first MSc in Neurology and Gerontology – an acknowledgement of wider demographic changes in Irish society.

In other changes, from 2003, ever-increasing numbers of RCSI graduates meant that conferring ceremonies were moved to the National Concert Hall (as it happens, directly across the road from the Irish Medicines Board – later the Health Products Regulatory Authority – whose premises were named Kevin O'Malley House in 2005, in recognition of Prof O'Malley's leadership in the regulation of medicine and medical devices).

GROWTH AND EVOLUTION: DEVELOPMENTS WITHIN THE FACULTIES AND THE ESTABLISHMENT OF THE FACULTY OF SPORTS AND EXERCISE MEDICINE

Throughout the period, the postgraduate Faculties grappled with the same issues of accreditation, training, assessment and professional development. Notable occurrences included the departure of the anaesthetists to form an independent entity, the College of Anaesthesiologists of Ireland (1998). The Faculty of Radiologists marked the centenary of their specialty with *A Century of Medication Radiation in Ireland* (1995); they also fostered connections with Kuwait and Malta, and conferred President McAleese with Honorary Fellowship (2006). When Max Ryan (Medicine 1993, FFRRCSI 1999) was appointed Dean (2016–18), he was following in the footsteps of his namesake father (Lic. 1951, FFRRCSI 1961; 1979–81).[95]

The Faculty of Dentistry launched the Fergal Nally lecture series in 2003, with Dr Nally himself as the inaugural lecturer; amongst subsequent non-dental contributors were the poet Brendan Kennelly and the explorer Tim Severin. When Dr Peter Cowan (FFDRCSI 1984) was elected Dean of the Faculty (2001–04), this was the first Faculty Deanship of *père et fils*, as his father, Adrian, a Founding Fellow, had been the second Dean (FFDRCSI 1963; 1966–69). The Faculty promoted collaboration with sister Colleges in the UK, with the Irish dental schools, and with the Dental Council through the Irish Commit-

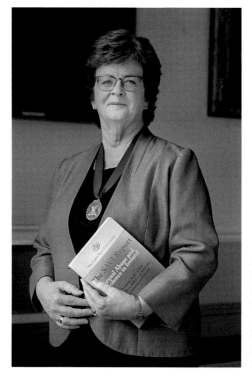

Prof Hannah McGee, holding a copy of the landmark *SAVI Report*. Photographed by Amelia Stein, 2020.

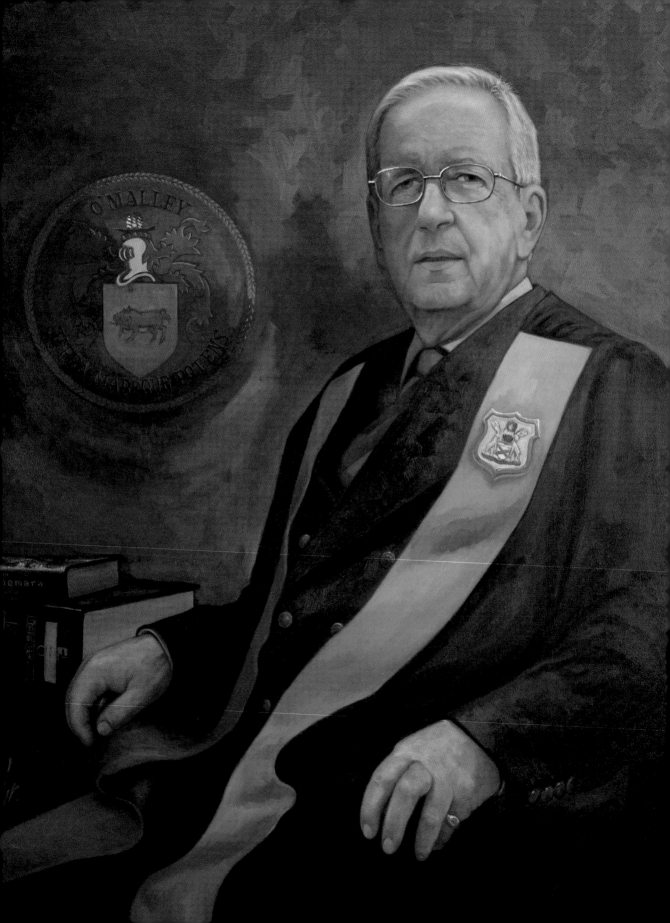

tee for Specialist Training in Dentistry (2001). Further afield, it examined and maintained standards in the Middle East – notably Kuwait – North Africa, Sweden and the USA.

Not least due to sheer numbers, the Faculty of Nursing and Midwifery was one of the most productive of College bodies. In 2001, under the aegis of the Faculty, RCSI established an undergraduate School of Nursing in partnership with St Michael's Hospital, Dún Laoghaire (this replaced a similar, short-lived late-1990s collaboration between RCSI, Dublin City University and Beaumont Hospital), with Prof Seamus Cowman as inaugural Head of School. Amongst the many specialist courses run by the Faculty, the Higher Diploma in Nursing Sexual Assault Forensic Examination (2009) stands out. In the year of the Ryan Report, the course can be seen as part of RCSI's contribution to a wider societal acknowledgment of some of the darkest aspects of Irish society – a process arguably ushered in by the landmark *SAVI Report: Sexual Abuse and Violence in Ireland* (2002) led by Prof Hannah McGee of the Department of Psychology.

In its choice of Honorary Fellows, the Faculty of Nursing and Midwifery consistently exhibited prescience and imagination, from President McAleese (1999) to Justice Mella Carroll, Ireland's first female High Court judge (2002), to Mary Davis of the Special Olympics (2004), and Mary Donohoe of the East Africa-based HIV/Aids charity, the Rose Project (2010).

Finally, there was the establishment of RCSI's first new faculty in almost thirty years, the Faculty of Sports and Exercise Medicine (2002). A first of its kind in Europe, this was a joint Faculty of RCSI and RCPI, with Prof Michael Molloy (Hon FRCSI 2007) – former Irish rugby international and Medical Officer to the IRFU since 1979 – as inaugural Dean. In recognition of his support in setting up the Faculty, the first Honorary Fellowship was awarded to Prof Kevin O'Malley (2004). That same year, the College awarded O'Malley its own highest honour. Delivering his citation for Honorary Fellowship, Vice-PRCSI Niall J. O'Higgins (FRCSI 1970, PRCSI 2004–06) pointed to O'Malley having transformed 'the educational and research life of this country':

> He is the quiet catalyst of progress. As a professor, he has played a large part in Ireland's scientific growth; as an educationalist, he has accelerated our cultural development; as an administrator, he has contributed to our social evolution; as diplomat, he has enhanced our international standing. Mr President, Kevin O'Malley has truly brought this country forward.

Facing page: Prof Kevin O'Malley, CEO/ Registrar and PRCSI Bahrain (2004-09) by Abbas Al Mosawi.

RCSI-MEDICAL UNIVERSITY BAHRAIN

By the time of this award, Prof O'Malley had stepped down as Registrar/CEO – he was succeeded in September 2004 by Michael Horgan – only to step up as Foundation President of RCSI-Medical University Bahrain. Without question, this was the key development of the decade. The first conversation on the subject took place at the College's Overseas Meeting in Penang in 2000. In attendance was Dr Faisal Al Mousawi, Bahrain's former Minister of Health and President of the Shura Council. Impressed by the fledgling Penang Medical College, he wondered aloud about a comparable venture in his country – or, verbatim, he asked: 'Why don't you do this in Bahrain?'[96]

The idea was supported in both Dublin and Bahrain. Following the signing of a Memorandum of Understanding (2003) and various feasibility studies, the new Medical School was officially opened in October 2004 by His Highness the Prime Minister of the Kingdom of Bahrain, Shaikh Khalifa Bin Salman Al Khalifa (Hon FRCSI 2003) and the Taoiseach of Ireland, Bertie Ahern TD. Twenty-seven students comprised the first intake, from Bahrain, India, Italy, Kuwait, Pakistan, Saudi Arabia, the United Arab Emirates, the USA and Yemen.

At this point, the school was in temporary accommodation, as planning progressed towards a permanent campus. Two particular questions presented themselves: where would the campus be located, and where would the students avail of clinical facilities? In the event, both questions had a single answer. Bahraini authorities were already planning the King Hamad General Hospital (KHGH) at Busaiteen on Muharraq Island – Bahrain is made up of thirty-three such islands – midway between the airport and the capital city, Manama. RCSI leased the land next door to the KHGH site. 'There was one problem,' noted Colin Stewart, Associate Director of Estate and Support Services: 'The land in question was on the sea bed of the Arabian Gulf.'[97]

Reclamation and infilling began, raising dry land above mean sea level by January 2005. A little over a year later, on 13 March 2006, the foundation stone was jointly laid by His Highness Shaikh Khalifa and the Tánaiste and Minister for Health and Children in Ireland, Mary Harney TD. The build faced difficulties – local shortages of cement and glass, the fact that the site was not connected to the public grid and a temporary power source had to be installed – but it was ready for the first students to begin taking classes in October 2008.

The official opening – by President McAleese, with Shaikh Khalifa and RCSI President Frank B.V. Keane (FRCSI *ad eundum* 1991, PRCSI 2008–10) in attendance – took place on 3 February 2009. 'Not only has RCSI moulded great medical graduates,' noted President McAleese on the occasion, 'it has also created a

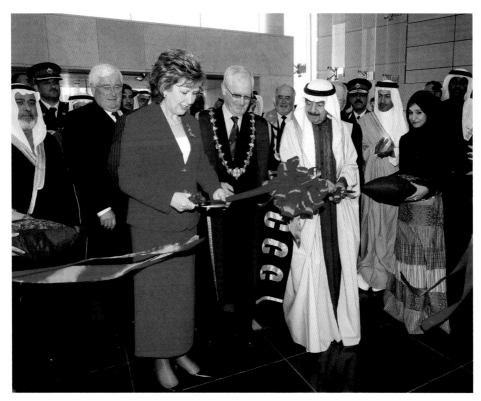

The official opening of RCSI-Medical University Bahrain, February 2009. (L–R) President Mary McAleese, Frank B.V. Keane (PRCSI 2008–10) and Shaikh Khalifa.

body of ambassadors, putting us on the map as a global leader in the delivery of healthcare education.'[98] PRCSI Keane called the occasion 'a landmark event signifying our commitment to Bahrain'.[99]

Conceptually, the new building drew equal inspiration from Ireland and Bahrain. Viewed from the south, the semicircular, sand-coloured building recalls the mound shape of the 5,200-year-old passage tomb at Newgrange, Co. Meath. Elsewhere – notably on a tall obelisk by the entrance – patterns from Newgrange's megalithic art are etched into the stonework. Inside, a tented, translucent fabric awning – reminiscent of fishing dhows or desert encampments – filters light into the vast atrium. The soft pink Jordanian sandstone panels and the glass balustrades bear similar decorative features. Up on the third floor, staff, students and visitors mingle in the 'St Stephen's Green Restaurant'.

The addition of a sports hall in November 2009 marked the end of the first phase of the $65 million project. The following June saw the first conferrals for seventy-two students in Medicine, Nursing and Healthcare Ethics and Law. As RCSI Bahrain – as it came to be called – was a constituent university of RCSI, their qualifications were the same as their contemporaries in Dublin – with, cru-

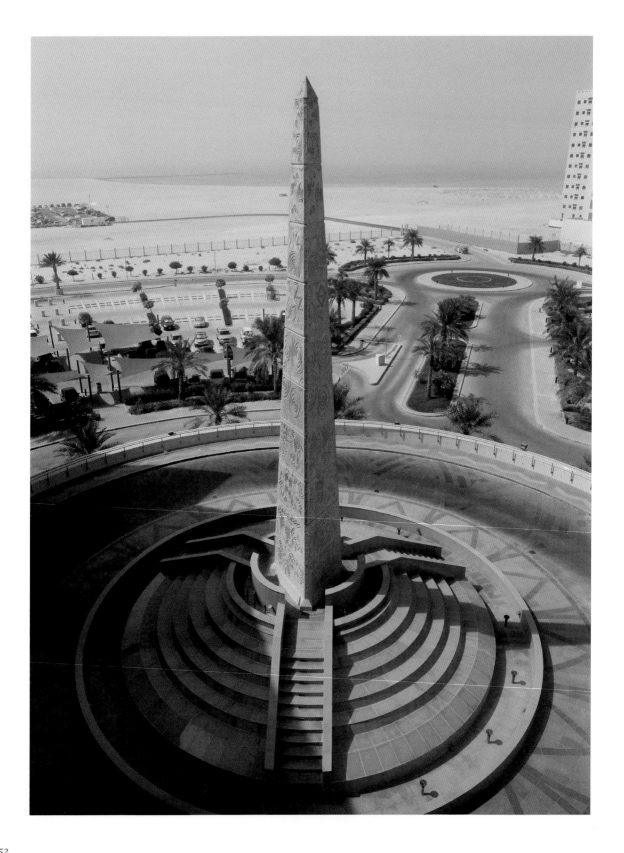

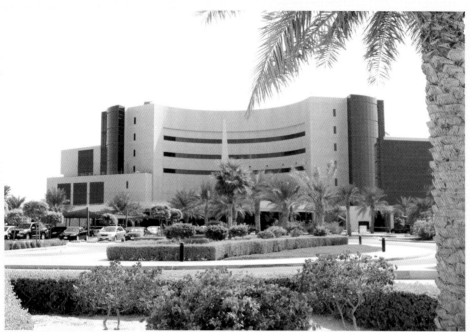

Facing page and left: RCSI Bahrain, inspired by East and West.

cially, the same international recognition. In 2009, Prof O'Malley completed his tenure as President, succeeded – appropriately – by Dr Faisal Al Mousawi, who had posed the original question in Penang.

Prof O'Malley stayed on, however, as a special advisor – principally to do what he had previously done in Dublin, develop a culture of research. That research would be conducted in laboratories and clinical settings – but also, unexpectedly, in the air: during his time in the region, Dr Brendan Kavanagh, Associate Professor of Human Biology and an experienced ornithologist, com-

piled his *Birds of Dilmun: an introduction to the birds of Bahrain* (2014).[100] Its publication was co-sponsored by RCSI and the Bahraini Supreme Council for the Environment.

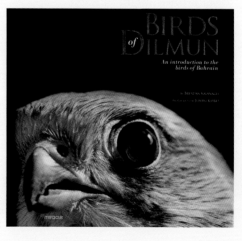

'BENCH TO BEDSIDE': RESEARCH STRATEGY AND COLLABORATION

In Dublin, since the first cycle of PRTLI funding, research had been identified as a core activity of RCSI – a declared pillar of its 'noble

Brendan Kavanagh's *Birds of Dilmun* (2014).

purpose'. In the five years following Cycle 1, RCSI's grant income increased at a rate of 37 per cent annually.[101] With PRTLI Cycle 2 funding (£7.4 million), RCSI established a Biopharmaceutical Sciences Network in collaboration with TCD, UCC and NUI Maynooth – in public funding, such intervarsity collaboration was the order of the day. RCSI-led projects were awarded in excess of €20 million in Cycle 3, notably for the Programme for Human Genomics.

This was a partnership between RCSI and the Dublin Molecular Medicine Centre (later known as Molecular Medicine Ireland). In Cycle 4, RCSI secured €13.3 million for proposals for clinician-scientist training and the National Biophontics and Imaging Platform.[102] From 2005 to 2006 alone, funding jumped by 61 per cent (to €18,145,000).[103] The following year, RCSI research funding came to €50.8 million, covering a broad spectrum of projects.[104]

Coordinating policy from 2004 was Prof Brian Harvey, Director of Research and Director of the RCSI Research Institute (for his promotion of Franco-Irish scientific collaboration, Harvey received a Gallic knighthood in 2006). The guiding principle of RCSI's research strategy was the promotion of 'translational' medical research – that is, 'Bench research informed by bedside problems, translated into diagnosis and treatment and into the community.'[105] Focused areas of inquiry were in the fields of neuroscience, cancer, cardiovascular biology, respiratory medicine, infection and immunity, and tissue engineering.

In what was something of a golden age for Irish research, RCSI's major funding bodies included the Health Research Board, the European Union, the Irish Research Council, Enterprise Ireland, Atlantic Philanthropies, the Irish Cancer Society, the Charitable Infirmary Trust, the Wellcome Trust and, perhaps most notably, Science Foundation Ireland (SFI). In 2003, Prof Jochen Prehn (Physiology and Medical Physics) joined RCSI as SFI's inaugural Fellow and Research Professor, an award specifically designed to bring world-class researchers to Ireland.

However, after the global financial crash of 2008, there were deep cuts everywhere; in 2010, RCSI's research funding dipped to €13 million. Despite this, the years of infrastructural investment still paid dividends in high-quality outputs: that year, RCSI was rated number one for citation impact in the clinical sciences amongst Irish higher educational institutions. In 2010 RCSI also launched its Research Summer School, seeding early awareness of research among undergraduate students; the same year, a small group of students founded ICHAMS (the International Conference for Healthcare and Medical Students), while an annual student-run scholarly journal – *RCSIsmj* (Student Medical Journal) – had been launched in 2008.

Supporting all of the above research activity was the Library. In her nineteen years as Head Librarian, Beatrice Doran had transformed the service into — in Prof Cathal Kelly's words — 'a flagship for medical libraries throughout the world'.[106] Doran retired in 2007, succeeded by Kate Kelly.

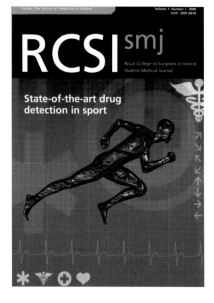

RCSIsmj (Student Medical Journal), 2008.

REACH AND OUTREACH

The ultimate beneficiary of research funding is the patient. Along the way, too, the recipient institution reaps reputational benefits. But while grants and awards cover the direct costs of research, the associated overheads will generally devolve to the institution. If this represents a good problem to have, it nonetheless demands a solution.

In 2003, RCSI launched its International Development Board, chaired by the financier Dermot Desmond, tasked with implementing RCSI's €60 million Development Plan — some fruits of which, such as the opening of York House, have been noted previously. In subsequent years, particularly during Michael Horgan's tenure as Chief Executive (2004–09, Order of Bahrain First Class 2006, Hon FRCSI 2009), RCSI fully embraced its corporate social responsibility. This manifested itself through donations, staff time and gifts in kind.

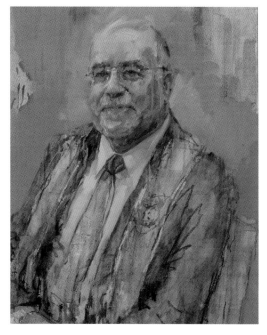

Michael Horgan, CEO/Registrar, by Cian McLoughlin.

One example was the joint programme between Our Lady's Hospital for Sick Children in Crumlin, the Christina Noble Children's Foundation and RCSI. This resulted in an annual visit by a paediatric, ENT, orthopaedic, surgical and anaesthetics team to the Children's Hospital, Ho Chi Minh City, to provide tertia-

Pride and Trans flags flying over St Stephen's Green.

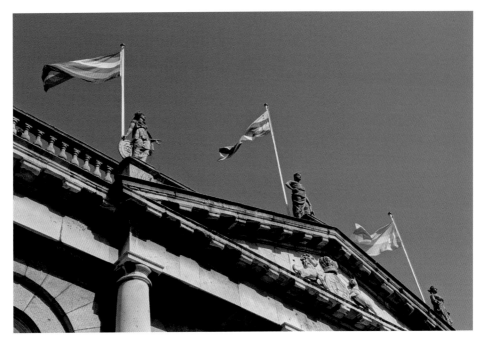

ry-level surgical exchanges and ongoing clinical and nursing education. Breast Cancer Ireland began under the aegis of RCSI Development, later becoming an independent charity in its own right; in this context, too, the central role of PRCSI Niall O'Higgins in instituting the national breast cancer screening programme may be noted.

In 2007, RCSI launched its REACH (Recreation, Education, and Community Health) programme, designed to increase third-level participation amongst the local community – in short, to be a good neighbour (especially during long-running building projects). The previous year saw RCSI initiate an access programme for members of the Traveller community. Further inclusivity efforts, at staff and student levels, date from this period too – early groundwork for the establishment of a dedicated Equality, Diversity and Inclusion (EDI) Unit (2017).

In January 2008, the first Mini Med School for Transition Year students began; in March, a sports day for local children was held at Dardistown, with help from RCSI students and Argentinian rugby star Felipe Contepomi (Medicine 2007). If most social responsibility programmes were long planned, others demanded a quick reaction: following the catastrophic earthquake in Haiti in 2010, RCSI coordinated a team of orthopaedic surgeons to provide on-the-ground expertise. It was not for nothing that the *Irish Times* had recently called RCSI 'an entrepreneurial rapid response unit'.[107]

RCSI AND THE GLOBAL FINANCIAL CRASH

Ever since the stark findings of a 1991 Financial Report – suggesting that RCSI could close within in a year or two if suddenly deprived of Gulf State student fees – RCSI had attempted to mitigate this dependence via property investment. As a result, by early 2008, the institution had amassed a net worth of nearly €500 million, with large land holdings in Ireland and around the globe.[108] The disadvantage, however, of behaving like a corporate entity is that the market can suddenly intervene like a *deus ex machina*.

In the global financial downturn of 2008, RCSI was exposed in ways that state-supported institutions were not. In late September 2008, the net assets of RCSI were €90 million, a decrease of 44 per cent on 2006/07; core activities operated at net deficit of €3 million, compared to a 2006/07 surplus of the same figure. Several long-cherished, ambitious projects – the hoped-for management contract for the King Hamad General Hospital in Bahrain, and an adjacent, vast Healthcare Oasis (with hotels, waterfront amenities, spas and 'wellness' facilities[109]) – did not come to pass.

Excavations on York Street that had already begun were suddenly halted, leaving RCSI with ownership of a large, literal and figurative hole in the ground. In time, following deep retrenchments – in both the financial and architectural senses of that word – the stately, student-oriented building, 26 York Street, would rise up in this place.

TWO HUNDRED YEARS ON THE GREEN, AND THE FIRST RCSI DEGREES

Despite such challenges – the serving RCSI President, Prof Frank Keane, spoke of 'a battening down of the hatches and the taking in of a few reefs of sail'[110] – in 2010, RCSI experienced two very significant milestones. In January, the College celebrated its 200th anniversary of taking up residence on St Stephen's Green; a reception was held, attended by the Lord Mayor, Councillor Emer Costello, neighbouring businesses on the Green, staff and student representatives.

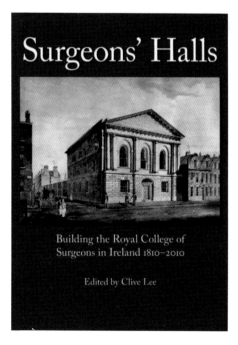

Surgeons' Halls (2011), edited by Clive Lee.

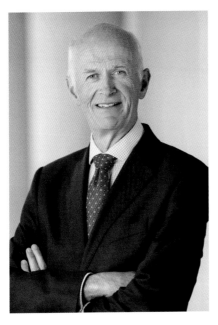

Prof Cathal Kelly, RCSI graduate, CEO/ Registrar and Vice Chancellor.

Soon after, on Charter Day, President McAleese unveiled a bicentennial plaque at the foot of the main staircase. A 2011 collection of scholarly essays – *Surgeons' Halls: Building the Royal College of Surgeons in Ireland 1810–2010* – also marked the anniversary. Edited by Prof Clive Lee (FRCSI 1989, Prof of Anatomy 2002–present), the title's plural 'Hall*s*' at once steals a march on Edinburgh's Surgeons' Hall, and acknowledges that RCSI had expanded internationally from its first permanent address.

January also began with something of a shock, when the outgoing Minister for Education and Science, Batt O'Keeffe TD, decided to dissolve the National University of Ireland – thereby jeopardising the hard-won degree-awarding arrangement that RCSI had enjoyed for the past

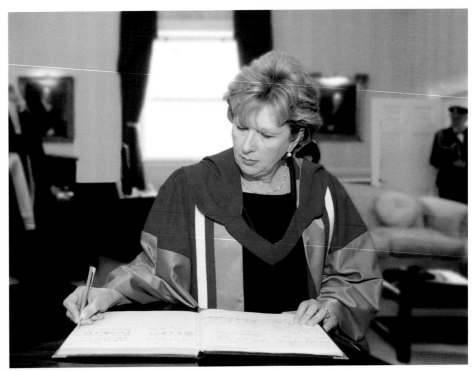

President Mary McAleese receives the first RCSI degree, May 2011.

thirty-two years.[111] Fortunately, the recent Charter changes had anticipated such an eventuality, so processes were now set in motion whereby RCSI could achieve degree-awarding status of its own.

What followed was a College-wide effort, albeit one led by the new Registrar/ CEO, Prof Cathal Kelly (appointed December 2009), and the new Dean of the Faculty of Medicine and Health Sciences, Prof Hannah McGee (appointed January 2010). Internally, a major assessment report was compiled, while rigorous external assessment came from the HEA, the National Qualifications Authority, and a panel of visiting – that is, once that the Icelandic ash cloud dissipated – international experts.

Finally, on 12 October 2010, the new Minister for Education and Skills, Mary Coughlan TD, issued formal notification of her decision to grant RCSI independent degree-awarding status. The first person to receive an RCSI degree was President McAleese, who was conferred with an Honorary Doctorate of Science on 30 May 2011. Before her conferral, she joined that year's graduands at their Conferring Dinner. They would be awarded the traditional NUI degree, and the historic RCSI/RCPI licences, in addition to their new RCSI degree. ∎

Chapter 9:
University Status, 2011-19

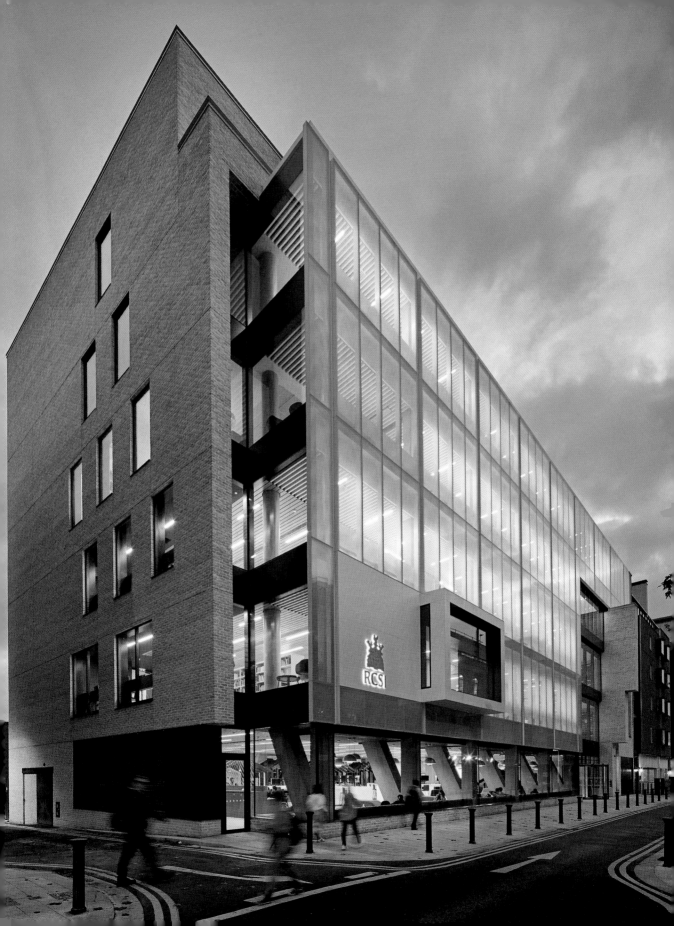

Chapter 9:
University Status, 2011–19

NEW GOVERNANCE AND A NEW 'MISSION STATEMENT'

As part of the 2010 application for degree-awarding powers, RCSI's governance structure came under close scrutiny. Recommendations from that time – and, in 2013/14, as part of wider institutional reviews of Irish universities – focused on the *sui generis* dual nature of RCSI as a health sciences higher education institution and a surgical Royal College. For nigh-on 240 years, this dual nature has been one of the great strengths of RCSI: the full gamut of medical education, from Foundation Year to specialist consultancy, thrives under one roof.

However, this combined identity also led to certain inherited, somewhat byzantine, governance structures, policies and procedures, which external reviewers now recommended be revised to align RCSI with its peers in the Irish university sector. One major upshot of this was the development of two parallel management strands: the Medicine and Health Sciences Board (MHSB) became the governing body for all RCSI educational programmes leading to degree awards in the health sciences, while the Surgery and Postgraduate Faculties Board (SPFB) dealt with all postgraduate and professional training and certification in surgery and related specialties.

Previous page: 26 York Street at dusk.

This distinction has in fact fostered greater harmony between the two strands, with certain SPFB courses managed and validated via the MHSB; conversely, some MHSB programmes actively incorporate SPFB strategies, notably in simulation-based training and quality assurance in clinical placements. In short, both sides of the RCSI coin are freer to focus on what they do best, while strategically profiting from the other.

The Council, meanwhile, remained as ever the overall governing body of RCSI, though the traditional complement of twenty-one surgical fellows is today augmented – in accordance with reviewers' recommendations – with two lay members, the first of whom (in 2014) were David B. Deasy, a chartered accountant and financial consultant, and the Honourable Mr Justice Peter Kelly, of the Court of Appeal.[1]

The other major development in governance was the establishment in 2013 of the College Advisory Board (CAB), to provide to Council and the Senior Management Team (SMT) external perspectives and guidance on critical strategic decisions. At its inauguration, this was a thirteen-member Board comprising seven Council members, including the President – Patrick J. Broe (FRCSI 1978, PRCSI 2012–14) – the CEO/Registrar, the Dean of the Medical Faculty, and four external members; in 2014, two of the last cohort were RCSI graduates: Lord Ara Darzi (Medicine 1984, FRCSI 1990, Hon Doctorate 2013), Chair of Surgery at Imperial College London, and Dr Michael Brennan (Lic. 1969, Hon FRCSI 2010), Professor of Medicine at the Mayo Clinic.[2]

As well as reporting to the Council, the CAB also advises the SMT, which, for all practical purposes, is the day-to-day decision-making body of RCSI (its relationship with the Council is not unlike that of the Dáil to the Seanad). Its current status dates from the late 2000s, when it comprised a core team of the Registrar/CEO, the Deputy CEO, the Dean of the Faculty of Medicine & Health Sciences, and the Directors of Finance, Research, Human Resources and Surgical Affairs. In the aftermath of the global financial crisis, a Director of Corporate Strategy was appointed (October 2010).

Reflecting the paramount importance of the digital domain, a Director of IT and Technology (later Chief Technology Officer) joined in 2015. Likewise reflecting the importance of RCSI's global alumni community (28,000 strong as of 2022), a Director of Development, Alumni Relations, Fellows and Members (also 2015) was appointed. Two further roles were also created – Managing Director of Healthcare Management (2016) and Director of International Engagement and External Relations (2020) – bringing the SMT complement to eleven at the time of writing.[3]

Taken collectively, all of the above developments – in train, to some degree, since the O'Flanagan era – have rendered RCSI a more equitable, modern institution, unbeholden to its specifically surgical origins. That tonal shift was also discernible in the updating of the somewhat unwieldy 'Noble Purpose' with the articulation, in 2013, of a new 'mission statement' for RCSI: 'to educate, nurture and discover for the benefit of human health'. Each element here underlines a priority: first and foremost, *education* is the core enterprise, generating some 82 per cent of RCSI's revenue;[4] *nurture* promises a culture of protective responsibility for students and staff alike; and *discovery* speaks to an ethical duty to advance medical endeavour through research.

THE TEN FLOORS OF 26 YORK STREET

The economic crisis of 2008 had a long tail in Ireland, despite politicians' optimistic talk of 'turning corners' and 'green shoots'. If there is a single moment that marks RCSI's recovery, however, it is the reimagining of the halted York Street development. Internally, the Corporate Strategy team turned their attention to the site in late 2011; the next two years saw multiple rounds of concept design, consultations, workshops and benchmarking against best practice elsewhere, until planning permission was secured in April 2014, and soon after, PRCSI Broe laid the foundation stone.[5]

Temporarily known as NAEB (New Academic Education Building), the design was by the Dublin- and Cork-based firm, Henry J. Lyons, with Peter McGovern – best-known for his striking circular Criminal Courts of Justice (2000) close to Phoenix Park – as lead architect. The contractors, Bennett Construction (founded in Mullingar in 1917, latterly with offices in the UK and Germany), took possession of the site in October. In this sensitive city-centre location, planning ordinances regulated the maximum permissible height – there was no chance, these days, of a thirteen-storey tower such as had been mooted in the late 1960s.

In order to achieve the desired – indeed, the required – interior space, the only option was to dig down – four floors down – rendering this the deepest building in Dublin. The significant challenge of descending so deep was dealing with the underground water table (the city has many hidden rivers, including the nearby Swan – from whence the name of the student-favourite pub at the end of York Street). Essentially, a four-storey-deep bathtub had to be created, in which the ten-storey (six above ground) new building stands. Topping out – by RCSI President Declan J. Magee (FRCSI 1977, PRCSI 2014–16) – took place in May 2016, with handover a year later. Now known as 26 York Street, the official opening – by RCSI President John Hyland (FRCSI 1976, PRCSI 2016–18) and Michael Bloomberg, media magnate, WHO Ambassador for Noncommunicable Diseas-

Facing page:
Cross-section of
the ten floors of
26 York Street.

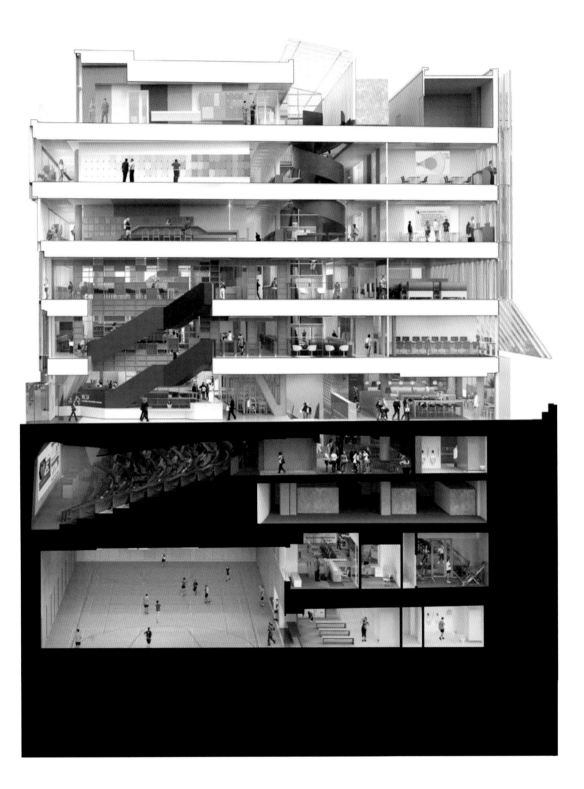

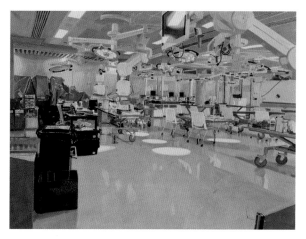

Laboratory by Colin Martin, 2022.

es and three-term mayor of New York City – took place on 5 June 2018. At that year's Royal Institute of the Architects of Ireland (RIAI) annual awards, 26 York Street was the winner in the 'Public Choice' and 'Educational Building' categories.

Costing €80 million – funded in part by a loan from the European Investment Bank – the facility represents a watershed moment not just for RCSI, but also for healthcare education in Ireland and Europe. The uppermost floors of the building are devoted to the state-of-the-art National Surgical and Clinical Skills Centre. Comprising a flexible wet lab (winner of Education Laboratory of the Year at the 2019 Irish Laboratory Awards), a mock operating theatre, clinical training wards, laparoscopic trainers, standardised patient rooms and task training rooms, it provides RCSI with 'the equivalent of an additional training hospital'[6] – albeit with much lower stakes.

Born out of the aviation industry, simulation-based learning has been part of RCSI training since 2003, utilising mannequins and role-playing actors;[7] in 2019, the appearance of an RCSI birthing mannequin on Irish television generated much wonder (and some complaints); in 2020 Prof Walter Eppich, whose earlier research led him to Antarctica, was appointed to the newly created Chair of Simulation. The SIM facilities are also used by the likes of the Dublin Fire Brigade, for whom RCSI has been providing a Diploma in Emergency Medical Technology since 2002. Promoting a more diverse learning experience, in 2022 RCSI SIM developed a range of skin tones for its models.

The Library is ostensibly spread across three lower floors, with multiple styles of learning spaces for individuals and group work. In truth, however, the Library has transcended its traditional definition as a bricks-and-mortar, or steel-and-glass, space: the vast majority of its offerings are digital, including ebooks, ejournals and (since 2008) RCSI's own institutional repository. In 2019, the new RCSI Library was selected by the Society of College, National and University Libraries (SCONUL) as a winner of one of its prestigious triennial Library Design Awards (the citation spoke of 'an exceptional example of transformative design... a significant contribution to the institution').

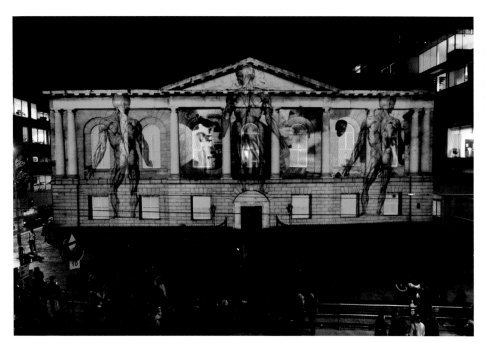

Light show as part of 'Surgeons & Insurgents', RCSI's centenary commemoration of the 1916 Rising.

In the Library's move from the Mercer Building, the extensive Heritage Collections stayed behind on the top floor. In 2010, a portion of the antiquarian stock that did not pertain to surgery or healthcare was sold, with the funds raised reinvested in preserving essential and unique collections, as well as allowing for the appointment of RCSI's first professionally qualified archivist, Meadhbh Murphy (2012) – in time for her to lead-curate the major national centenary exhibition, 'Surgeons & Insurgents: RCSI and the Easter Rising' (2016).

In 26 York Street, a vast central Atrium channels natural light all the way down to the first underground floor and the doors to a 540-seat auditorium, where in any given week students, staff and – crucially – the public might attend talks by the likes of oncologist Siddhartha Mukherjee (Hon Doctorate 2018) or former US ambassador to the United Nations, Samantha Power (Emily Winifred Dickson Award 2019). One wall of the atrium features a 'time capsule' installation by the artist Vanessa Donoso López and curator Clodagh Kenny. It consists of clay bullae made from the soil of three locations: the site of the Elephant Tavern, where it was believed the Dublin Society of Surgeons first met; the Rotunda Hospital, where the first RCSI meeting took place; and 26 York Street itself.

Inside each of the bullae is a message etched on a wafer-thin metal scroll by students and trainees from the graduating class of 2017. The capsules will be opened, and the messages within revealed, in 2057. Below the auditorium, the deepest

The 'time capsule' bullae in the Atrium of 26 York Street.

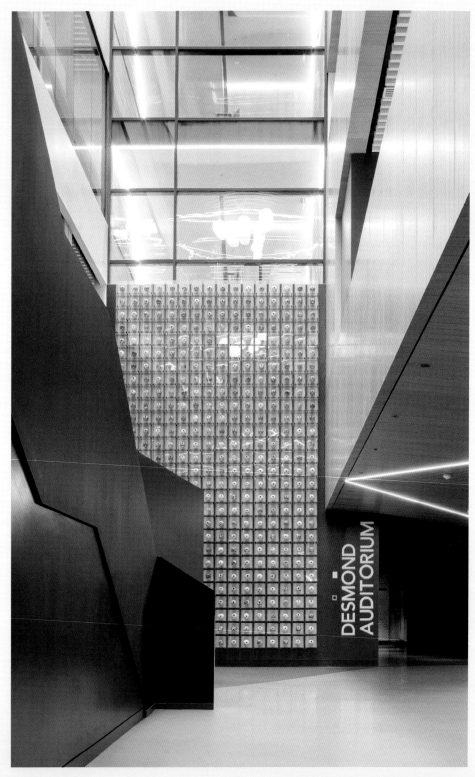

floors of 26 York Street house a gym suite (including a ladies' gym) and the full-size intervarsity regulation Al Mutchnik (Lic. 1953) Sports Hall. A project on the scale of 26 York Street involves countless contributors, but specific mention is necessary for Michael McGrail (Director of Corporate Strategy) for steering the on-time and on-budget delivery of the building. Likewise, the project's duration benefitted from guidance exemplified by successive PRC-SIs Broe, Magee and Hyland.

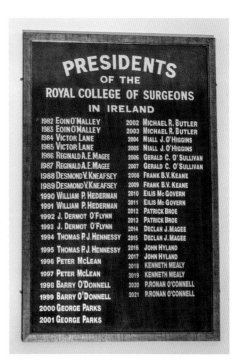

The Presidents of RCSI, 1982–2021.

'MEDICINE MAKES LIFE POSSIBLE, ART MAKES IT WORTHWHILE'

The bullae installation is part of a new tradition. In recent years, RCSI has fostered art on campus — notably under the aegis of anatomy. One of the major works is Robert Jackson's *The Anatomy Lesson of the Irish College of Surgeons* (2009). 'Most anatomy lesson paintings show medics around a cadaver,' explains Prof Clive Lee:

> but this one has them grouped around a surface anatomy model to emphasise the importance of living anatomy... In Rembrandt's *The Anatomy Lesson of Dr Nicolaes Tulp* (1632), there is an anatomical error, as the forearm flexor muscles take origin from the lateral epicondyle of the humerus. In Jackson's painting, Dr Faraz Khan is shown dissecting a forearm with the flexors arising from the anatomically correct medial epicondyle.[8]

Following the acquisition of Jackson's painting, the Anatomy Room has evolved into a gallery of contemporary Irish art, with contributions from talented students as well as the likes of Eithne Jordan, Harry Kernoff, Patrick Scott (who also donated his body to RCSI), Camille Souter, Imogen Stuart and Catherine Greene. Perhaps the most striking installation is *The Ever Present Dead* by Mick O'Dea: life-sized figures tumbling from the high ceiling. Prof Lee continues: 'When the students, trainees and teachers look up from their labours in the Anatomy Room, they can

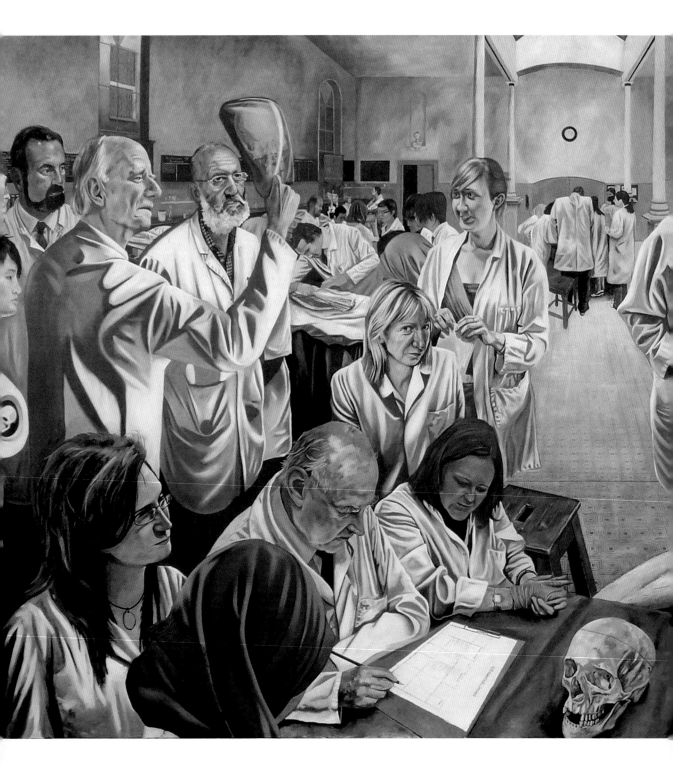

The Anatomy Lesson of the Irish College of Surgeons by Robert Jackson, 2009.

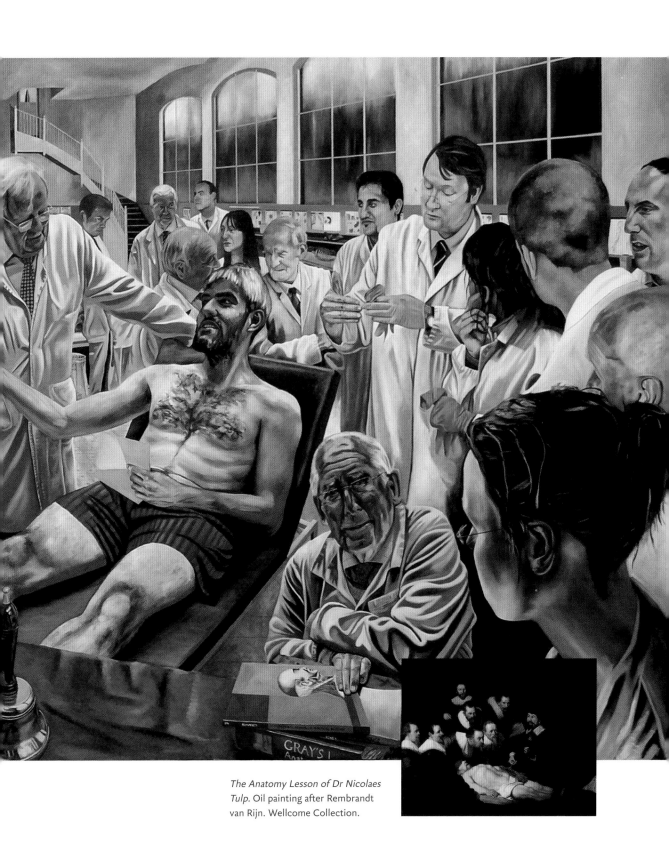

The Anatomy Lesson of Dr Nicolaes Tulp. Oil painting after Rembrandt van Rijn. Wellcome Collection.

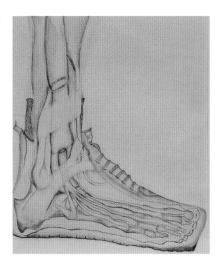

Behind the Seams by Ali Hazari (2nd Med), 2014.

now see gifts of drawings, paintings and sculptures that inspire and help them realise that, while medicine makes life possible, art makes it worthwhile.'[9]

In 2016, PRCSI Declan J. Magee launched the annual RCSI Art Award, in collaboration with the Royal Hibernian Academy and the *Irish Times*; the inaugural winner of the Award was Remco de Fouw.

HIGH-IMPACT RESEARCH

In 2017, art, science and technology were fused in a graphical interpretation of Twitter posts concerning breast cancer.[10] The image – winner of a Wellcome Trust award – is a striking visualisation of just one aspect of RCSI's ever-expanding research activity. From a pre-crash high, external research funding dropped precipitously: from €50.8 million (2007/08) to €10.4 million (2011/12); thereafter a new, jagged climb begins, reaching a recent high of €38.4 million (2017/18).[11]

Major funding bodies in the period included the HEA, the HRB and Science Foundation Ireland. In the first half of the 2010s, RCSI core research areas were: neuroscience; neurodegeneration and stroke; epilepsy; cardiovascular disease;

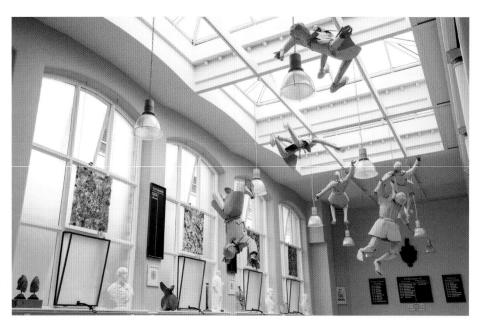

The Ever Present Dead by Mick O'Dea, 2015.

cancer (especially breast cancer); respiratory illnesses and cystic fibrosis; and bioengineering.[12] Major collaborations with other universities included the 3U Partnership (with DCU and Maynooth University, launched 2012) and the SPHeRE Programme (Structured Population and Health-services Research Education; with UCC and TCD, launched 2014).[13]

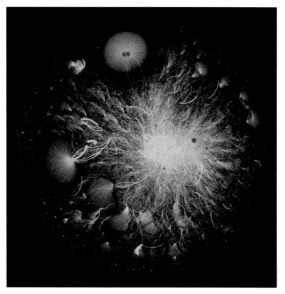

Award-winning visualisation of Twitter conversations about breast cancer, 2016. The image was created by Richard Arnett, Jane Burns and Eric Clarke.

Coinciding with the infrastructural rebirth of 26 York Street, RCSI invested a further €11 million to extend and improve the ERC Building at Beaumont. Moreover, from 2015, RCSI began a major €50 million investment in attracting new talent with the StAR (Strategic Academic Recruitment) Programme; this would lead to significant numbers of research lectureships and associate professorships, alongside methodological and biostatistics supports, and PhD and MD studentships. Expansion continued with the establishment of a new Centre for Vascular Biology and an SFI Research Centre, FutureNeuro, to diagnose, monitor and treat chronic and rare neurological conditions.

By any metric, RCSI research – directed by Prof Ray Stallings from October 2012, and subsequently from September 2019 by Prof Fergal O'Brien – was and is thriving.[14] Meanwhile, all of the above research resulted in high-impact publications: in 2017, RCSI articles were cited more than twice as often as the average publication in their field; in 2018, RCSI was the most highly cited educational institution in Ireland.[15] From 2018, six key areas for research were identified: cancer, regenerative medicine (in 2019, the Department of Anatomy was renamed the Department of Anatomy and Regenerative Medicine), neurological and psychiatric disorders, surgical science and practice, population health and health services, and vascular biology.

Considerations of data management and storage, and patient and public involvement (PPI), were increasingly to the fore. The commercialisation of research, including spinout companies such as the award-winning pioneer in regenerative medicine, SurgaColl Technologies (2010), was supported by the Office of Research and Innovation (ORI).[16]

TRANSFORMING HEALTHCARE EDUCATION, RESEARCH AND SERVICE

Undergraduate research thrived too. There was the ongoing Research Summer School – which went International in 2015, as part of wider RCSI collaborations with Soochow University in China – while the annual *RCSIsmj* and ICHAMS conference had become staples of the academic calendar. If such extracurricular activities were fixed points, the actual curriculum itself was in a state of flux. In the aftermath of the economic crash, higher education reform was in the air (notably, there was the HEA's 2011 *National Strategy for Higher Education to 2030* – aka 'the Hunt Report' – many of whose recommendations RCSI already had in place[17]).

Separately, the 2015 CanMEDS framework, developed by the Royal College of Physicians and Surgeons of Canada, influenced thinking in Dublin. In 2018, following a long consultation process, RCSI published its 2018–22 Strategic Plan, entitled *Transforming Healthcare Education, Research and Service*. Envisaged as part of the undergraduate education 'pillar' of this plan was 'the most radical overhaul of our curriculum in the history of the College'.[18]

Academic excellence was of course a key component of this substantial, multi-stranded document, but two particular points of focus set it apart: first, a deep commitment to what might once have been a pastoral afterthought – that is, attention at every step of the student's journey to building character and well-being. (Further expressions of this thinking at RCSI include: the launch of a Centre for Mastery: Personal, Professional and Academic Success (CoMPPAS); the establishment of the country's first Chair in Medical Professionalism (Dubhfeasa Slattery, 2017); and the foundation of the RCSI Centre for Positive Psychology and Health (2019).) The second area that felt fresh was the wholehearted embrace of IT in every aspect of healthcare education.

LIVING IN A DIGITAL LANDSCAPE

By now, Information Technology was well-established as a traditional strength of RCSI, dating back to the 1990s laptop scheme, then piloted via Technology Enhanced Learning (TEL) schemes of the mid-2010s, jointly curated by the Health Professions Education Centre (HPEC, whose inaugural chair (2013) was Prof Teresa Pawlikowska). From 2017, the IT Department achieved a decade's-worth of digital transformation in five years, including an entirely new website; a personalised student portal for tracking one's progress and feedback; further automation (for assessment, OSCEs and University-wide administration); quantum computing capabilities for researchers; and the fit-out of a recording studio to produce in-house content.

IT also implemented new Customer Relationship Management software to facilitate vital global and local Reputation, Recruitment and Clinical Engagement departments. More than ever, too, all aspects of cybersecurity required constant vigilance and revision.[19] Unbeknownst to everyone, this was the groundwork that made possible RCSI's wholesale digital pivot when the Covid-19 pandemic interrupted on-campus life.

RCSI HOSPITALS GROUP AND THE PHYSICIAN ASSOCIATES PROGRAMME

For all this digital connectedness, there are aspects of healthcare education that are ineluctably 'hands-on'. In 2013, the Minister for Health, Dr James Reilly (Medicine 1979), reorganised Irish hospitals into six (later seven) largely autonomous groups, each with an academic partner. Established two years later, the RCSI Hospitals Group comprises Beaumont Hospital; Connolly Hospital; Our Lady of Lourdes Hospital, Drogheda; Louth County Hospital, Dundalk; Cavan General Hospital; Monaghan Hospital; and the Rotunda Hospital. Since 2015, PRCSI Patrick J. Broe has been Group Clinical Director of the RCSI Hospitals Group. RCSI students also attend a wide variety of other public, private and specialist clinical sites, notably at Waterford University Hospital, where a €4.2 million RCSI academic centre opened in 2008.

From 2016, students of Medicine, Nursing,[20] Physiotherapy and Pharmacy were joined in clinical sites by a new postgraduate cohort: Physician Associates. In the UK and US, PAs represented a well-established professional grouping, but RCSI's MSc in Physician Associate Studies was a first for Ireland.[21] Perhaps unsurprisingly, in the mid-2010s, RCSI's larger conferring ceremonies outgrew the National Concert Hall and moved to the new Convention Centre Dublin on the Liffey quayside.

MILESTONES IN PENANG AND PERDANA

Looking further afield, there were landmark events for RCSI's international campuses. In Malaysia, Penang Medical College celebrated its twentieth anniversary in the academic year 2016/17, with its 1,500th student graduating in the summer. From 2018 it became RCSI & UCD Malaysia Campus (RUMC), graduating its 2,000th student in 2021, including postgraduates from 2016.[22] Further south, in Kuala Lumpur, RCSI began a medical programme in conjunction with Perdana University in 2011, with Prof Anthony J. Cunningham (Anaesthesia[23]) as Foundation Dean. Unlike the Penang model, Perdana students – seventy of whom began that September – remained in Malaysia throughout their studies, with Kuala Lumpur General Hospital as the principal clinical site. When the first cohort graduated in 2016, RCSI was now awarding exactly the same undergraduate medical degree, from start to finish, in three time zones.

RCSI'S RESPONSE TO UNREST IN BAHRAIN

In 2010 and 2014, the RCSI-Medical University of Bahrain marked auspicious achievements: the graduation of its first medical and nursing students and a tenth anniversary, respectively. The period in between, however, was marked by grave occurrences. In February 2011, as part of a wider movement in the region, a series of political demonstrations took place; in response, in March, the authorities declared a state of emergency, part of which included the order for all educational institutions to cease operations temporarily – impacting the 922 students and 117 staff at RCSI Bahrain.

RCSI CEO Prof Cathal Kelly immediately travelled to the campus, where contingency plans were put in place to ensure that final year students would graduate on time. Despite delayed exams, this goal was achieved. Meanwhile, Amnesty International, the United Nations and the Royal College of Surgeons of England were amongst many organisations who criticised the Bahraini authorities for 'targeting medical personnel in its crackdown on popular protests and for proposing military trials'.[24]

Initially, RCSI's official position was that it 'does not comment publicly on a political situation, or individual cases' – a stance that met with vociferous complaint, not least from a number of RCSI graduates.[25] Prof Kelly was obliged to comment further: 'The RCSI approach in Bahrain is appropriate to our circumstances and we believe our approach has been influential and effective.' On the subject of a widely perceived conflict of interests, he said: 'RCSI does not put financial concerns above human rights and our investment in Bahrain will not compromise this position.'[26]

The matter was raised in the Dáil, where Tánaiste Eamon Gilmore TD underlined the distinction between the Bahraini authorities' actions and RCSI's training of medical personnel, 'which I would regard as entirely positive'.[27] On 25 June, RCSI (and RCPI[28]) responded to mounting pressure with substantial public statements. Prof Kelly's 'Letter to the Editor' is quoted here in full:

Sir –

The Royal College of Surgeons in Ireland (RCSI) fully respects the unequivocal right of all doctors to practise as enshrined in the Geneva Convention. We are very aware of and concerned about the plight of those detained in Bahrain.

RCSI is a not-for-profit organisation. Our mandate is to focus on education in the health sciences. We are internationally focused, working in Africa, the Middle East and Far East as well as in Ireland. Many of the countries have very different cultures and are at different stages in their political evolution. This diversity is a challenge that faces all organisations that work overseas.

Since the beginning of these events we have endeavoured to ensure the safety of our 900 students and 100 staff in Bahrain, to enable our students to complete their programmes and to advocate for the rights of the arrested healthcare professionals. Our approach has been guided by what we have judged to be most effective in Bahrain. In support of this approach we have chosen to minimise public statements in Ireland.

We have attached considerable importance to ensuring the continuity of the education of our students. When the situation first escalated in February, we temporarily suspended teaching and staff continued to attend the university maintaining it as a focus for our students. We developed an evacuation plan and when the situation deteriorated we evacuated students and staff who wished to leave. A core group of staff remained in Bahrain to maintain the university and to set up and staff a temporary A&E unit for the local population in Muharraq. We developed contingency plans to ensure that irrespective of political unrest, our final medical year students would graduate on time. A delay in graduation for this class would mean a full year of lost employment at a pivotal time in their careers.

Last week 53 medical doctors and 70 nurses graduated as originally scheduled. It was important that the graduation take place as a tribute to the commitment and courage of these young people. Many of these students are the first members of their family to attend a university and to obtain a degree. This degree is an avenue to an infinitely better future for them and their families.

Medical practice is a privilege which carries rights and responsibilities. Doctors have a responsibility to treat all patients, irrespective of their background, to the highest possible standard, under all circumstances.

Hospitals must be politically neutral. Society has a responsibility to allow doctors and nurses to treat all patients in need. The protection and care of people wounded in conflict is a basic right guaranteed by the Geneva Convention. Punishing doctors or nurses for treating patients, irrespective of their backgrounds, is completely unacceptable. The World Medical Association's International Code of Medical Ethics Manual define the duties of physicians as including the administration of emergency care and adhering to principles of non-discrimination. Governments should not infringe upon the duties of medical professionals and should not target or punish those who seek to uphold these internationally recognised principles.

On six separate visits to Bahrain since February, I have met senior Bahraini government ministers. The focus of these meetings was to express our deep concerns for the rights of the detained medical personnel.

The future for Bahrain has to be one of dialogue and reconciliation. Our own national story tells us that this will not be resolved quickly. We will continue to contribute through education and continue to advocate for just outcomes. – Yours, etc,

Cathal J. Kelly[29]

This diagnosis of a slow resolution was accurate. In November 2011, the 513-page Bahrain Independent Commission of Inquiry (BICI) itemised human rights abuses by Bahraini security forces. This document was welcomed by the UN, the EU, the international community in general and RCSI in particular. In December, RCSI formally wrote to the King of Bahrain 'asking him to drop all outstanding charges against all those who were charged, including medical personnel', a number of whom held RCSI qualifications. RCSI also corresponded with the BICI, pointing out that the medical profession in Bahrain had become 'deeply polarised to the extent that public trust in the profession is now seriously compromised'.[30] In early 2012, Prof Kelly also addressed the Oireachtas to reiterate these points: 'As an international organisation, it is critical that RCSI helps build bridges rather than contribute to greater fracturing.'[31]

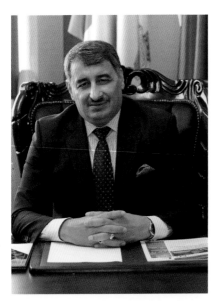

Prof Sameer Otoom, PRCSI Bahrain, 2014–present.

As the publication of the BICI report pointed towards a new openness by the authorities, in early 2013 RCSI Bahrain proposed a two-day conference, in conjunction with *Médecins sans frontières* (MSF), on the subject of 'medical ethics and dilemmas in situations of political discord or violence'. However, in March, it was made known to RCSI that this event should not proceed, under the pretext that 'the timing was not right'.[32] Shortly thereafter, Prof Tom Collins – President of RCSI Bahrain since September 2011 – resigned. Prof Sameer Otoom – formerly Dean (2009) – was appointed as Prof Collins' successor.

In June 2013, speaking as a member of the advisory board of the Bahraini Rehabilitation and Anti-Violence Organisation (BRAVO), Prof Collins commented that RCSI was 'extraordinarily powerless' in the situation but that its continued presence was a means of keeping the 'eye of the world on Bahrain'. What is needed, he continued, 'is a debate and agreement between higher educational institutions from all over the world... about how they can reconcile the values of academic freedom and personal liberty and freedom of expression with regimes in which they find themselves located'.[33] In December 2014, after some delays – not least caused by the protests and ensuing crackdown – RCSI Bahrain was fully accredited by the Irish Medical Council.

Further east, from 2008, RCSI Dubai offered its well-established Institute of Leadership and Healthcare courses from its own campus, officially opened by the Tánaiste Mary Coughlan TD; subsequently, it relocated to Sheikh Mohammed Bin Rashid Academic Medical Centre in Dubai Healthcare City, where it now operates as a hub for RCSI in the region. In its first ten years – that milestone was reached in November 2016 – RCSI Dubai graduated more than 600 health professionals in leadership, quality, education and healthcare management. Another noteworthy success was the launch in 2013 of an annual Women in Leadership Programme, designed for senior female healthcare leaders across the Middle East, Turkey and Africa.

SEE IT TO BE IT: THE WOMEN ON WALLS PORTRAITS

Back in Dublin, the role of women at RCSI – past and present – was being imaginatively reassessed. Under the auspices of the Equality, Diversity and Inclusion (EDI) Unit (established 2017, with Dr Avril Hutch as inaugural Head of EDI), and in partnership with Accenture, RCSI launched its 'Women on Walls' campaign. Six artists were commissioned to create eight portraits of pioneering RCSI women, thereby making visible a previously overlooked contribution. Some of those eight women have been mentioned so far: Dr Mary Josephine Hannan (Lic. 1890), Dr Emily Winifred Dickson (Lic. 1891, FRCSI 1893), Dr Margaret (Pearl) Dunlevy (Lic. 1932) and Dean Mary Frances Crowley (FFNRCSI 1974). The remaining four were Dr Mary Somerville Parker Strangman (Lic. 1896, FRCSI 1902; portrait by Mick O'Dea), the College's second female Fellow, a committed suffragist and Waterford's first female councillor (1912); the paediatrician and researcher Dr Victoria Coffey (Lic. 1936, Dip. Child Health 1943; portrait by Molly Judd); Dr Barbara Maive Stokes (Dip. Child Health 1946, Senior Demonstrator in Pharmacy and Physiology; portrait by Catherine Creaney), a pioneering disability campaigner, closely associated with St Michael's House; and Sr Dr Maura Lynch (FRCSI 1985; portrait by Enda

Griffin) of the Medical Missionaries of Mary, who revolutionised obstetric fistula care in Uganda. The portraits were unveiled in the Board Room in March 2019. One year later, a new collection of nine contemporary photographic portraits of leading female academic RCSI staff by Amelia Stein (winner of the RCSI Art Award 2018) was also unveiled.[34]

Similarly under the auspices of the EDI Unit, in 2018 RCSI was accredited with an Athena SWAN Bronze award in recognition of positive gender practice in higher education (linked to HEA funding, Athena SWAN is the body to whom the government delegated reform of gender inequality). EDI at RCSI goes further, however, advocating for fair treatment for students and staff regardless of 'ability, age, civil status, family status, gender, membership of the Traveller community, race, religion, sexual orientation or socioeconomic status'.[35] As far back as 2012, RCSI had quietly celebrated the first graduate from its Traveller Access Programme, while in November 2021, RCSI was the first higher education institution in Ireland to publish a Race Equality Action Plan.

GLOBAL AND LOCAL SURGICAL AFFAIRS

The pursuit of greater equality was likewise to the fore in RCSI's establishment of its Institute of Global Surgery (2018): five billion people worldwide are unable to access safe, affordable surgical care when needed. The inaugural O'Brien Chair of Global Surgery, Prof Mark Shrime, co-author of the groundbreaking *Lancet* Report on Global Surgery, was appointed in June 2020. The Institute evolved out of the success of a range of RCSI projects such as SURG-Africa (Scaling up Safe Surgery for District and Rural Populations in Africa; formerly COST-Africa), led by Prof Ruairi Brugha (Epidemiology and Public Health), which operates in Malawi, Zambia and Tanzania; and the flourishing COSECSA collaboration, which logged its 150,000th operation in 2019 (this was an e-logbook, custom-built by RCSI for COSECSA).

Historically, women were a rarity in African surgery, but by 2019 they represented 14 per cent of COSECSA graduates and 23 per cent of trainees. April 2019 saw the Institute's launch of a new project 'Akazi' ('women' in Chichewa). Funded by the Irish Research Council (to the tune of €350,000), this is an integrated screening package for breast and cervical cancer for rural women in Malawi. Alongside these surgical projects, RCSI's commitment to African health is expressed in two clean water projects (WATERSPOUTT and PANIWATER); and through the research and activities – encompassing disease control, surveillance and vaccination – of the Department of International Health and Tropical Medicine.

Facing page: Top left: Mary Somerville Parker Strangman by Mick O'Dea, 2019. Top right: Victoria Coffey by Molly Judd, 2019. Bottom left: Barbara Maive Stokes by Catherine Creaney, 2019. Bottom right: Sr Dr Maura Lynch by Enda Griffin, 2019.

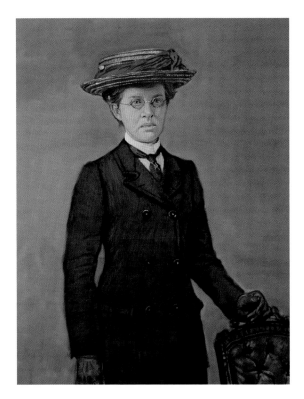
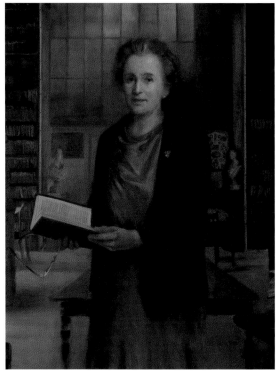
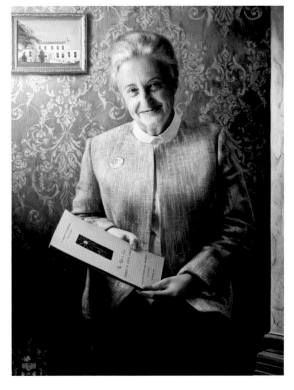
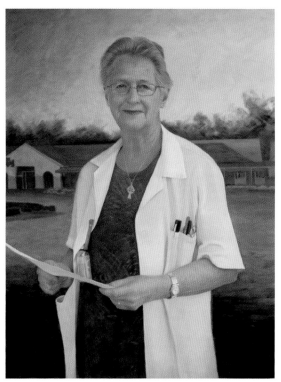

At home, Surgical Affairs had for some time been looking to improve conditions for its trainees. In the first instance, this involved streamlining the Basic Surgical Training (BST) years; later, the advent of the Equivalent Standards Route (ESR) added further flexibility. In between, in the mid-2010s, the need to support a gender-balanced surgical workforce became a priority. 'If surgery is less appealing to women than men,' asked Prof Deborah McNamara (FRCSI 1997, VPRCSI 2022–24), chair of a Working Group on the subject, 'we need to know why and remove the obstacles.'[36]

From 2012 to 2018, the numbers of female surgical trainees entering higher surgical training programmes increased from 34 per cent to 41 per cent; those advancing into Core Surgical Training remained at 30 per cent. In February 2020, the recipient of the first PROGRESS Women in Surgery Award, designed to support female surgeons' advancement towards consultant, was announced. Separately, if not entirely unrelated, from 2012, the newly established National Office of Clinical Audit (NOCA) was located at RCSI, with a brief to improve patient outcomes and promote patient safety in hospitals.

Funded by the HSE, but administered by RCSI, NOCA's vast data harvest both informs the general public about how Irish hospitals are performing and identifies for healthcare professionals opportunities for improvement. During the Covid-19 pandemic, NOCA's real-time monitoring of ICU bed capacity and occupancy was nightly news. In a separate pharmacological development, in 2015 the Irish Institute of Pharmacy (IIOP) was established at RCSI to manage CPD for Irish pharmacists.

ENGAGEMENT INITIATIVES AND INTERNATIONAL RANKINGS

In February 2015, RCSI opened its own hospital – for teddy bears. This annual charity event – proceeds have gone to St Michael's House and the Jack & Jill Foundation, amongst others – is hosted by Medicine, Physiotherapy and Pharmacy students of the RCSI Paediatrics Society. As furry patients rotate through triage, X-ray and MRI, and surgery, their young owner-carers learn about healthy diet and active lifestyle and have any fears of hospitals and healthcare alleviated. This is of a piece with RCSI's 'Engage' Strategy, supporting education and health at local and national levels. This ranges from one-to-one grinds for local schoolchildren, hands-on workshops, a Transition Year MiniMed School, Young Men's Health and Fitness Programme (RCSI sponsors the local Aungier Celtic FC team) to free health checks and an annual 'Ballroom of Romance' for local senior citizens.

In addition, RCSI runs access scholarships (such as the alumni-funded Aim High Medicine Scholarship, the Kiran Pathak Pharmacy Scholarship and the Traveller Community Access Programme) and contributes to national conversations via the RCSI MyHealth public lecture series, expert directory and an associated app (launched 2015) — in partnership with charities such as Aware, Breast Cancer Ireland, the Alzheimer Society of Ireland and more than a dozen others — to provide free, easy access to credible healthcare information. In purely fiscal terms, RCSI annually contributes in the region of €25 million to the Irish economy through employment and other taxes, with an equivalent amount

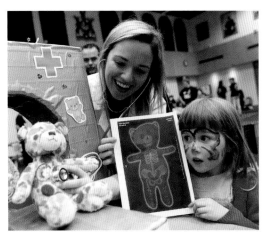

MRI time at the teddy bear hospital.

accruing from the multiplier effect of international students' presence.[37]

In the context of international reputation, rankings of higher education institutions carry increasing weight in a competitive global market. In late 2014, the *Times Higher Education* (THE) World University Rankings listed RCSI in the first 400 institutions in the world; finer detail followed in January, putting RCSI in the top fifty institutions in the world for 'International Outlook'. In subsequent years, RCSI has risen consistently within the same metrics, from #251–300 bracket in 2016, to #201–250 in 2017, and maintained since — that is, in the top 250 of universities worldwide, or joint second out of the nine universities included from the Republic of Ireland.

This high ranking was largely due to the strong citation rate of RCSI research papers. Under the rubric of 'International Outlook', RCSI rose from 49th (2015) to 46th (2016). In 2020, THE ranked RCSI as number one worldwide for 'Good Health and Well-Being', one of the United Nations' declared 'Sustainable Development Goals', to which RCSI is a signatory. To further foster RCSI's global reputation, the role of Director of International Engagement and External Relations, a member of the SMT, was created in 2020.[38]

If RCSI impresses external reviewers, it also looks after its own most important cohort: in November 2021, RCSI was named University of the Year for Student Engagement in *The Sunday Times* Good University Guide 2022. Beyond the curriculum, students now have the activities of almost ninety different clubs and societies to squeeze into their timetables. Cultural Diversity Month culminates in International Night, where student groups compete for the Parnell Keeling trophy (an intern award at Connolly Hospital is also named for Keeling (Lic. 1974, FRCSI 1978)).

Since the completion of 26 York Street, RCSI can now host intervarsity basketball, volleyball, fencing, table tennis and archery, as well as provide city-centre training for its soccer, cricket, netball and GAA teams (in 2017 and 2021, RCSI Men's GAA team won its first ever All Ireland Final; in 2011 and 2018, the RCSI Ladies' GAA team won the Donaghy Cup). Field sports and tennis are also played at Dardistown and, increasingly, at Railway Union in Sandymount. In 2017, the RCSI-Beaumont rugby team won the 129th Dublin Hospitals Cup.

THE ACHIEVEMENT OF UNIVERSITY STATUS

A photo outside the York Street Sports Hall shows the first RCSI basketball team, with Al Mutchnik (captain, Lic. 1953) holding the All Ireland University Champions trophy for 1952–53. The fact that Mutchnik and his teammates won a 'university' championship sixty-plus years ago points to a longstanding anomaly: RCSI has often been treated as a *de facto* university, and has often acted like one – since 1978, its graduates earned university degrees, and from 2010 RCSI was awarding its own degrees – without in fact being a university *de jure*.

In truth, until the 1990s, RCSI's existence was still predicated on the original Charter function of the training and oversight of surgical practice, augmented by the activities of the postgraduate Faculties, with the Medical School having the status of, essentially, a vocational college. The ambition to expand the range of educational offerings came about during Prof Kevin O'Malley's registrarship. With the subsequent addition of new Schools of Pharmacy and Physiotherapy, plus a newfound commitment to research, RCSI began to take the shape of a health sciences university. However, in Ireland, the title 'university' is protected by the University Act (1997). This legal framework defines universities as bodies which receive their funding from the state. By definition, then, RCSI could not be a university – unless the definition changed.

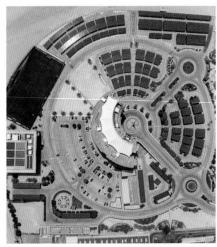

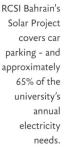

RCSI Bahrain's Solar Project covers car parking - and approximately 65% of the university's annual electricity needs.

In 2015, an initial, subtle change was made. The Education (Miscellaneous Provisions) Act allowed that, provided they offered degrees to at least doctoral level – which RCSI now did – an Irish education provider 'may apply to the Minister for authorisation... to describe the provider as a university outside the State'.[39] RCSI applied for and duly received this authorisation from the Minister, Jan O'Sullivan TD. Welcome as this was, it was not enough; indeed, the oddity of the restriction meant that RCSI in fact downplayed its external 'university' designation.

The Department, meanwhile, busied itself with legislation to allow Technological Universities to be established. Once the way was clear, RCSI was invited to submit a benchmarking analysis against key university criteria, as well as to indicate how the lack of university status negatively impacted RCSI's international reputation. A long, searching course of action ensued, with many exchanges between RCSI, its advisors and the Department.[40]

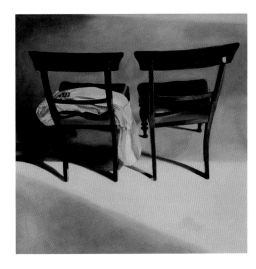

Inspired by RCSI's White Coat Ceremony. *I make these promises solemnly, freely, and upon my honour* ©2020, Mary A. Kelly. By kind permission of the artist.

As with the earlier, related achievement of degree-awarding status, the final chapter in the complex advance towards University status was led by CEO Cathal Kelly and Dean Hannah McGee. Their efforts were rewarded when the key piece of legislation – the Qualifications and Quality Assurance (Education and Training) (Amendment) Act – came in July 2019. This amended the existing Universities Act, removing the proviso that Exchequer funding must be an education provider's main income for it to be a university. (In point of fact, RCSI receives about 2 per cent of its income from this source, largely in the form of payments for services rendered – that is, its contribution to medicine, pharmacy and physiotherapy education for Irish and EU students; in addition, public funding comes to RCSI by way of competitively secured research grants.)

RCSI was now free to make its application for university status.[41] On 10 December 2019, Minister for Education and Skills, Joe McHugh TD, and Minister of State with responsibility for Higher Education, Mary Mitchell O'Connor TD, announced that RCSI was henceforth authorised to use the title of university both in Ireland and around the world. RCSI thus became at once Ireland's ninth university and its first health sciences university. This represented, as CEO Cathal Kelly said, 'a significant milestone in our journey'.[42]

In certain respects, the new designation finally caught up with the breadth of activity – that is, every branch of the healing art – already embraced, nationally and internationally, at RCSI. The year, and the decade, ended on this high note. Under normal circumstances, celebrations for the achievement of university status ought to have continued into the New Year – but as 2020 came round, circumstances the world over turned into anything but normal. ∎

Coda:
On the Horizon, 2020 to the Present

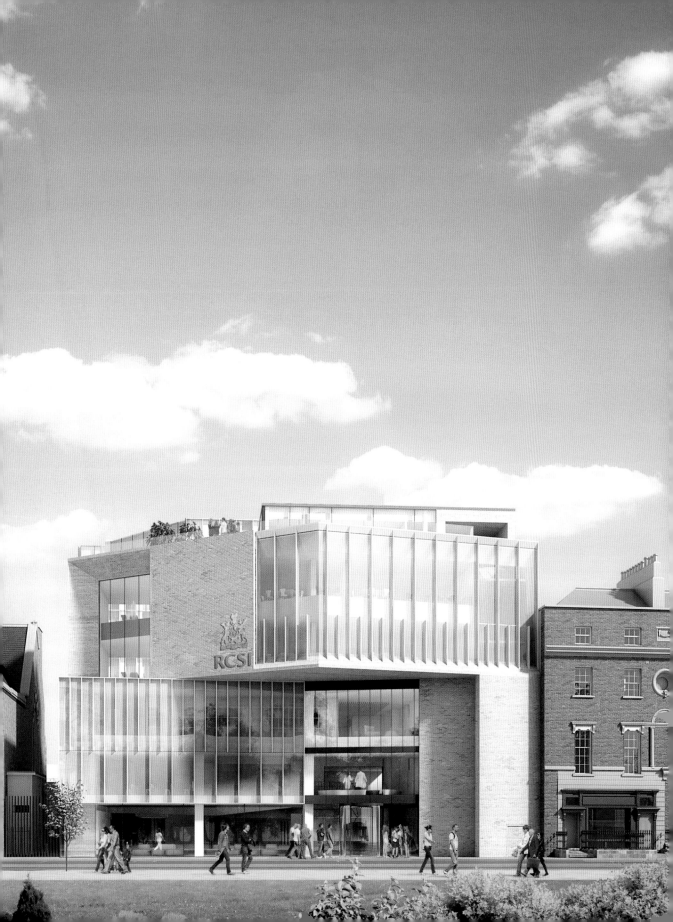

Coda:
On the Horizon, 2020 to the Present

IN AN EXTRAORDINARY TIME: THE COVID-19 PANDEMIC

'We are living through the most extraordinary health crisis we have ever experienced.'[1] In these simple, declarative words addressed to the RCSI community, RCSI President Kenneth Mealy (FRCSI 1985, PRCSI 2018–20) offered a reading of a moment in time that, under normal circumstances, would await the verdict of history. But the instant impact of the Covid-19 coronavirus pandemic upended all normal circumstances and these days – and weeks, and months – were recognised as the stuff of which history is made. The long-term effects of the pandemic – be they physical, psychological or societal – are yet to be revealed, but certain key dates and, for RCSI, emblematic responses, may be recorded here.

That ever-eloquent expression of RCSI's vital signs, the Charter Day Meeting, took place on 11–15 February 2020. As PRCSI Mealy noted in welcoming delegates, RCSI's recent attainment of University status lent a celebratory air to proceedings. Other elements of the meeting would have, in retrospect, faintly prescient overtones: there was the annual conference of the National Office of Clinical Audit (NOCA), a body soon to feature in nightly news reports; there was

Previous page:
RCSI's new civic
front door: 118
St Stephen's
Green.

('a novel event') a demonstration by the RCSI Emergency Medicine Programme of an 'emergency crisis simulation'; and Dr Olle Ten Cate of UMC Utrecht came to ask the question, 'What is a 21st Century Doctor?' One year later, the Charter Day Meeting would be an entirely virtual event, while in 2022, the event was deferred at the last minute owing to a resurgent wave of infections, eventually taking place in a hybrid format in April.

EXTRAORDINARY MEASURES: RCSI'S RESPONSE

Covid-19 was by no means unheard of at the time of the 2020 Charter Day. On the last day of 2019, the World Health Organization (WHO) Country Office in China was informed of several cases of a pneumonia of unknown etiology with symptoms including shortness of breath and fever occurring in Wuhan, China. On 30 January, the WHO described this spreading virus as a 'public health emergency of international concern'. On 11 February, the WHO announced the official name for the disease causing the 2019 Novel Coronavirus outbreak: Covid-19 (an abbreviation of 'Coronavirus Disease 2019'). One month later, on 11 March, the WHO declared Covid-19 to be a pandemic. By this time, more than 118,000 cases, and 4,291 deaths, had been recorded across 114 countries.[2]

Individual countries – and institutions – were already taking action. In January, at RCSI in Dublin, SMT acted on early in-house advice to establish a Business Continuity Plan in case the outbreak reached Ireland.[3] On 26 February, the Bahraini government closed all educational campuses; RCSI Bahrain's own Business Continuity Plan Committee set about managing and maintaining the University's operations remotely; within weeks, final medical OSCE and Long Case examinations were successfully completed. In short order, Bahrain's pioneering example was followed in Dublin, following the announcement by Taoiseach Leo Varadkar that all Irish schools, colleges and childcare facilities were to close at 6 p.m. on Thursday, 12 March. (Initially, this was to be for a two-week period; in the event, entirely in-person teaching would not resume at RCSI until January 2022.) On the Monday following the Taoiseach's announcement, RCSI reopened for business as (un)usual in an entirely virtual world.

RCSI's history of progressive IT investment now paid dividends on previously unimaginable levels, across all College and University activities. To synecdochically point to just two examples among countless others: less than three weeks into 'lockdown', the Faculty of Dentistry conducted its first ever exclusively online, proctored, synchronised and secured FFD in Paediatric Dentistry Exams in Qatar, strictly following the examination regulations – with examiners some 5,600km away, in Ireland and Scotland; and within the School of Medicine, clinical teaching staff donned Realwear smart glasses to simultaneously record and transmit patient interactions to students. For all the tech marvels, no one lost sight of what was lost: 'Students come to university for both the experience of learning and the experience of living.'[4] The cyberattack on the HSE (May 2021), just as life was returning to normal, was a reminder of the unpredictability of the digital realm.

The ambition to bring together learning and life in a disrupted world found expression in the adopted motto of 'one step closer to graduation'. This applied to all students in all programmes in all years – but it was the various Classes of 2020 who found themselves at the sharp end of the history unfurling alarmingly around them. Medicine students saw their final clinical exams brought forward; instead of having six weeks to prepare, they had six days. 'This is what we've been training for over the last five years,' said one, Dr Anthony Javid Machikan: 'To abandon ship now just wouldn't be right... The system needs all the support it can get.'[5]

Across all courses, RCSI introduced 1,426 graduates on to the 'frontline'.[6] For those students continuing in September, the new concept of 'social distancing' created novel logistical issues – so RCSI established a satellite campus for certain cohorts within the vast precincts of the GAA's Croke Park stadium.[7] This was at once a practical, student-serving development and, by the by, a pleasing nod to RCSI's 137-year-old connection to the GAA via Prof Auckinleck. In Penang, RUMC celebrated its silver anniversary (2021), albeit in a somewhat subdued, pandemic-inflected fashion. Student recruitment (and retention) across all campuses was probably never more important – nor challenging.[8]

Behind the scenes, and facing laptop screens, the entire RCSI community supported their 'frontline' colleagues, whether as educators, trainers or researchers. This ranged from senior staff offering best-practice advice to the government, to in-house experts countering the concomitant 'infodemic'; their faces and voices rapidly became trusted authorities on the national airwaves.[9] In addition, 26 York Street became the country's largest HSE Caller Training Hub for those undertaking contact tracing;[10] the Faculty of Nursing and Midwifery fast-tracked the registration process for overseas nurses to increase workforce capacity by 40 per cent; and new guidelines were made avail-

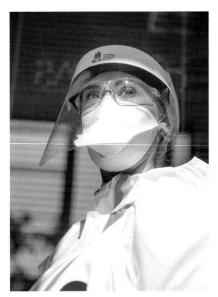

On the frontline in the time of Covid-19.

able for specialist surgery, for community pharmacists, for wound care related to sedated Covid-19 patients (and, indeed, facemask-wearing clinicians) and for ethical decision-making in end-of-life situations.

Entire new systems, headquartered in RCSI, were set up to optimise the usage of ICU beds nationwide and to connect GPs with surgeon advisors so as to safely minimise hospital referrals (the first volunteer to contribute to this service was PRCSI Kenneth Mealy). Meanwhile, as the streets of the city emptied, Mercer's Medical Centre provided its usual comprehensive service, in particular to local residents, hostel-dwellers and other socially disadvantaged groups. The Library collated the latest publications and worked with researchers to maximise the impact of their findings.[11] RCSI laboratories produced for the HSE enough swab buffer fluid to make possible an additional 10,000 tests for Covid-19.[12]

As the pandemic wore on, PRCSI P. Ronan O'Connell (FRCSI 1983, PRCSI 2020–22) could speak of collective fortitude and resilience: 'Notwithstanding major bed capacity issues and a severe shortage of ICU beds, the health service did not implode, and we were spared the worst ravages of the pandemic. Great credit is due to the healthcare workers across the nation who put themselves in harm's way and demonstrated extraordinary fortitude in the initial phases of the pandemic.' But it also fell to him to address other grave consequences: 'On behalf of RCSI, I wish to express our gratitude to those who put their own lives at risk and to remember those who sadly died. Their sacrifice will not be forgotten.'[13] The news that Dr Amged el-Hawrani (Medicine 1993) was the first confirmed NHS hospital frontline worker to die after testing positive for coronavirus, on 28 March 2020, provoked widespread grief amongst the RCSI community, especially his fellow alumni.

PRCSI O'Connell also noted how the pandemic highlighted global inequalities: 'RCSI is particularly mindful of the difficulties faced by our alumni and colleagues around the world especially in locations where healthcare infrastructure has been overwhelmed. While in Ireland almost 90 per cent of the adult population is now vaccinated, this is not the case in middle- and low-income countries. As an institution with a global healthcare remit, RCSI will advocate for equitable distribution of vaccines.'[14]

In December 2021, RCSI called on the Irish government to support the TRIPS (Trade-Related Aspects of Intellectual Property Rights) Waiver to enable equality of access to Covid-19 vaccines and treatments. 'No one is safe until everyone is safe,' said Mike Ryan, Executive Director of the WHO Health Emergencies Programme, and – drawing a line between the 1918 pandemic and the present one – in March 2021, Ryan received the inaugural Sir Charles A. Cameron Award for Population Health.[15]

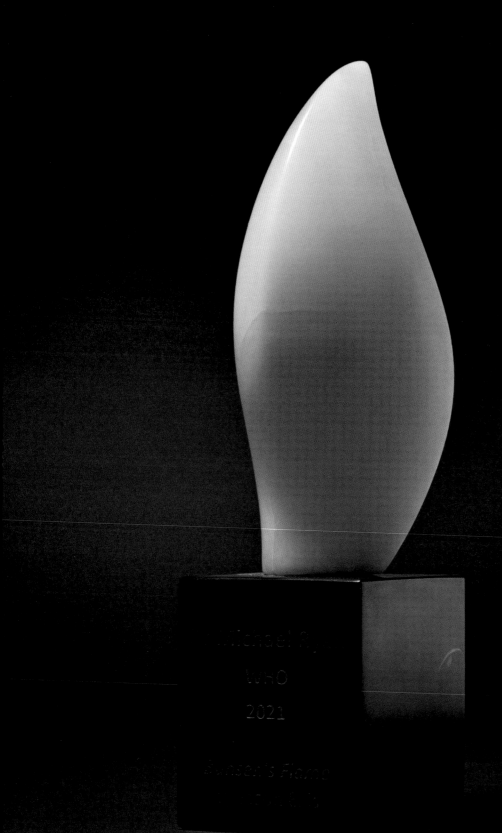

A little later, in June 2021, Cameron's contemporary equivalent, Chief Medical Officer Dr Tony Holohan, was awarded Honorary Fellowship of RCSI. Relatedly, in February 2020, at a ceremony in Geneva, WHO Director-General Dr Tedros Adhanom Ghebreyesus had been made an Honorary Fellow of the RCSI Faculty of Nursing and Midwifery.

Facing page: The Cameron Award: 'Bunsen's Flame' by Jason Ellis, 2021.

RCSI AFTER THE PANDEMIC: A SNAPSHOT OF A GLOBAL COMMUNITY IN PERPETUAL MOTION

No crisis comes without its opportunities. Students and trainees alike benefitted from the accelerated introduction of transformative educational formats. Some of these had been long-planned, such as the small-group ethos of the Copernican – or, in time for his 250th birthday, Colles-ian? – reimagining of the curriculum known as THEP (Transforming Healthcare Education Project; launched in September 2022); others were born out of the disruption, such as the launch in February 2022 of the digital-only – and therefore, *inter alia*, environmentally responsible – postgraduate course platform, RCSI Online (February 2022).

Other milestone developments of the pandemic period include the establishment – a world first – of the RCSI Centre for Positive Psychology and Health (October 2020); the launch of the RCSI Institute of Global Surgery (March 2021); a

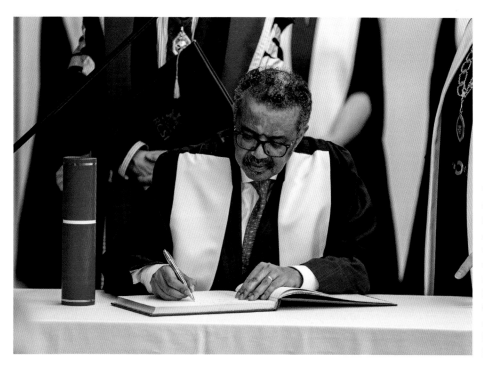

WHO Director-General Dr Tedros Adhanom Ghebreyesus awarded Honorary Fellowship of the RCSI Faculty of Nursing and Midwifery, February 2020.

reimagined RCSI Graduate School of Healthcare Management (October 2021); and the advent of the Centre for Professionalism in Medicine and Health Sciences (May 2022). October 2022 saw the foundation of the new School of Population Health (combining under one banner the Department of Public Health and Epidemiology, Department of Health Psychology, Data Science Centre, Healthcare Outcomes Research Centre, Institute of Global Surgery and SPHeRE).

Another new School created out of fusion was that of Pharmacy & Biomolecular Sciences (July 2019). In September 2022, the School began RCSI's first new BSc degree programme (Advanced Therapeutic Technologies) in two decades. The School also curated RCSI's first international 'university to university' part-

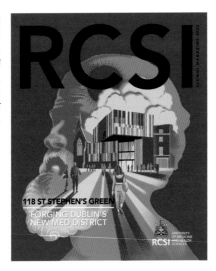

An ongoing global conversation: *RCSI Alumni Magazine* (2022), featuring an illustration of Asclepius by Eoin Ryan.

nership, with longstanding collaborator, Soochow University (SUDA) in China, including development of a new 1,200-student Joint Education Institution (JEI).[16]

Further strengthening ties in the region, during the (virtual) Charter Week of 2021, Prof C.M. Lo, Chief Executive of HKU-Shenzhen Hospital, Shenzhen, was conferred with an Honorary Fellowship of RCSI. Elsewhere, the pandemic further concentrated RCSI researchers, as evidenced by €37.5 million in grant income, 1,739 PubMed-indexed articles,[17] and four new spin-out companies.[18] Other numeric indices of RCSI's vitality at the time of writing include, across five campuses (Dublin, Dubai, Bahrain and two in Malaysia) 28,000 alumni in ninety-eight countries; 10,000 Fellows and Members in eighty-seven countries; in Dublin alone, 534 surgical and emergency medicine trainees, 4,647 students (undergraduate, postgraduate and other), availing of eighty-seven clubs and societies; and 1,311 staff.[19]

A NEW FRONT DOOR – AND NEW FRONTIERS

In 2022, the world remained unstable: following the invasion of Ukraine, RCSI's Surgical Affairs teams enrolled Ukrainian doctors in Ireland as Affiliate Members, providing them with free CPD courses; RCSI also joined the Scholars At Risk network to protect scholars and promote academic freedom; in this grim context, one story that raised spirits was the award in 2019 of the William C. Campbell Bursary to RCSI medical student – and refugee from Syria – Suaad Alshleh. Sub-

Facing page: Another vision of Dublin's emerging medical quarter.

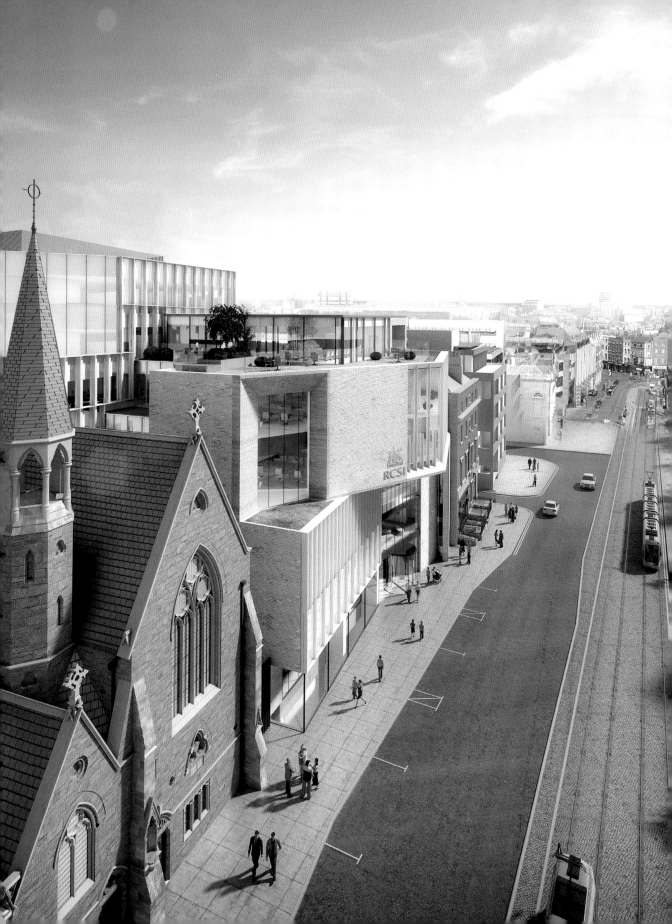

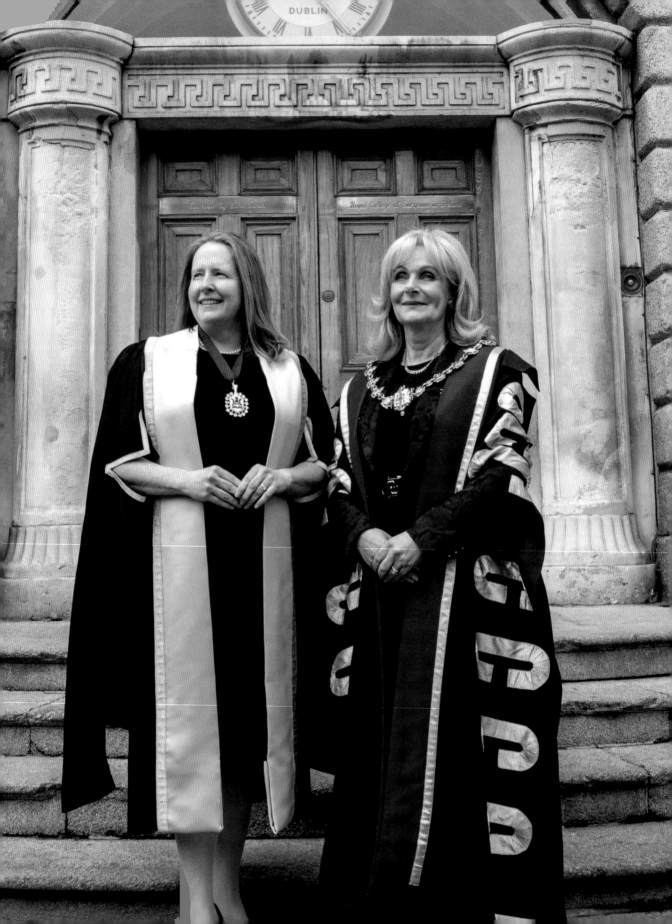

sequently, Alshleh's remarkable journey was prominently noted by the incoming President of the European Commission, Ursula von der Leyen, in her first State of the Union address.

Amid turmoil, RCSI invested in new foundations: in January 2022, PRCSI O'Connell and Vice-Chancellor (a new title) and CEO/Registrar Cathal Kelly jointly signed the contract for a new €22 million Education and Research Centre at Connolly Hospital in Blanchardstown, joining the ERC at Beaumont as RCSI's second clinical centre of academic excellence in Ireland. An even more ambitious project followed soon after, in May, when work began on RCSI's most significant capital investment to date (€95 million) at 118 St Stephen's Green. Rising to five storeys on the Green-side, seven at the rear, the new building – temporarily known as Project Connect for its physical link to 26 York Street[20] – will expand RCSI's Dublin campus by 12,700 square metres. With a public-engagement space at pedestrian level, it is also envisaged as an open invitation for locals and visitors alike to step through RCSI's newest front door.

In June 2022, Prof Laura Viani (FRCSI 1987, PRCSI 2022–24) was elected President of RCSI, and Prof Deborah McNamara (FRCSI 1997, VPRCSI 2022–24) was elected Vice-President – marking the first time in RCSI's history that two women have occupied these roles. Two hundred and thirty-eight years – and counting – after the original Charter was fought for and secured, history is still being made at the Royal College of Surgeons in Ireland. ∎

Prof Laura Viani, PRCSI 2022-24 (*right*), and Prof Deborah McNamara, VPRCSI 2022-24.

Acknowledgments, Notes and Index

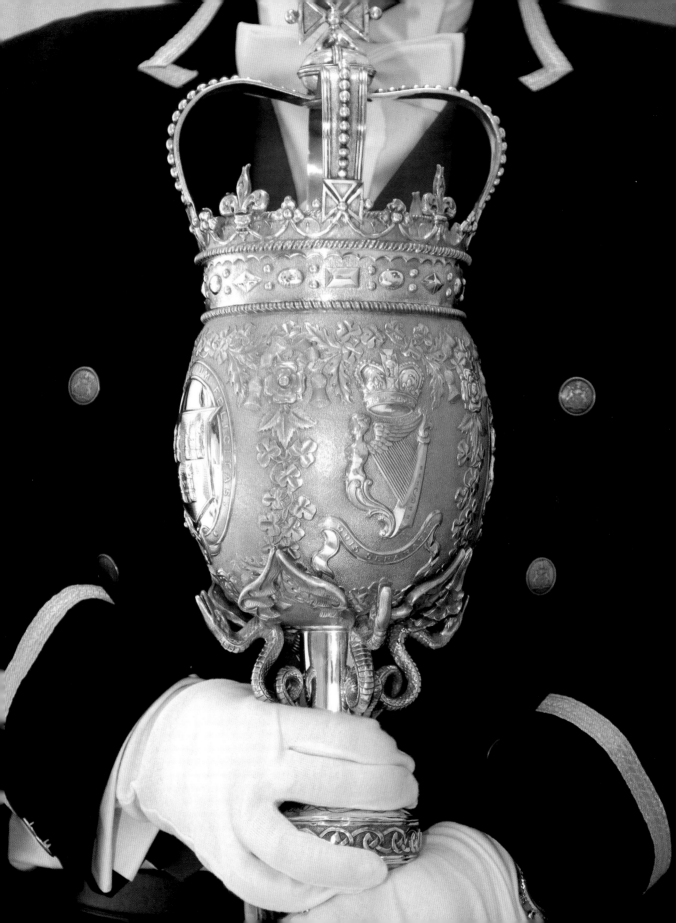

About the Author

Ronan Kelly holds a BA and a PhD from Trinity College, Dublin, an MFA from University College Dublin, and a DipLIS from Aberystwyth University. A former Fulbright Fellow, his first book, *Bard of Erin: the Life of Thomas Moore* (2008) was an *Irish Times* and *Times Literary Supplement* Book of the Year. He works in RCSI Library's Heritage Collections.

Previous page: In safe hands. Head Porter Frank Donegan holds the RCSI Mace.

Acknowledgments

My first thanks go to Prof Cathal Kelly, who initiated this project and entrusted it to me. To assist me, Prof Kelly convened an Editorial Board comprising Dr Maurice Manning (Chair), Prof Kevin O'Malley, Mr Michael Horgan, Ms Aíne Gibbons and Prof Clive Lee. We met for the first time on 11 March 2019, the day before Covid-19 wrote itself into the narrative; the next time we were in a room together was October 2022. In between – and since – the Board have been unflagging in their energy, interest and commitment and I am indebted to each of them for their vast expertise and ever-generous encouragement. A particular word of thanks goes to Clive, not only as my line manager and mentor, but for nominating me as the potential author of this history in the first instance. I am indebted, too, to all of the members of the RCSI community, past and present, who provided countless points of information and much-needed assistance – none more so than my close colleagues in RCSI Library, Carol Creavin, Anne Gregg, Jessica Handy, Susan Leyden, Grainne McCabe and Mary O'Doherty. Ronan Colgan and Fiona Murphy at Wordwell and the designer Fiachra McCarthy have at all stages been a joy to work with. No one has been more interested in this book's progress than my father, Peter Kelly; in working at RCSI, as in so much else, it is my great fortune to get to follow in his footsteps. Finally, this book is dedicated to Emilie Pine, without whom there would be no words.

Endnotes

CHAPTER 1 ORIGINS, BEFORE 1784

1 One striking feature of the 1577 Charter is that it allowed women to join the guild. How long this obtained, and how successfully, is unclear.

2 This statistic is from an anonymous pamphlet entitled *Reasons for Regulating the Practice of Surgery in the City of Dublin, by Making the Surgeons a distinct Society from the Barbers, Peruke-makers, etc.* The document is undated, but Widdess estimates its publication as being 'about 1703' (J.D.H. Widdess, *The Royal College of Surgeons in Ireland and its Medical School 1784–1984* (3rd ed. 1984); henceforth, simply, Widdess), p. 4.

3 See Zachary Cope, *The History of the Royal College of Surgeons of England* (1959) and Helen Dingwall, 'A Famous and Flourishing Society': The History of the Royal College of Surgeons of Edinburgh, 1505–2005* (2005).

4 The date of the first meeting was 29 March 1780; the location was not recorded. The second meeting took place in the Elephant Tavern, Essex Street – so named because an elephant was accidentally burned alive, and subsequently dissected, on the site in 1681.

5 RCSI/MS/37.

6 Quoted in Charles A. Cameron, *History of the Royal College of Surgeons in Ireland, and of the Irish Schools of Medicine, including a Medical Bibliography and a Medical Biography* (2nd ed., revised and enlarged, 1916); henceforth, simply, Cameron; p. 132.

7 Atul Gawande, 'Two Hundred Years of Surgery', *New England Journal of Medicine* (2012), vol. 366, pp. 1716–23.

8 See Harold Ellis, *The Cambridge Illustrated History of Surgery* (2009).

9 In addition, a shallow brass dish with a rounded notch in its lip often hung from the pole. These dishes were used to collect the blood, the notch allowing its close fit to the limb in question. The exact meaning of the two colours is debated by scholars. In Widdess's reading, 'the pole represents a phlebotomists' staff, which was grasped by the patient while an arm vein was incised. Alternate relaxation and tightening of the grip promoted blood flow. The red stripe represented the fillet, a bandage which was put around the arm above the elbow to constrict the veins, and them to fill lower down. The white stripe signifies the bandage applied when sufficient blood had been withdrawn' (p. 3).

10 Tony Farmar, *Patients, Potions and Physicians: A Social History of Medicine in Ireland* (2004), p. 21.

11 Clement Archer, *A Course of Lectures on Natural History, Composition, Operations, Doses, etc. of Various Medicines used in the Practice of Surgery Compiled for the use of Pupils of the Royal College of Surgeons in Ireland* (Dublin, 1791), pp. 2–3.

12 This summary of the work of Alexander Read is by Andrew Wear in his *Knowledge and Practice in English Medicine, 1550–1680* (Cambridge: Cambridge University Press, 2000), p. 213.

13 See Serge J. Dos, *French Surgery of the Eighteenth Century: the Royal Academy of Surgery (1731–1793)* (2021). Dos notes

that the motto was inspired by the Jesuit heraldist Claude-François Ménestrier.

14 Quoted in Cameron, p. 38.

15 O'Halloran's *Proposals* appeared as an appendix to his treatise on gangrene.

16 Hereafter, 'Lic.' and 'MRCSI'. For the transition from MRCSI to FRCSI, see Chapter 4, pp. 112.

17 Arthur Jacob, *The Introductory Lecture Delivered by Dr Jacob at the Royal College of Surgeons for the Session 1844–45* (1844), p. 11.

18 For the history of RCPI's name – and the history of that institution generally – see Alf McCreary, *The Healing Touch: An Illustrated History of the Royal College of Physicians of Ireland* (2015), p. 6.

CHAPTER 2 FOUNDATIONS, 1784-1820

1 Cameron, p. 143.

2 Cameron, p. 145.

3 Cameron, p. 145.

4 Cameron (p. 149) and Widdess (p. 16) both record further minutiae regarding the date of Birch's examination and qualification.

5 Cameron, pp. 149–50.

6 Smollett, *The Adventures of Roderick Random* (1745), Chapter 17. Other famous fictional ship's surgeons of the time include Jonathan Swift's Lemuel Gulliver and Patrick O'Brian's Stephen Maturin. Low as the bar was, the writer Oliver Goldsmith (1728–1774) failed in his attempt to clear it in London in 1758.

7 Cameron, p. 348.

8 Widdess, p. 50. Exams for naval surgeons were instituted in 1797. The date of the raising of standards to Licence-level is unclear, but a similar process took place in Edinburgh in 1816 (Dingwall, p. 118).

9 Cameron, p. 154.

10 The sources for dates and durations of professorships in the early years are inconsistent. The given dates largely follow Widdess. See also Cameron, p. 570.

11 My thanks to Rónán Conroy for this last point.

12 Quoted in Widdess, pp. 17–18.

13 Quoted in Widdess, p. 19.

14 Quoted in Cameron, p. 153.

15 Quoted in Widdess, p. 20.

16 See J.B. Lyons, *The Quality of Mercer's: the Story of Mercer's Hospital, 1734–1991* (1991).

17 Quoted in Widdess, p. 23.

18 See Martin Fallon, *Abraham Colles, 1773–1843, Surgeon of Ireland* (1972), p. 191. Unless otherwise stated, Fallon is the source for all references to Colles.

19 Or possibly five years old: the exact date of William Colles' death is not known.

20 RCSI/IP/Colles/3/2.

21 See Davis Coakley, *Medicine in Trinity College Dublin: An Illustrated History* (2014), p. 78; p. 110.

22 Fallon, *Colles*, p. 29.

23 Cameron, p. 421.

24 RCSI/IP/Colles/3/1.

25 Quoted in Widdess, p. 42.

26 Quoted in Fallon, *Colles*, p, 43.

27 Alexander Monro *secundus* was followed by Alexander Monro *tertius* (1773–1859), Colles' classmate. Between them, the Monros held the Chair of Anatomy at Edinburgh for 126 years – not necessarily on merit. In his *Autobiography*, Charles Darwin said, 'Dr. Munro made his lectures on human anatomy as dull, as he was himself, and the subject disgusted me. It has proved one of the greatest evils in my life that I was not urged to practice dissection, for I should soon have got over my disgust; and the practice would have been invaluable for all my future work.'

28 Cameron, p. 129.

29 His poetic confrère Percy Shelley was also a surgeon *manqué* – see Sharon Ruston *et al.*, 'Vegetarianism and Vitality in the Work of Thomas Forster, William Lawrence and P.B. Shelley', *Keats-Shelley Journal* vol. 54 (2005), pp. 113–32; p. 115). Another tantalising connection, yet to be explained, is Shelley's signature on a copy of the *Bye-Laws, Ordinances, Rules and Constitutions of the Royal College of Surgeons in Ireland* (n.d.) – see the Catalogue for the exhibition *The Golden Era of Irish Medicine with Predecessors and Successors* (2016), at the Kevin M. Cahill MD Study Centre, Lenox Hill Hospital, New York City.

30 Quoted in Cameron, p. 392.

31 Quoted in Fallon, *Colles*, p. 152.

32 Quoted in Bartlett, Dawson and Keogh, *The 1798 Rebellion* (1998), p. 54.

33 This was the clergyman and statistician James Whitelaw (1749–1813), quoted in Widdess, p, 21.

34 See Farmar, p. 35. As Cameron noted, 'At a time when the Municipal Corporations and many Public Boards rarely appointed a Roman Catholic to any office of honour or profit, the College of Surgeons elected Roman Catholics to be their Presidents and Professors' (p. 211). Indeed, in RCSI's first seventy-five years, he counted eleven PRCSIs who were Roman Catholic (p. 212).

35 Quoted in William J. Fitzpatrick, *Secret Service under Pitt* (1892), p. 393, n. 17.

36 Quoted in Cameron, p. 413.

37 Quoted in Widdess, p. 45.

38 For an account of this ceremony, see Journal of the Irish Colleges of Physicians and Surgeons (henceforth JICPS), vol. 25, no. 25 (April 1996), pp. 146–47.

39 See Cameron (p. 371) and Widdess (pp. 44–45).

40 Quoted in Coakley, p. 140.

41 See Fallon, *Colles*, pp. 109–10.

42 Quoted in Fallon, *Colles*, p. 126.

43 Cameron, p. 373.

44 See Fallon, *Colles*, p. 115.

45 In both chairs he had as co-professor Richard Dease (*c*.1774–1819, Lic. 1795, MRCSI 1795, Prof of Anatomy and Physiology 1798–1819, Prof of Surgery 1799–1819, PRCSI 1809), son of the late William.

46 Quoted in Fallon, *Colles*, p. 63.

47 Quoted in Martin Fallon (ed.), *The Sketches of Erinensis: Selections of Irish Medical Satire 1824–1836* (1979), p, 18, p. 21, pp. 24–25. 'Erinensis' was (mis)named by Charles Cameron as 'Dr Herris Greene' (p. 397). As Fallon clarifies, this should have been 'Dr Peter Hennis Green' (p. 9).

48 See Mary O'Doherty, 'The medical connections of Dublin's York Street', *JICPS* vol. 30, no. 2 (April 2001), pp. 107–13.

49 Quoted in Colin Brennan, 'The Royal College of Surgeons in Ireland, St Stephen's Green, West, Dublin: An Architectural History, 1805–1997', unpublished MA thesis, UCD (1997); henceforth, simply, Brennan; p. 6. See also Patricia McCarthy, '"Simply elegant" – the original building of the Royal College of Surgeons in Ireland', in Clive Lee (ed.), *Surgeons' Halls: Building the Royal College of Surgeons in Ireland 1810–2010* (2011), pp. 24ff. Also conveyance deed, RCSI BF LO/An/1.

50 See McCarthy, 'Simply elegant', p. 17.

51 McCarthy, 'Simply elegant', p. 17 and following.

52 Cameron, p. 166.

53 As Brennan puts it: 'the British government footed the entire bill for the new Royal College of Surgeons and its School' (p. 11). The total building cost up to 1810 was £29,139 1*s* 7*d* – of which £1,421 0*s* 7*d* was Parke's commission; £9,100 went on the purchase of land, and the building work itself ran to £18,618 1*s* 0*d* (the earlier estimate was £15,467 10*s* 7*d*, the price fluctuation owing to wartime shortages). There was additional construction in 1812, parts of which survive, notably the south wall of the current Anatomy Room (p. 13).

54 Quoted in Fallon, *Colles*, pp. 64–65.

55 Quoted in Fallon (ed.), *Erinensis*, p. 17.

56 According to Brennan, 'it is clear that from the outset the new buildings violated the terms of the purchase agreement' (p. 7). Widdes concurs that 'the agreement was broken, perhaps in the belief that the Quakers would not take legal action' (p. 62), but he does not say when this took place. Cameron dates the violation to the extensions of 1825 and 1836 (p. 165, see also p. 264). Patricia McCarthy suggests that '[T]he agreement seems to have been honoured up to 1875' ('Simply elegant', p. 24). Some of this difference of opinion may rest on the fact that the *College* was not built on the reserved land –

though of course the *School* buildings were.

57 Quoted in Widdess, p. 63.

58 J.B. Lyons, *A Pride of Professors: the Professors of Medicine at the Royal College of Surgeons in Ireland 1813–1985* (1999), p. 102.

59 Quoted in Lyons, *Pride*, p. 104.

60 Cameron, p. 556.

61 Quoted in Fallon (ed.), *Sketches*, pp. 21–22.

62 Abraham Colles, *A Treatise on Surgical Anatomy* (1811), 'Preface'.

63 See Fallon, *Colles*, p. 70.

64 Colles, p. 27.

65 Colles, p. 24.

66 Colles, p. 25.

67 Colles, p. 26.

68 Colles makes this bid for the novelty of his approach: 'While systems of anatomy are multiplied beyond number, we have scarcely any elementary treatise, the sole object of which is, to describe the relative position of the parts, or point out the subserviency of anatomical knowledge to surgical practice. To supply that defect for the pupils of this school, is the design of the present work' (p. 28). As Fallon notes, a more complete history of regional anatomy would include the names of Pierre Dionis, Jean-Louis Petit and Marie Bichat in Paris; John Bell in Edinburgh; Astley Cooper in London; and James Macartney at Trinity College, Dublin (*Colles*, p. 71).

69 Colles, 'Preface', p. v.

70 Quoted in Fallon, *Colles*, pp. 185–86.

71 John Cheyne, 'Autobiographical Sketch', in his *Essays on Partial Derangement of the Mind* (1843), p. 6.

72 Cheyne, p. 8.

73 Cheyne, p. 12.

74 Cheyne, p. 14.

75 Quoted in Lyons, *Pride*, p. 7.

76 Quoted in Lyons, *Pride*, p. 15.

77 Widdess, p. 128

78 Cheyne, p. 19.

79 See Lyons, *Pride*, pp. 18–19, and Masha Gessen, '"The Death of Stalin" Captures the Terrifying Absurdity of a Tyrant', *The New Yorker*, 6 March 2018. For a time, William Stokes was a student at RCSI, but he earned his qualification in Edinburgh. His father, Whitley Stokes (1763–1845), succeeded Cheyne as Professor of Medicine (1819–28) – see Lyons, *Pride*, pp. 46–79.

80 See Cameron, pp. 171–73.

81 This quote refers to a separate proposal concerning 'surgeon apothecaries', but the inference is widely applicable. See Cameron, pp. 172–73, who writes: 'The wording of the petition – a lengthy document – shows that the College did not wish to be placed in the position occupied by the sister Colleges, but, on the contrary, desired that all

candidates for surgical qualifications should be obliged to study their profession during a reasonably long period.'

82 Cameron, p. 402. See also Widdess, pp. 46–47.

83 Quoted in Widdess, p. 47. See Colles, 'Fatal Consequences resulting from slight wounds received in dissection', *Dublin Hospital Reports* (1822), vol. 3, p. 203.

84 See Lyons, *Pride*, pp. 131–32. The paper was Charles Benson's 'Fatal Effects of a light Wound received in Dissection', *Dublin Journal of Medical and Chemical Science* (1835), vol. 7, pp. 189–97.

CHAPTER 3 EXPANDING AMBITION, 1821-43

1 College Minutes, quoted in McCarthy, 'Simply Elegant', p. 37.

2 Warburton, Whitelaw and Walsh, *History of the City of Dublin* (1818), vol. 2, pp. 751–52, quoted in McCarthy, 'Simply Elegant', p. 37, pp. 38–39.

3 The quote – and the wider point – belongs to Brennan (p. 16).

4 For his service, the Lord Lieutenant was presented with a commemorative silver trowel (cost: £26 6*s* 7*d*) – see Cameron, p. 178.

5 Part of the logic of this was to enlarge the floor area of the library, which was located on the corner of St Stephen's Green and York Street (currently, the CEO's office). In the event, that did not happen: Parke's Entrance Hall stayed intact where it was, albeit converted into an office. It is now the Robert Smith Room.

6 See McCarthy, 'Simply Elegant', pp. 49–51.

7 Brennan and McCarthy describe the Greek-key frieze as 'unorthodox' (p. 18) and 'unusual' (p. 50), respectively. McCarthy notes that the main entrance railings were also added in 1827 (p. 50).

8 Owing to a mistake by Widdess (p. 68), for many years this was believed to be Hippocrates. The College Minutes (RCSI/COL/5, 1825–28, Saturday, 6 January 1827) make clear that the figure is Asclepius.

9 The short story in question is 'Two Gallants'.

10 Dexter means on the right hand of the shield, but the left as viewed; likewise sinister.

11 John Smyth, AHRA (*c.*1773–1840). See also Alan Browne and Beatrice Doran, 'The external statuary of the Royal College of Surgeons in Ireland' in *JICPS*, vol. 17, no. 4, October 1988, pp. 177–79.

12 Quoted in Brennan, p. 20.

13 Quoted in McCarthy, 'Simply Elegant', p. 51.

14 The originally agreed completion date was 1 October 1827. Work was delayed by a builders' strike in August 1826. The contractor was a firm called 'Murray, J. Dwyer & Son' – the Murrays here being Edward and Arthur – brothers of William, the architect.

15 This figure is based on disparate figures given by Cameron, Brennan and McCarthy.

16 Cameron, pp. 179–80.

17 Cameron, p. 180.

18 Cameron, p. 174.

19 See Fallon, *Colles*, p. 72.

20 Fallon, *Colles*, p. 72.

21 See Coakley, *Medicine in Trinity College*, p. 25.

22 [Corrigan – though the paper was published anonymously], 'Reminiscences of a Medical Student prior to the Passing of the Anatomy Act', *British Medical Journal* (11 January 1879), pp. 59–60. See also John Fleetwood, *The Irish Body Snatchers: A History of Body Snatching in Ireland* (1988).

23 See Coakley, *Medicine in Trinity College*, p. 105.

24 Erich Brenner, 'Human Body Preservation – Old and New Techniques', *Journal of Anatomy*, vol. 224, no. 3 (March 2014), pp. 316–44.

25 Quoted in Brennan, p. 13. A similar wall was erected around the School of Physic at Trinity. As Coakley writes, 'The board had been more comfortable when medicine was largely book-based like other subjects and it became increasingly uncomfortable as anatomical dissection, vivisection and chemical experimentation began to assume such importance', *Medicine in Trinity College*, pp. 100–01.

26 [Corrigan], 'Reminiscences', p. 60.

27 Quoted in Farmar, *Patients, Potions and Physicians*, pp. 55–56.

28 Elsewhere around the city and environs – at Killester, Kilbarrack, Drumcondra or Kilgobbin – watchmen were easily distracted with a quick bribe.

29 [Corrigan], 'Reminiscences', p. 60. See also Eoin O'Brien, *Conscience and Conflict: A Biography of Sir Dominic Corrigan, 1802–1880* (1983).

30 As Cameron notes, 'After the Mercer Street premises had been procured, one guinea was deducted from the fee paid by each pupil, and was retained by the College; but in 1793 the professors of anatomy were allowed to retain the entire fee, as they undertook to supply subjects and to pay the superintendents of dissections, as the demonstrators of anatomy were then termed' (pp. 553–54).

31 Widdess, p. 35.

32 See Cameron, pp. 649–50.

33 See Cameron, p. 171.

34 Quoted in Widdess, p. 37.

35 Widdess, p. 37.

36 See Neville M. Goodman, 'The Supply of Bodies for Dissection: a Historical Review', *British Medical Journal* (23 December 1944), pp. 807–11.

37 See Fallon, *Colles*, p. 74. Fallon is likely basing his figure on Erinensis' calculations, also quoted in Widdess, p. 37. In London, Astley Cooper suggested that about 450 bodies were dissected per season (Goodman, p. 808) – almost all coming from Dublin.

38 John F. Fleetwood, 'The Dublin Body Snatchers: Part One,' *Dublin Historical Record*, vol. 42, no. 1 (December 1988), p. 38. As Fleetwood notes: 'Cameron's History of the College makes no reference to this, nor does Kirby in his brief manuscript autobiography. However, as he had 16 children, of whom seven predeceased him he may have overlooked one in the count' (p. 38).

39 'Irish cheddar', 'limestone' – John F. Fleetwood, 'The Dublin Body Snatchers: Part Two', *Dublin Historical Record*, vol. 42, no. 2 (March 1989), p. 50; 'salted herring' – Fallon, *Colles*, p. 75; 'pianos' – Widdess, p. 40.

40 See Widdess, p. 38.

41 Widdess, pp. 39–40.

42 Quoted in Farmar, *Patients, Potions and Physicians*, p. 57.

43 Quoted in Widdess, p. 40.

44 Widdess, p. 40.

45 Widdess, p. 40.

46 Quoted in Shane McCorristine, 'Bodysnatching in the Name of Science', *Times Higher Education*, 26 September 2019, p. 45.

47 Quoted in Fallon, *Colles*, p. 75. As Coakley notes, Macartney 'endeavoured to promote private donation and he persuaded over three hundred people to sign a mass pledge empowering their surviving relatives and friends to donate their bodies for dissection' (p. 105).

48 John F. Fleetwood, 'The Irish Resurrectionists', *Irish Journal of Medical Science* (July 1959), p. 321.

49 Quoted in Fallon, *Colles*, p. 77.

50 Fleetwood, 'The Irish Resurrectionists', *Irish Journal of Medical Science* (July 1959), p. 314.

51 The 'first' is claimed by Widdess (p. 72), though his parameters – in Ireland, Britain, worldwide? – are unclear.

52 Quoted in Widdess, p. 72.

53 Quoted in Charles Mollan, *It's Part of What We Are: Some Irish Contributors to the Development of the Chemical and Physical Sciences* (2007), p. 458.

54 James Apjohn, 'Combustion, Spontaneous Human', *Cyclopedia of Practical Medicine* (1832), vol. 1, pp. 449–55.

55 See Mollan, *It's Part of What We Are*, p. 464.

56 Cameron, p. 657. The other two founders were Samuel Cusack, brother of James William Cusack, and Robert Graves.

57 Roy Porter, *Blood and Guts: A Short History of Medicine* (2005), p. 144.

58 To be accurate, the Institute was in fact co-founded by Marsh with Charles Johnson, formerly Master of the Rotunda, and Sir Philip Crampton.

59 The most invaluable study of Jacob is L.B. Somerville-Large, 'The First Irish Ocular Pathologist, Arthur Jacob (1790–1874)', *British Journal of Ophthalmology*, vol. 32, no. 9 (September 1948), pp. 601–17.

60 This was in the journal *Philosophical Transactions* (1819), pp. 300–07.

61 See Somerville-Large, 'The First Irish Ocular Pathologist', p. 606. A rodent ulcer of the lids is also known by the eponym 'Jacob's Ulcer'.

62 Quoted in Somerville-Large, 'The First Irish Ocular Pathologist', pp. 608–09 (some punctuation amended).

63 Quoted in Helen Andrews, 'Arthur Jacob', *Dictionary of Irish Biography* (2009). See also Ann Daly, 'The *Dublin Medical Press* and Medical Authority in Ireland, 1850–1890', unpublished PhD thesis, NUI Maynooth (2008). The *Press* merged with the *Medical Circular* in 1866 to become the *Medical Press and Circular*, finally ceasing publication in 1961. A centenary history of it was published in 1939 by Robert Rowlette (Prof of Pharmacy, 1921–26). The elder *Journal*, meanwhile, continues as the *Irish Journal of Medical Science* (1832–).

64 Cameron, p. 455.

65 Quoted in Somerville-Large, p. 616. Jacob was persuaded to accept the medal a year later.

66 Quoted in Lyons, *Pride*, pp. 105–06.

67 Kirby raised this at a meeting in February 1825 – see Lyons, *Pride*, p. 106.

68 John T. Kirby, *Observations on the intended Motion for Connecting a National Surgical Hospital with the Royal College of Surgeons in Ireland, addressed to the Members and Licentiates* (Dublin, 1825).

69 Quoted in Lyons, *Pride*, p. 107 (emphasis added).

70 Quoted in Davis Coakley, *Baggot Street: A Short History of the Royal City of Dublin Hospital* (1995), p. 12.

71 See Coakley, *Baggot Street*, pp. 12–13. Lyons suggests that White and Kirby may plausibly be considered founders, too (*Pride*, p. 109, n. 21).

72 Quoted in Lyons, *Pride*, p. 112.

73 Quoted in Lyons, *Pride*, p. 113. For further controversy following Kirby's second retirement, see pp. 113–14.

74 The commentator was Samuel Haughton, quoted in Coakley, *Medicine in Trinity College Dublin*, p. 169.

75 R.G. Butcher, 'Memoir of Dr. Houston', *Dublin Quarterly Journal of Medical Science*, new series, vol. 2 (1846), pp. 294–302; p. 295.

76 John Houston, 'Observations on the Mucus Membrane of the Rectum', *Dublin Hospital Reports*, vol. 5 (1830), pp. 158–65.

77 John Houston, 'On the Microscopic Pathology of Cancer', *Dublin Medical Press*, vol. 7 (1844), p. 14; p. 4.

78 See Cameron, p. 340. Clouzot was a hernia specialist, while Tiedemann was an expert on brain anatomy who debunked racist theories of intelligence.

79 John Houston, *Descriptive Catalogue of the Preparations in the Museum of the Royal College of Surgeons in Ireland, vol. 1* (1834), p. 13.

80 See also John Houston, *An Essay on the Structure and Mechanism of the Tongue of the Chameleon* (1828).

81 Houston, *Descriptive Catalogue*, vol. 1, p. 135.

82 Cameron, p. 332.

83 RCSI/COL/07.

84 See Lee TC, Allen E., 'Anatomical wax modelling and the Northumberland Museum of the Royal College of Surgeons in Ireland', *JICPS*, vol. 21, no. 3 (July 1992), pp. 213–18.

85 R.G. Butcher, 'Memoir of Dr. Houston' (1846), pp. 294–302.

86 *Annual Report* 1937, p. 10.

87 This was gifted by Houston's sister, Mrs Denny – see Cameron, p. 262.

88 Cameron, p. 317.

89 Cameron, p. 318.

90 See J.D.H. Widdess, J D. 'William Wallace (1791–1837)', *The British journal of venereal diseases*, vol. 41, no. 1 (1965), pp. 9–14.

91 Certain illustrations were also by Wallace's daughters – see Morton, R., 'Dr. William Wallace (1791–1837) of *Dublin*', *Medical History*, vol. 10, no. 1 (1966), pp. 38–43.

92 See Gore, Surgeon-Major Albert A., 'Maister John Arderne. Some account of an old MS. Presented to the Royal College of Surgeons in Ireland by Sir John Lentaigne, CB.', *Dublin Journal of Medical Science*, vol. 76, no. 4 (1883), pp. 269–77.

93 Quoted in Widdess, p. 150.

94 Widdess, p. 152.

95 See Stanley McCollum, 'The Lentaigne manuscript: an account by John of Arderne of his treatment of fistula-in-ano', *JICPS*, vol. 25, no. 3 (July 1996), pp. 214–16.

96 See Cameron, p. 218; *JICPS* vol. 14, no. 1 (January 1985), p. 12; Farmar, *Patients, Potions and Physicians*, p. 87. The Association has a complex subsequent history. Carmichael's version of it foundered in the 1840s; then it was re-established as the Irish Medical Association in 1853, becoming 'incorporated' in 1882. In 1936, the IMA merged with the Irish branch of the British Medical Association to become the Irish Free State Medical Union – later the Medical Association of Eire (IMA & BMA), which reverted to the IMA name in 1950. A breakaway group formed the Irish Medical Union in 1962; both came together in 1984 to form the Irish Medical Organisation (while consultants formed their own Irish Hospital Consultants Association).

97 Quoted in Cameron, p. 218.

98 Quoted in Cameron, p. 198.

99 Quoted in Fallon, *Colles*, pp. 90–91.

100 Richard Carmichael, *Plan of Medical Reform and Reorganization of the Profession, without subverting the existing Colleges of Physic and Surgery* (1841), p. 12.

101 This was 1836, when he was succeeded by William Henry Porter (1790–1861, Lic. 1814, MRCSI 1817, Prof of Surgery 1836–47, PRCSI 1838). Colles had already stepped down from the Chair of Anatomy and Physiology in 1827.

102 Quoted in Fallon, *Colles*, pp. 89–90.

103 Quoted in Fallon, *Colles*, p. 168.

104 See Fallon, *Colles*, p. 161.

105 Quoted in Fallon, *Colles*, pp. 165–66.

106 See Cameron, p. 398. An eponym, Colles' Law, derived from the *Observations* ('It is a curious fact, that I never witnessed nor ever heard of an instance in which a child deriving the infection of syphilis from its parents has caused an ulceration of the breast of its mother'), but this has since been refuted. For other Colles eponyms, see Fallon, *Colles*, pp. 177–89.

107 Cameron suggests that this refusal was owed to the fact that the offer came too late (p. 397).

108 See William Stokes, 'Observations on the case of the late Abraham Colles', *Dublin Quarterly Journal of Medical Science*, vol. 1, no. 2, pp. 303–22; p. 309.

109 See Fallon, *Colles*, p. 211. PRCSI O'Beirne had a distinguished career – he was the first person to hold the honorary office of Surgeon Extraordinary to the King in Ireland, and he published widely on colorectal surgery. And yet he died penniless in London, the local bishop paying his funeral expenses (see Cameron, pp. 461–62). The Library had already paid him £525 for his collection of 3,000 volumes – which, according to Cameron, was an over-the-odds price (p. 319).

CHAPTER 4 INVENTION AND INNOVATION, 1844-85

1 Quoted in Widdess, p. 79.

2 Lyons, *Pride*, p. 144.

3 Quoted in Cameron, pp. 234–35.

4 The current mace featues the post-1907 coat of arms in bas-relief, suggesting this is a twentieth-century replacement.

5 James Joyce, *Ulysses*, p. 114.

6 This is 'Erinensis' again, quoted in Fallon, *Colles*, p. 123.

7 Quoted in Cameron, p. 417.

8 *Irish Times*, 27 November 1950.

9 See an overview article in the *Irish Times*, 18 July 1962, p. 8.

10 Cliodhna Cussen's 'Stein of Long Stone' (1986) now occupies the spot.

11 Richard Gregory, 'Neuralgia – introduction of fluid to the nerve. By Mr. Rynd' (1845), *Dublin Medical Press*, vol. 13, pp. 167–68.

12 D. Brunton, 'A question of priority: Alexander Wood, Charles Hunter and the hypodermic method', *Journal of the Royal College of Physicians of Edinburgh*, vol. 30, no. 4 (2000), pp. 349–51.

13 Francis Rynd, 'Description of an instrument for the subcutaneous introduction of fluids in affections of the nerves' (1861), *Dublin Quarterly Journal of Medical Science*, vol. 32, no.

1, p. 13.

14 In fact, the patient – Edward Gilbert Abbott – said afterwards that he had experienced 'considerable pain but it was mitigated', quoted in Declan Warde, Joseph Tracey and John Cahill, *Safety as We Watch: Anaesthesia in Ireland 1847–1998* (2022), p. 9.

15 George Hayward, *Some Account of the First Use of Sulphuric Ether by Inhalation in Surgical Practice* (1847), p. 4.

16 The dialogue here is from Harold Ellis and Sala Abdalla, *A History of Surgery* (2019). For a (rare) patient-centred account of the operation, see Guenter B. Risse, *Mending Bodies, Saving Souls: A History of Hospitals* (1999).

17 See Harold Ellis, *The Cambridge Illustrated History of Surgery* (2009), pp. 78–79.

18 Quoted in Widdess, 'The Introduction of Ether and Chloroform to Dublin', *Irish Journal of Medical Science*, vol. 21 (1946), pp. 649–55.

19 Tufnell himself, who had extensive military experience, was the inventor of a self-explanatory 'bullet scoop'. He was appointed as RCSI's first (and only) Regius Professor of Military Surgery. His lectures were praised – and particularly recommended to potential surgeons of the East India Company – but the chair was abolished in 1860 with the opening of a vast military hospital at Netley, near Southampton.

20 For the quoted lines, Butcher is specifically referring to operations on the jaw, where there was the danger of blood going down the throat – see Farmar, *Patients, Potions and Physicians*, pp. 78–79.

21 Cameron, p. 481.

22 Richard Butcher, 'Mr. Butcher's cases of amputation – use of a new saw', *Dublin Quarterly Journal of Medical Science* (1851), vol. 12, no. 23, pp. 209–23.

23 Quoted in Widdess, 'The Introduction of Ether', p. 652.

24 J. Harbison, "The old guessing tube": 200 years of the stethoscope', *QJM: An International Journal of Medicine*, vol. 110, no. 1 (January 2017), pp. 9–10.

25 Arthur Leared, 'On the self-adjusting double stethoscope', *The Lancet* (1856), vol. 2, p. 138.

26 Cammann's instrument was manufactured by George Tiemann & Co.

27 See Leonard F. Peltier's introduction to an abridgement of Smith's work in *Clinical Orthopaedics and Related Research*, vol. 245 (August 1989), pp. 3–9.

28 Quoted in L.M. Geary, 'William Wilde (1815–76) as historian – a bicentenary appraisal', *History Ireland* (2015), 23 (5).

29 J.W. Cusack and W. Stokes, 'On the Mortality of Medical Practitioners from Fever in Ireland', *Dublin Quarterly Journal of Medical Science*, vol. 4, no. 7 (1847) – first article – pp. 134–45; p. 134.

30 Cusack and Stokes (1848), vol. 5 – second article – pp.

111–28; p. 119.

31 Cusack and Stokes (1848) – second article – p. 127.

32 Cusack and Stokes (1848) – second article – p. 128.

33 Cameron, p. 447.

34 For RCSI's involvement in this commemoration, see *JICPS* vol. 27, no. 3 (July 1998), p. 199. The sculpture of Cusack is by Anne Buckley.

35 The phrase is Coakley's, *Medicine in Trinity College Dublin*, p. 143.

36 Quoted in Cameron, p. 245.

37 Coakley, *Medicine in Trinity College Dublin*, p. 143.

38 Quoted in Widdess, pp. 103–04.

39 From 1880, CUMS students took their degrees from the Royal University of Ireland, the successor body to the Queen's University of Ireland.

40 For the finer points of the 1858 Medical Act, see Andrew Hull and Johanna Geyer-Kordesch, *The Shaping of the Medical Profession: the History of the Royal College of Physicians and Surgeons of Glasgow, 1858–1999* (1999), especially pp. 6–47.

41 See Cameron, p. 455.

42 Arthur Jacob, *The Introductory Lecture Delivered by Dr Jacob at the Royal College of Surgeons for the Session 1844–45* (1844), p. 11.

43 See Rawdon Macnamara, *Observations on the Position Occupied by the Corporation of the Royal College of Surgeons in Ireland: with Reference to the Board of Trinity College, Dublin, and the Senate of the Queen's University in Ireland* (1859).

44 Henry Maunsell, *Political Medicine; being the substance of a discourse lately delivered before the Royal College of Surgeons in Ireland, on medicine, considered in its relations to government and legislation* (1839), p. 21.

45 Maunsell, p. 4.

46 Maunsell, p. 45.

47 Maunsell, p. 2.

48 Quoted in Widdess, p. 76.

49 Robert McDonnell, 'Remarks on the Operation of Transfusion and the Apparatus for its Performance', *Dublin Quarterly Journal of Medical Science*, vol. 50, no. 2 (1870), pp. 257–65.

50 The biennial Presidency was introduced in 1890–91.

51 Bram Stoker, *Dracula* (1897), Chapter X.

52 The inventor of the ophthalmoscope, Hermann von Helmholtz (1821–1894), was conferred with Honorary Fellowship in 1881. In his acceptance speech, von Helmholtz referred to this invention as 'an accident – a lucky accident' (Cameron, p. 269).

53 Cameron, p. 247.

54 Widdess, p. 160.

55 Cohen, R.A. 'A general history of dentistry from the 18th century, with special reference to Irish practitioners', *Irish Journal of Medical Science*, vol. 27 (1952), pp. 128–35.

56 See Stanley Gelbier, '125 years of developments in dentistry, 1880–2005 Part 2: Law and the dental profession', *British Dental Journal*, vol. 199 (2005), pp. 470–73.

57 See Gerard Kearns, 'A strong tradition of dentistry', *Journal of the Irish Dental Association* (December 2013/January 2014). See also the work of John B. Lee, especially *The Evolution of a Profession and of its Dental School in Dublin* (1992).

58 Cameron, p. 560.

59 Cameron, pp. 560–61.

60 See Pat O'Donohoe, *150 Years of Stewarts Care – The Pathway to the Present* (2020).

61 Quoted in Cameron, pp. 286–87. Cameron mistakenly calls this the 'Second Supplemental Charter'.

62 Quoted in Laura Kelly's invaluable book on this subject, *Irish Women in Medicine, c.1880s–1920s: Origins, Education and Careers* (2012), p. 21.

63 See Clara Cullen, '"Starry Eyed" Women and Science in Nineteenth-Century Ireland', in Brendan Walsh (ed.), *Knowing Their Place? The Intellectual Life of Women in the Nineteenth* Century (2014), pp. 18–36; p. 34.

64 *The Englishwoman's Review of Social and Industrial Questions* (15 Dec. 1885), p. 534.

65 Cameron (1886), p. 453. In his later (1916) edition, he continues the sentence: 'but many ladies have been educated in it since that year' (p. 561).

66 RCSI/STR/16 (1879–99).

67 Dowson had trained at the London School of Medicine for Women, founded in 1874 by Blackwell, Garrett Anderson and Jex-Blake. In February 1885, RCSI voted to recognise lectures given at the LSMW (Cameron, p. 278).

68 *British Medical Journal*, 12 June 1886, p. 1124.

69 *Dublin Medical Press*, 8 June 1886, p. 524.

70 *The Cambridge Guide to Woman's Writing in English* (1999) describes Dowson as 'a religious writer associated with the Roman Catholic modernist movement'. She was prolific as a writer, a translator (of the philosopher Henri Bergson) and editor, often under the pseudonym W. Scott Palmer. In the 1895 Medical Register, Dowson was listed as a member of the British Medical Association and the Association of Registered Medical Women (the forerunner of the Medical Women's Federation). Dowson died in Hartfield, Sussex, on 2 September 1941, aged 93.

71 Hannan's forenames on the baptismal register of St Werburgh's church are 'Mary Wilhelmina'. It is not known when she became known as 'Mary Josephine'. Her mother, Grace Hannan, gave birth to her youngest son, Benjamin Jocelyn Hannan, on 25 April 1863; she died five days later on 30 April, when Mary Josephine was four years old. Hannan's family home was attached to a branch of La Touche's Bank at 14 Castle Street, where her father, Benjamin Bloomfield Hannan (d. 1900), was Manager. For the Rotunda and Salvation Army connections, see the *Medical Directory* (1891, 1897). *Times of India*, 1 October 1891. Two photographs of Hannan from her time in India are in the Wellcome Collections (14898i, 14899i).

72 See the Medical Register 1896 and 1898. The allusion to ill health is from *Contemporary portraits and biographies: men and women of South Wales and Monmouthshire: Cardiff section* (Cardiff, 1896).

73 The Census of 1901 records a curiosity: Hannan gives Roman Catholic as her religion, though she had originally been baptised into the Church of Ireland.

74 For the South African connection, see M.D. Nash, *The settler handbook: a new list of the 1820 settlers* (Johannesburg: Chameleon Press, 1987). For Hannan's various appointments, see the *British Medical Journal*, 18 March 1905, p. 620, and the *Medical Directory* 1914 ('Med. Off. Native Females; Lect. Midw. Probationers Vict. Matern. Hosp.') and 1918 ('Temp. att. Med. Sect. Union Defence Force'). For the 'champion of unmarried ladies' quote, see the *Western Mail*, 23 November 1918 (in which Hannan is described as a 'former Cardiff lady medical practitioner'). The Girl Guides information is from an obituary of Hannan in the *South African Medical Journal*, vol. 10, no. 14 (July 1936), p. 515.

75 *Handbook on child health education and kindred subjects for South African parents and school teachers* (Cape Town and Johannesburg: Juta & Co., 1924). Hannan writes: 'I have been actuated to prepare these two little handbooks, for the use of South African Parents and Teachers, by personally realizing the benefits and advantages [of] American experiences, from faithfully following the plans which I have herein set forth, and which I have culled from a generous supply of literature given me by the Secretary of the Child Health Organization of America, when I was in New York last year' ('Preface'). For Hannan's journalism, see the *Medical Directory* 1922: 'Author, "Venereal Dis. among Natives", *Women's Outlook*, 1920; Arts. on "Venereal Dis. in connection with Publ. Health", *Star*, 1921.'

76 See *South African Medical Journal*, vol. 10, no. 14 (July 1936), p. 515. The quoted lines are attributed to 'A colleague'.

77 In fact, a Conjoint Licence with the RCPI – discussed below.

78 RCSI/IP/Dickson/4/1/1.

79 *The Medical Women's Federation Quarterly Review* (July 1944), p. 31; the friend was Mary Griscom.

80 In 1898, Dickson applied unsuccessfully for the position of Professor of Obstetrics. The post went to Frederick William Kidd (1857–1917, Lic. 1881, Prof of Obstetrics 1898–1917).

81 See *Irish Times*, 29 January 1892, quoted in Kelly (2012), p. 95; p. 98.

82 'A short account of the school of medicine for men and women, RCSI', quoted in Kelly (2012), p. 89.

83 Kelly (2012), p. 100.

84 *JRCSI* vol. 5, no. 2 (1969), p. 70.

85 Quoted in Kelly (2012), p. 167.

CHAPTER 5 REVOLUTIONS, 1886-1923

1 Quoted in Farmar, *Patients, Poisons & Physicians*, p. 123.

2 Unfortunately, these honorees did not visit RCSI for the occasion. Only Sir James Paget (1814–1899) – also honoured – was in attendance.

3 *Reminiscences of Sir Charles A. Cameron, C.B.* (1913), p. 28.

4 Cameron, *Reminiscences*, p. 71.

5 Cameron, *Reminiscences*, p. 32.

6 For Cameron's biography generally – but especially his public health activities – see Claudia Carroll, *In the Fever King's Preserves: Sir Charles Cameron and the Dublin Slums* (2011).

7 Before Mapother's appointment, the Chair of Hygiene or Political Medicine had been vacant since Maunsell vacated it in 1846. When Mapother resigned as Prof of Anatomy and Physiology, the Chair became that of Physiology only. For Mapother's public service career, see Mary O'Doherty, 'Salus Populi – the Endeavours of Edward Dillon Mapother (1835–1908)', *JICPS* vol. 28, no. 3 (July 1999), pp. 169–73.

8 Cameron gives the date as 1868 in his *Reminiscences*, p. 75. Elsewhere – in his *History* of RCSI – 1867 is posited. Cameron had many strengths, but dates were not his forte. See also Carroll, *In the Fever King's Preserves*, p. 31.

9 Cameron, *Reminiscences*, p. 30.

10 Quoted in Carroll, p. 32.

11 See also J.B. Lyons, *Surgeon-Major Parke's African Journey 1887–89* (1994).

12 *British Medical Journal*, 16 February 1884, p. 334.

13 Cameron, *Reminiscences*, p. 83; p. 86.

14 Cameron, p. 293.

15 At this point the longstanding association of the College of Physicians and Trinity College began to wane – see Coakley, *Medicine in Trinity College*, p. 161.

16 Cameron, p. 764.

17 See Widdess, pp. 95–96; p. 182.

18 Only the rear block here dates to the Carmichael School era. The more elaborate terracotta-coloured front section – a coffeeshop at the time of writing – was erected in 1905.

19 Quoted in Widdess, p. 106.

20 'The scheme [of amalgamation] was finally approved by the College of Surgeons on 1 November 1888, and the transaction completed on December 19. Work under the amalgamation was actually begun on the former date' (Widdess, p. 107). Cameron states: 'The terms of the amalgamation agreed on by all the interested parties were embodied in a deed signed on the 19th September, 1889.

Subsequently it was frequently discussed as to the meaning of some of its provisions' (p. 565).

21 Cameron, p. 566. Widdess says these represent five-year averages (p. 109).

22 *Irish Times*, 29 January 1892.

23 In 1889, the Chair of Descriptive Anatomy was renamed the Chair of Anatomy, retaining this designation until 2019, when it became the Chair of Anatomy and Regenerative Medicine.

24 Quoted in Lyons, *Pride*, p. 206.

25 Auchinleck's daughter Sydney (1884–1970), whom Cameron praised for her poetry (p. 580), would become the first female chemistry graduate of TCD.

26 Both were co-authored with Leonard Strangways.

27 *British Medical Journal*, 7 March 1925, p. 485.

28 *British Medical Journal*, 17 June 1871. The correspondent was future Prof of Ophthalmology, Henry Swanzy.

29 Rubber surgical gloves were introduced by Caroline Hampton and William Halsted at Johns Hopkins Hospital in 1889 – see KP Lee, 'Caroline Hampton Halsted and the origin of surgical gloves', *Journal of Medical Biography*, vol. 28, no. 1 (2020), pp. 64–66.

30 See, for example, Widdess, p. 110.

31 Cameron, p. 270.

32 Quoted in Mary McAuliffe, *Surgeons & Insurgents: RCSI and the Easter Rising* (2016), p. 16.

33 Quoted in Lyons, *An Assembly of Irish Surgeons*, p. 20. Ormsby had a particualr interest in orthopaedic surgery and the diseases of children, which led him to establish the National Orthopaedic and Children's Hospital (1876), a rather grand name for a modest, two-room institution located at 7 Upper Kevin St. Nonetheless, it was the direct forerunner of the National Children's Hospital, Harcourt Street – of which Ormsby was a senior surgeon.

34 This was Cameron's idea – RCSI/COU/21, p. 165, p. 175 (1 and 15 December 1910).

35 RCSI/COU/18, pp. 294–95 (13 July 1904).

36 RCSI/COU/20, p. 195 (6 February 1908).

37 RCSI/COU/20, p. 219 ff. (2 April 1908).

38 *Reports to Council* 1908–09, p. 16.

39 RCSI/COU/21, p. 179 (22 December 1910).

40 *Reports to Council* 1909–10, p. 16.

41 This document can be found in RCSI/NEWS/01.

42 These were Myles' sentiments, quoted in a newspaper – see RCSI/NEWS/01.

43 Blake served as Registrar from 1889 to 1911. He died suddenly a year later, in the Salthill Hotel in Monkstown, an event which made newspaper headlines: 'Found Dead in Bed – Dublin Man's Sudden End'.

44 RCSI/COU/22, p. 11 (31 July 1912).

45 See RCSI/COU/21, pp. 375–79 (20 June 1912).

46 RCSI/COU/20, p. 36, 5 July 1906. All of the referenced

changes took place in the period 1901–08, with the exception of daylight saving, which was introduced in 1916 and appeared in the Council Minutes on 7 June 1917.

47 RCSI/COU/20, p. 188 (16 January 1908); see also J.B. Lyons, *An Assembly of Irish Surgeons* (1984), p. 36.

48 Quoted in RCSI/COU/22, p. 86, 1 May 1913.

49 *Reports to Council* 1910–11, p. 22.

50 RCSI/COU/22, p. 106, 5 June 1913.

51 James Joyce, *Ulysses* (1922; rpr. 1992), p. 300.

52 Quoted in Carroll, *In the Fever King's Preserves*, p. 167.

53 Charles Alexander Cameron, *Reminiscences* (1913), p. 106.

54 See Carroll, *In the Fever King's Preserves*, p. 47.

55 Quoted in Carroll, *In the Fever King's Preserves*, p. 227.

56 *Who Was Who 1916–28* (1929), p. 165.

57 See Carroll, *In the Fever King's Preserves*, p. 51.

58 For TCD's OTC, 1908 is the date given by David Durnin, *The Irish Medical Profession and the First World War* (2019), p. 68; in his *Trinity in War and Revolution* (2015), Tomás Irish points to 1910.

59 *Irish Times*, 10 May 1910, p. 10.

60 See Greta Jones, '"Strike Out Boldly for the Prizes that are Available to You": Medical Emigration from Ireland 1860–1905', *Medical History*, vol. 54, no. 1 (2010), pp. 55–74.

61 See P.J. Casey, K.T. Cullen, and J.P. Duignan, *Irish Doctors in the First World War* (2015), p. 1.

62 See Durnin, *The Irish Medical Profession*, p. 8.

63 In December 2022, the Faculty and School of Nursing and Midwifery unveiled a bust of Nightingale to mark the fortieth anniversary (2021) of their Research and Education Conference. A second bust, marking the same occasion, was of Elizabeth O'Farrell.

64 Casey *et al.*, *Irish Doctors*, p. 12.

65 Quoted in Barry O'Donnell, *Irish Surgeons and Surgery in the Twentieth Century* (2008), p. 315.

66 In particular, in Casey, Cullen and Duignan's *Irish Doctors in the First World War* (2015). My personal thanks to Joseph P. Duignan (FRCSI 1978) for his help.

67 Quoted in Durnin, *The Irish Medical Profession*, p. 54.

68 The women received the rations and pay of temporary commissioned officers; a uniform was introduced after April 1918 – see maltaramc.com.

69 Ahern later received an OBE (1936) for her contribution to child welfare in Malaysia – my thanks to Antonia Lehane (Medicine 1982) for this information about her relative.

70 Quoted in Durnin, *The Irish Medical Profession*, p. 52.

71 See Durnin, *The Irish Medical Profession*, p. 27.

72 Quoted in Durnin, *The Irish Medical Profession*, p. 58.

73 For a table of awards to RCSI personnel, see Casey *et al.*, *Irish Doctors*, p. 19.

74 See Casey *et al.*, *Irish Doctors*, p. 177.

75 This point is from Casey *et al.*, *Irish Doctors*, p. 135.

76 Quoted in Durnin, *The Irish Medical Profession*, p. 74.

77 Quoted in Joseph Harbison, 'The 13th Stationary/83rd (Dublin) General Hospital, Boulogne, 1914–1919', The *Journal of the Royal College of Physicians of Edinburgh*, vol. 45, no. 3 (January 2015), pp. 229–35 p. 231.

78 When Fullerton's successor as PRCSI, T.E. Gordon, died in office (24 July 1929), Fullerton was asked to resume duties until June 1930.

79 Quoted in O'Donnell, *Irish Surgeons and Surgery*, p. 280.

80 O'Donnell, *Irish Surgeons and Surgery*, p. 606.

81 See Sylvie Kleinman, 'Dublin Castle's Viceregal Apartments as Red Cross Military Hospital', *History Ireland*, vol. 24, no. 4 (July/August 2016), pp. 6–7.

82 Quoted in Durnin, p. 107.

83 The first recorded use of X-rays in Ireland was by Richard Bolton McCausland (1864–1933, Lic. 1885, FRCSI 1895) in 1896, just four months after their discovery by Conrad Röntgen.

84 Magaret Skinnider, *Doing My Bit for Ireland* (1917), p. 126.

85 John Freeman Knott, *The Mistletoe* (1908).

86 The wife Knott left running the family farm died of dysentery just as he was completing his studies. Knott married again in 1881; the couple's daughter, Eleanor (1886–1975), a Celtic scholar, became the first woman elected MRIA (1949).

87 Quoted in McAuliffe, *Surgeons & Insurgents*, p. 66, no. 2.

88 Frank Robbins, *Under the Starry Plough* (1977), passim.

89 Skinnider, *Doing My Bit*, p. 118.

90 Quoted in McAuliffe, *Surgeons & Insurgents*, p. 26.

91 The witness was the writer James Stephens – quoted in Fintan O'Toole and Shane Hegarty, *The Irish Times Book of the 1916 Rising* (2006), p. 69.

92 Max Caulfield, *The Easter Rebellion* (1963), p. 154.

93 Skinnider, *Doing My Bit*, p. 116.

94 Amongst ffrench-Mullen's team was Rosie Hackett (1893–1976), later commemorated by a bridge – the first named after a woman – over the Liffey.

95 Quoted in Widdess, p. 154.

96 Patrick Pearse preferred profile poses too, being self-conscious of his strabismus in one eye – see Brian Crowley, *Patrick Pearse: A Life in Pictures* (2013), p. 63.

97 Quoted in McAuliffe, *Surgeons & Insurgents*, p. 42.

98 Quoted in O'Toole and Hegarty, *The Irish Times Book of the 1916 Rising*, p. 82.

99 Quoted in McAuliffe, *Surgeons & Insurgents*, p. 38.

100 Quoted in McAuliffe, *Surgeons & Insurgents*, p. 39.

101 Quoted in McAuliffe, *Surgeons & Insurgents*, p. 44.

102 Quoted in Barry O'Donnell, *Irish Surgeons and Surgery*, p. 198.

103 Cameron, *Autobiography* (1920), pp. 157–58.

104 This was William Oman – see NAI BMH WS 421, p. 11.

105 Quoted in McAuliffe, *Surgeons & Insurgents*, p. 34.

106 Skinnider, *Doing My Bit*, p. 187.

107 NAI BMH WS 1666 (Thomas O'Donoghue), p. 27.

108 Skinnider, *Doing My Bit*, p. 133. Robbins' recollection was of eighty-nine rifles and about 24,000 rounds of ammunition (*Starry Plough*, p. 114).

109 Robbins, *Starry Plough*, pp. 107–08. A bust of Laurence Kettle's brother, the poet and politician Thomas Kettle, killed at the Somme in September 1916, stands in the Green. Skinnider also mentions two other British army officers held captive (p. 140).

110 Quoted in McAuliffe, *Surgeons & Insurgents*, p. 49.

111 Robbins, *Starry Plough*, p. 120.

112 In December 2022, the Faculty and School of Nursing and Midwifery unveiled a bust of O'Farrell to mark the fortieth anniversary (2021) of their Research and Education Conference. A second bust, marking the same occasion, was of Florence Nightingale.

113 Quoted in McAuliffe, *Surgeons & Insurgents*, p. 50.

114 Robbins, *Starry Plough*, p. 122.

115 McAuliffe, *Surgeons & Insurgents*, p. 74, n. 62.

116 Quoted in O'Toole and Hegarty, *The Irish Times Book of the 1916 Rising*, p. 151.

117 See Maynooth University's Letters 1916–1923 collection – items 3640 and 3802.

118 Quoted in Harry Nicholls, NAI BMH WS 296, p. 10.

119 Quoted in Carroll, *In the Fever King's Preserves*, p. 230.

120 Quoted in McAuliffe, *Surgeons & Insurgents*, p. 62.

121 Quoted in Carroll, *In the Fever King's Preserves*, p. 231.

122 The following section is particularly indebted to Ida Milne's *Stacking the Coffins: Influenza, War and Revolution in Ireland* (2018).

123 See Guy Beiner, Patricia Marsh and Ida Milne, 'Greatest killer of the twentieth century: the Great Flu of 1918–19', *History Ireland*, vol. 17, no. 2 (March–April 2009).

124 Shanks, G. Dennis *et al.*, 'Low but highly variable mortality among nurses and physicians during the influenza pandemic of 1918–1919', *Influenza and other respiratory viruses*, vol. 5, no. 3 (2011), pp. 213–19.

125 Milne, *Stacking the Coffins*, p. 95.

126 *Irish Times*, 28 October 1918, p. 6.

127 Milne, *Stacking the Coffins*, p. 33.

128 *Irish Times*, Thursday, 31 October 1918, p. 2.

129 Milne, *Stacking the Coffins*, p. 134.

130 The phrase is Milne's (*Stacking the Coffins*, p. 120).

131 Price, quoted in Milne, *Stacking the Coffins*, p. 120.

132 Quoted in Milne, *Stacking the Coffins*, p. 132.

133 Quoted in Milne, *Stacking the Coffins*, p. 131.

134 Carroll, *In the Fever King's Preserves*, p. 232. The table is also reproduced by Carroll.

135 Quoted in Carroll, *In the Fever King's Preserves*, p. 232.

136 Liam Ryan, 'The Liffey Swim: Dublin's hardy annual has its 100th outing', *Irish Times* (27 July 2019). See also: https://www.hse.ie/eng/services/list/1/public-analyst-laboratory/about-us/history/

137 Quoted in Beiner, Marsh and Milne, 'Greatest killer of the twentieth century', *History Ireland*, vol. 17, no. 2 (March–April 2009).

138 Milne makes the point that there is no mention of the disease in Trinity's muniments (*Stacking the Coffins*, p. 194, n. 7).

139 See also Guy Beiner (ed.), *Pandemic Re-Awakenings: The Forgotten and Unforgotten 'Spanish' Flu of 1918–1919* (2021).

140 See RCSI/IP/Cameron/2/2.

141 Quoted in Lyons, *Pride*, p. 229

142 Lyons, *Pride*, p. 230.

143 Quoted in Lyons, *Pride*, p. 230. On the subject generally, see also Brendan Kelly, *'He Lost Himself Completely': Shell Shock and its Treatment at Dublin's Richmond War Hospital, 1916–1919* (2014).

144 Harvey Cushing, *From a Surgeon's Journal, 1915–1918* (1936), pp. 359–61. The visit occurred in May 1918. On a related note, the French surgeon René Leriche (1879–1955) was scheduled for the same honour in early 1956. During the First World War, he instituted the convention of blue walls and blue gowns to denote surgical environments. But alas, he died a few weeks before he could accept his award.

145 See Lyons, *Assembly*, p. 37.

146 RCSI/COU/24, 2 December 1920, p. 320.

147 See Lyons, *Assembly*, p. 53.

148 Quoted in Durnin, *The Irish Medical Profession*, p. 201.

149 'Reports on Wounded in Dublin Hospitals', *BMJ*, 3139, no. 1 (1921), p. 319.

150 'Wounded in Hospital', *BMJ*, 3143, no. 1 (1921), p. 477.

151 RCSI/COU/24, 3 March 1921.

152 See Barry O'Donnell, *Irish Surgeons and Surgery*, p. 229.

153 See Eunan O'Halpin and Daithí Ó Corráin, *The Dead of the Irish Revolution* (2020), pp. 358–59. See also NAI BMH WS 1361 (Gerald Davis) for references to Darcy and another Republican RCSI student, Thomas Lawless (p. 8). My thanks to Kevin Finnan for this information.

154 'Arrests of Medical Men', *BMJ*, 3139, no. 1 (1921), p. 319.

155 RCSI/COU/24, 7 July 1921, p. 362.

156 RCSI/COU/24, 6 October 1921, p. 368.

157 RCSI/COU/26, 20 July 1922. When (Anti-Treaty) soldiers visited RCSI, they asked to see 'the vulnerable danger points which particularly needed the defenders' attention'. They were shown around by Christy O'Toole, who had joined RCSI in 1919 as a technician in the Department of Pathology. In 1964, O'Toole became resident caretaker in the Medical School (*Yearbook* 1970, p. 128). He died in 1972, after fifty-three years in continuous RCSI employ.

158 Eoin Neeson has suggested RCSI as the location ('So,

once and for all, who did shoot Michael Collins?', *Irish Times*, 22 August 2003); Ulick O'Connor suggests Trinity College. A larger consensus points to St Vincent's, not least as Collins' body lay in the chapel there before being brought to City Hall.

159 Dáil debates, 'Nominations for the Senate', 25 October 1922.

160 Quoted in Lyons, *Assembly*, p. 66.

161 Quoted in Lyons, *Assembly*, p. 63. Healy was a first cousin of T.F. Higgins (senior, mentioned above), who was killed in February 1923 (the Council sent a note of sympathy to his widow); his son Kevin O'Higgins was killed in 1927 (the family added the 'O' in 1921). In 1932, T.F. O'Higgins (junior, the Licentiate of RCSI and RCPI) was appointed leader of the Army Comrades Association, better known as 'the Blueshirts' – see Maurice Manning, *The Blueshirts* (1970, 3rd ed. 2006).

162 *Freeman's Journal*, 27 February 1923.

CHAPTER 6 IN ADVERSITY, 1924-61

1 See Laura Kelly, *Irish Medical Education and Student Culture, c.1850–1950* (2017), p. 247.

2 *Irish Times*, Friday, 21 December 1923.

3 See J.B. Lyons, 'Irish medicine's appeal to Rockefeller, 1920s', *Irish Journal of Medical Science* (Jan, Feb, Mar 1997), pp. 50–56; and Greta Jones, 'The Rockefeller Foundation and medical education in Ireland in the 1920s', *Irish Historical Studies*, vol. 30, no. 120 (November 1997), pp. 564–80.

4 Quoted in Farmar, *Patients, Potions & Physicians*, p. 138.

5 Quoted in Kelly, *Irish Medical Education*, p. 204.

6 Quoted in Lyons, 'Irish medicine's appeal to Rockefeller', p. 52.

7 Quoted in Farmar, *Patients, Potions & Physicians*, p. 138.

8 Quoted in Lyons, 'Irish medicine's appeal to Rockefeller', p. 52; p. 55.

9 See Jones, 'The Rockefeller Foundation and medical education in Ireland', pp. 577–79.

10 The proposal was first mooted in August 1923 – see Jones, p. 573. Cosgrave was the President of the Executive Council of the Irish Free State – the precursor to Taoiseach.

11 These particular figures are from the *Irish Times*, Monday, 17 February 1935. Farmar puts the 'export' figure at 80 per cent (*Patients, Potions & Physicians*, p. 137).

12 Quoted in Kelly, *Irish Medical Education*, p. 202.

13 Quoted in Jones, 'The Rockefeller Foundation and medical education in Ireland', p. 574.

14 Quoted in Jones, 'The Rockefeller Foundation and medical education in Ireland', p. 575.

15 RCSI/COU/26, 13 February 1924.

16 RCSI/COU/26, 8 May 1924, p. 101.

17 RCSI/COU/26, 11 February 1926, p. 150

18 *RCSI Reports to Council, 1917–35*, p. 226.

19 Hugh Hampton Young, *A Surgeon's Autobiography* (1940), p. 488.

20 RCSI/COU/26, 10 January 1929, p. 218.

21 RCSI/COU/26, 10 July 1930, p. 244; 11 December 1930, pp. 249–50.

22 *Irish Times*, 21 February 1927, p. 7.

23 See Lyons, *Assembly*, p. 78.

24 RCSI/COU/26, 11 January 1934, p. 299.

25 *Irish Times*, 14 July 1927, p. 4. Future PRCSI Henry Sords Meade was one of those who attempted to save O'Higgins (O'Donnell, *Irish Surgeons and Surgery*, p. 199).

26 RCSI/COU/26, p. 152, 11 March 1926.

27 Following Cameron's retirement (1920), the Chair of Hygiene or Political Medicine was united with that of Medical Jurisprudence.

28 Coakley, *Medicine in Trinity College*, p. 216.

29 Quoted in Lyons, *Pride*, p. 248.

30 Quoted in Lyons, *Pride*, p. 250.

31 Quoted in Lyons, *Pride*, p. 248.

32 *Irish Times*, Monday, 8 February 1932, p. 6.

33 *Irish Times*, Monday, 8 February 1932, p. 6.

34 *Weekly Irish Times*, 13 February 1937, p. 9.

35 See Marie Coleman, *The Irish Sweep: A History of the Irish Hospitals Sweepstake, 1930–87* (2009).

36 Quoted in Kelly, *Irish Medical Education*, p. 159.

37 Worth noting too, in 1898, as a student at Trinity, Francis Carmichael Purser (RCSI Prof of Medicine, 1917–29), played for Ireland three times.

38 See Philip O'Halloran, 'The Dublin Hospitals Rugby Cup', *RCSI SMJ*, vol. 1, no. 1 (2008), pp. 10–11. See also Conleth Feighery, Michael Farrell and Morgan Crowe, *The Hospital Pass – 140 Years of Dublin Hospitals Rugby* (2019).

39 Kelly, *Irish Medical Education*, p. 157.

40 Quoted in Kelly, *Irish Medical Education*, p. 159.

41 Quoted in Billy O'Riordan, 'The Doc: Remembering Pat O'Callaghan – Ireland's first Olympic hero', *Irish Examiner*, 1 August 2018.

42 *Irish Times*, Monday, 24 October 1932, p. 2.

43 He was a son of Andrew Daniel Clinch (1867–1937, Dip. Public Health 1912), who was capped for Ireland ten times. Clinch senior was President of the IRFU (1904–05) and a founder of the Hermitage Golf Club. Both Clinches toured with the Lions.

44 RCSI/COU/28, 10 December 1942, p. 73. Some twenty-four years later, attitudes had changed: in her vivid memoir, *The Women's Doc: True Stories from My Five Decades Delivering Babies and Making History* (2021), Caroline de Costa recollects that an atmosphere of the utmost respect was cultivated in the Anatomy Room, and there was 'no possibility of anyone who was not a student, doctor, teacher or technician being admitted' (p. 42).

45 *Irish Times*, 1 June 1939, p. 13.

46 RCSI/COU/26, 8 February 1928, p. 197.

47 See O'Donnell, *Irish Surgeons and Surgery*, p. 268. See also Lyons, *Assembly*, pp. 40–42, especially for Purefoy's Joycean connections.

48 RCSI/COU/26, 17 June 1937, p. 360.

49 See *Irish Times*, 30 January 1990, 16 February 1990, 24 February 1990; *JICPS* vol. 19, no. 2 (April 1990), p. 151. For Caroline de Costa's role in this repatriation, see her memoir, *The Women's Doc* (2021), pp. 51–52. De Costa writes: 'Over the past 30 years, more than 1,500 Australian Indigenous ancestral remains have been repatriated from institutions, and even private collections... Until the last one is returned, this stain on our [Australian] history will remain' (p. 52).

50 RCSI/COU/26, 10 December 1936, p. 350, and passim until 14 April 1938, p. 376.

51 *Irish Times*, Monday, 19 June 1939, p. 7.

52 My thanks to Joseph Duignan (FRCSI 1978) for these figures. For further research, gathered for the first time, see also Patrick Casey, Kevin Cullen and Joseph Duignan, *Irish Doctors in the Second World War* (forthcoming).

53 My thanks, again, to Joseph Duignan for this point.

54 See Cathy Hayes, *Dictionary of Irish Biography*.

55 Lyons, *Assembly*, p. 150.

56 In addition, Wilson wrote biographies of Jonathan Swift and William Wilde.

57 From the same era, RCSI holds two more stained-glass windows, both by Terence Clarke (nephew of Harry Clarke): *Crucified Christ* (1953) and *Blessed Virgin with the Christ Child and St John the Baptist* (1954); both are in the basement-level Serenity Room in 123 St Stephen's Green, having been presented to RCSI by Mary and John Clarke in June 1983.

58 Quoted in Coakley, *Medicine in Trinity College Dublin*, p. 226.

59 This Pringle was a cousin of his PRCSI namesake, who had served in the First World War (1879–1955, FRCSI 1905, PRCSI 1934–36).

60 RCSI/COU/28, 10 October 1940, pp. 39–40.

61 After the first edition, only Reilly and Rae were the named co-authors.

62 See Declan Warde, Joseph Tracey and John Cahill, *Safety as We Watch: Anaesthesia in Ireland 1847–1998* (2022), p. 403.

63 RCSI/COU/28, 28 March 1946, p. 133.

64 Lyons, *Assembly*, p. 104.

65 Lyons, *Assembly*, p. 106.

66 Quoted in Lyons, *Assembly*, p. 121.

67 Established in 1912, the annual Mary Louisa Prentice Montgomery Memorial Lecture in Ophthalmology – named for a bequest by Robert Montgomery (1897–1912, FRCSI 1889) in memory of his mother – rotates between TCD and RCSI every five years. It is now curated by the Irish College of Ophthalmologists.

68 RCSI/COU/28, 14 December 1944, p. 107.

69 *Irish Times*, Saturday, 18 December 1943, p. 4.

70 See Greta Jones, *'Captain of All These Men of Death': The History of Tuberculosis in Nineteenth and Twentieth Century Ireland* (2001), p. 189.

71 *Irish Times*, Monday, 10 July 1944, p. 3.

72 Greta Jones, *Captain of All These Men of Death*, p. 187.

73 Greta Jones, *Captain of All These Men of Death*, p. 194.

74 See Lyons, *Pride*, pp. 190–91.

75 RCSI/OH/2/1 (W.A.L. MacGowan).

76 *Irish Medical Times*, 26 February 1982.

77 See *Irish Medical Times*, 18 June 1982.

78 RCSI/EDC/8 (1948–1959), 11 and 13 May 1953.

79 Quoted in Lyons, *Assembly*, p. 110.

80 *Irish Times*, 29 October 1945, p. 2. See also photo, p. 1.

81 *Irish Times*, 15 November 1954, p. 5.

82 *Irish Times*, 30 April 1962, p. 6.

83 'The training of doctors: report by the Goodenough Committee', *British Medical Journal*, 22 July 1944, p. 121.

84 Quoted in *Irish Times*, 26 April 1952, p. 6.

85 *Irish Times*, 15 May 1946, p. 7.

86 Information on students prior to 1828 is scanty, but after that point the Roll of Licentiates (RCSI/LIC/01/01, 1828–74) records Licentiates who gave home addresses in, *inter alia*, India (1830), Canada (1833), Brazil (1838), Turkey (1865), USA (1866), Australia (1866), Jamaica (1867), the West Indies (1867), Mauritius (1869), Macao (1877), Argentina (1883) and New Zealand (1883). My thanks to Jessica Handy for this research.

87 *Irish Times*, 8 February 1955, p. 6.

88 *Irish Times*, 8 February 1955, p. 6.

89 *Irish Times*, 18 December 1953, p. 1.

90 Harry O'Flanagan, 'The Immediate Past', in J.B. Lyons, H. O'Flanagan and W.A.L. MacGowan, *The Irresistible Rise of the RCSI* (n.d., [1984?]), p. 21.

91 Stacey B. Day, *The Idle Thoughts of a Surgical Fellow* (1968), p. 18. Day later enjoyed a remarkable career with the WHO in New York and Nashville, and in Nigeria, Czechoslovakia and Japan; he is also the author of a Joycean novel, *Rosalita* (1968) and multiple collections of verse and drama.

92 In 1936, the late Mrs M.C. Nolans bequeathed £1,000 to fund this prize in memory of her husband, Francis Nolans (FRCSI 1900). See RCSI/COU/26, 12 March 1936, p. 340.

93 RCSI/EDC/8, 13 December 1950.

94 For this entire debate, see Greta Jones, '"A Mysterious Discrimination": Irish Medical Emigration to the United States in the 1950s', *Social History of Medicine*, vol. 25, no. 1 (2011), pp. 139–56.

95 This came to light in the run-up to the subsequent inspection – see *Irish Times*, 22 July 1953, p. 1.

96 RCSI/COU/28, 13 December 1951, p. 241.

97 RCSI/EDC/8, 8 July 1953.

98 Quoted in Coakley, *Medicine in Trinity College Dublin*, p. 252.

99 *Irish Times*, 7 November 1953, p. 4.

100 *Irish Times*, 5 December 1953, p. 9.

101 These figures are quoted in the *Irish Times*: 31 May 1949, p. 1; 7 December 1950; 4 March 1953, p. 4.

102 *Irish Times*, 5 December 1953, p. 9.

103 'The American Visit', *Journal of the Irish Medical Association*, vol. 33, no. 197 (November 1953), pp. 149–50.

104 See Greta Jones, '"A Mysterious Discrimination": Irish Medical Emigration to the United States in the 1950s', *Social History of Medicine*, vol. 25, no. 1 (2011), pp. 139–56. ECFMG stands for Educational Commission for Foreign Medical Graduates.

105 *Irish Times*, 9 November 1953, p. 9.

106 The phrase is from Jones, 'A Mysterious Discrimination', p. 144. In the period, that word 'unstructured' also applied to the wider relationship between the Irish medical establishment and the neophyte Department of Health (operational since 1947, Ireland was one of the last countries in Europe to set up such a separate entity). On the (in)famous occasion when the Irish Medical Association and the Catholic Church jointly set themselves against Minister Noël Browne's 'Mother and Child scheme', the IMA convened an EGM at RCSI to hear that their members' vote on the proposal resulted in 'an overwhelming rejection' (*Irish Times*, 24 November 1950, p. 1).

107 Abrahamson's birthplace and date of birth given here are from Helen Andrews' entry in the *Dictionary of Irish Biography*. In Lyons' portrait, he points to Newry, Co. Down and the year 1897 (*Pride*, p. 255).

108 This was Patrick Bofin (Prof of Forensic Medicine and Toxicology 1972–1990), quoted in Lyons, *Pride*, p. 261.

109 Quoted in Lyons, *Pride*, p. 260.

110 Lyons, *Pride*, p. 261.

111 Day, *Idle Thoughts*, p. 26.

112 During the 'Mother and Child' imbroglio, Abrahamson's position was that 'the medical profession did not want any State control of medical services because it felt that it would destroy the doctor–patient relationship' (quoted in Farmar, *Patients, Potions & Physicians*, p. 177). In 1961, Mervyn Abrahamson was appointed to his father's former Chair of Materia Medica (1961–74). The filmmaker Lenny Abrahamson is his namesake's grandson.

113 RCSI/COU/28, 14 April 1949, p. 190. Thereafter, Doolin became to colleagues less and less a surgical consultant and more and more a man of letters. He had been editor of the *Irish Journal of Medical Science* since 1925; from 1954, he was also the editor of the *Journal of the Irish Medical Association*.

114 Report to Council 1947, 14 November.

115 *Irish Times*, 9 July 1960, p. 7.

116 See Richard Clarke's chapter in O'Donnell, *Irish Surgeons and Surgery*, especially pp. 582–84.

117 This was rectified in 1986, with the appointment of Tony Cunningham as Gilmartin's successor.

118 For these developments in greater detail, see Declan Warde, Joseph Tracey and John Cahill, *Safety as We Watch: Anaesthesia in Ireland 1847–1998* (2022).

119 Quoted in David McInerney's chapter in O'Donnell, *Irish Surgeons and Surgery*, p. 610.

120 For these developments in greater detail, see J.C. Carr (ed.), *A Century of Medical Radiation in Ireland – An Anthology* (1995).

121 *Irish Times*, 12 February 1962, p. 9.

122 RCSI/COU/28, 8 June 1950, p. 218.

123 Dublin Distillers and Arthur Guinness and Sons also made donations.

124 RCSI/COU/28, 14 December 1944, p. 107.

125 RCSI/COU/28, 12 April 1951, p. 230.

126 The student was John O'Hagan Ward (Lic. 1937), quoted in J.D. Garry, *A Dublin Anatomist* (revised ed. 1998), pp. 30–31.

127 *Irish Times*, 13 August 1956, p. 7.

128 Pressed on the subject himself, Garry was known to reply: 'Mind your own f****** business' (Garry, *A Dublin Anatomist*, p. 43).

129 Quoted in Garry, *A Dublin Anatomist*, p. 23.

130 Quoted in Garry, *A Dublin Anatomist*, p. 46.

131 Garry, *A Dublin Anatomist*, p. 46.

132 AK Henry, *Extensile Exposure*, p. 8.

133 RCSI/COU/28, 10 February 1949, p. 187.

134 Relatedly, when William John Edward ('W.J.E.') Jessop (1902–1980, Prof of Physiology 1929–53, PRCPI 1972–74) was appointed to the Senate in 1952 for his nutritional expertise, the joke went around RCSI that this was the time to press for 'an improvement in the standard of their commons!' (*Irish Times*, 13 March 1952, p. 7).

135 Joan Briscoe (Lic. 1946), Brian Briscoe (1956) and Joe Briscoe (Lic. Dent. 1952). My thanks to Brian and Ben for their recollections. Thanks, too, to Daniel Briscoe (Medicine 1987) for his recollections of a later era.

136 *Irish Times*, 7 February 1956, p. 3.

137 The name 'Doherty', as opposed to 'Docherty', appears in the Medical Register.

138 The Basketball Club was 're-established' in 1963 by Jack Kearney (Lic. 1969), with help from Dr Seamus Gallen, Superintendent of the Schools. The star player of this era was Jack Prendergast (Lic. 1972). Without a regulation court of their own, all RCSI's game were 'away', usually in Cathal Brugha Barracks, Rathmines. Practice time — and hot showers — was provided by sneaking into Trinity's gym (information provided by Jack Kearney). The Ladies' Basketball Club was founded by Anne Rigney (Lic. 1972).

139 *Surgeons Log: Annual of the Schools of Surgery, Royal College of Surgeons in Ireland* [1948], pp. 123–24. Edited by L.E. Mc-Loughlin, this was produced under the auspices of the Literary and Dramatic Society. It appears to have lived for a single issue only.

140 Subsequently, Dr Terence Bradshaw (Lic. 1938) took over, guiding the society through 'an exceptionally good year' (*Surgeons Log* [1948], p. 134).

141 In the late 1960s, the Emile Stone Cup went missing; it was found again in 2020.

142 This particular department went through several identity and nomenclature shifts before and after the war.

143 RCSI/COU/34, 9 November 1961, p. 36. In truth, Gaffney's association with RCSI predates her official appointment; when her husband was an external examiner for RCSI, it was she who corrected the scripts (see Phyllis Gaffney's recollections of her mother in *Irish Chemical News* no. 5 (December 2017), pp. 53–55).

144 Quoted in Lyons, *Assembly*, p. 100.

145 W.J.E. Jessop, 'The Medical Schools in the Republic of Ireland', *Journal of Medical Education*, vol. 36 (September 1961), pp. 1,102–19.

146 As it happens, Mercer's became exclusively a Trinity hospital later that year.

CHAPTER 7 RENAISSANCE, 1962-84

1 Hereafter, birth and (post-2000) death dates are not recorded, except where particularly relevant.

2 Harry O'Flanagan, 'The bombing of Dresden: Shrove Tuesday / Ash Wednesday – February 13–14th, 1945', *JICPS*, vol. 21, no.3, July 1992, pp. 185–88. The quoted lines in this section are from this text.

3 See O'Flanagan's essay, 'The Immediate Past – the RCSI from 1961–1981', in *The Irresistible Rise of the RCSI*, p. 17.

4 For a compelling argument for preservation, see Frank McDonald (Hon FRCSI 2019), *The Destruction of Dublin* (1985). With specific reference to the Bolton Street and Fenian Street disasters, McDonald makes the point that 'almost any building, no matter how old, will survive as long as it is well-maintained' (p. 24).

5 These details, and the paragraphs below, are drawn from O'Flanagan's 1981 account ('The Immediate Past', pp. 22–24). Widdess' slightly different version (pp. 121–23) draws on correspondence with O'Flanagan dated September 1980.

6 RCSI/COU/34, 1960–63, 16 March 1961, p. 20; 8 June 1961, p. 30.

7 The Council Minutes record the donation being £10,000 (RCSI/COU/34, 14 June 1962, p. 55).

8 See O'Donnell, *Irish Surgeons and Surgery*, pp. 569–70. See also O'Donnell's biography, *Terence Millin: A Remarkable Surgeon* (2002).

9 Following President O'Ceallaigh (1958) and Rupert Guinness, 2nd Earl of Iveagh (1961), President De Valera was only the third non-medical Honorary Fellow (1964).

10 'The Immediate Past', p. 23.

11 The sitting tenants were rehoused by the Corporation. Late in the day, RCSI was obliged to deal directly with three landlords, who in the event, said O'Flanagan, 'proved to be quite reasonable' (p. 24).

12 The name of the company that O'Flanagan gives is 'The Mineral Water Company'; Taylor Keith's ownership of the site is reference in RCSI/COU/36, 1963–68, 8 April 1965, p. 46.

13 RCSI/COU/36, 14 January 1964, p. 39; 11 February 1965, p. 42. The price for the 7.5 acres was £16,500 plus costs.

14 Goodwin's memoir quotes, 'Come back when they're green' – but elsewhere (*Yearbook* 1972, p. 27), Kane's word is the more plausible 'brown'.

15 Robert C. Goodwin, 'You Had to be There, RCSI 1965–1971', *JICPS* vol. 13, no. 2 (April 1984), pp. 96–98.

16 'Geographic Distribution of Graduates, 1964–73', Lyons, 'Irresistible Rise', p. 14.

17 For example, in 1965 and 1970, respectively, eight and nine Irish students qualified – see O'Flanagan, 'The Immediate Past', p. 21.

18 *Irish Times*, Tuesday, 8 December 1964, p. 4. For the record, seventeen said there was a 'colour bar', four said there wasn't; twelve found it 'fairly difficult' to make contact with locals, twelve said it was 'fairly easy'.

19 As Medical Director of St Patrick's Hospital (1946–79), Moore led that institution, as well as much Irish psychiatric practice, out of the Victorian age. He was also an early advocate of Alcoholics Anonymous in Ireland.

20 RCSI/COU/34, 12 July 1962, p. 58.

21 See *JICPS* vol. 5, no. 3 (January 1976), p. 102. The history of this department is told by Prof Cahill in *A Dream in Dublin* (2016).

22 *Irish Times*, 27 March 2004.

23 *Irish Times*, 11 December 1972, p. 16.

24 RCSI/COU/40 (1969–72), 8 May 1969, p. 18.

25 This was at Bofin's presidential address to the Biological Society – see *Irish Times*, 7 November 1972, p. 9.

26 *JRCSI* vol. 1, no. 1, (1963), p. 67.

27 *Irish Times*, 2 May 2006.

28 RCSI/COU/34, 13 June 1963, p. 83.

29 The phrase is O'Flanagan's; *Irish Times*, 6 November 1967, p. 7.

30 RCSI/COU/36, 13 October 1966, p. 102.

31 *Journal of the Royal College of Surgeons in Ireland*, vol. 5, no. 3 (January 1970), p. 115.

32 Quoted in O'Flanagan, 'The Immediate Past', p. 20.

33 Quoted in O'Flanagan, 'The Immediate Past', p. 20.

34 Charles Mulvey, *The Medical School of the Royal College of Surgeons in Ireland: A Cost-Benefit Study* (Dublin: Institute of Public Administration, 1971).

35 Mulvey, *A Cost-Benefit Study*, p. 45.

36 Mulvey, *A Cost-Benefit Study*, pp. 1–2.

37 *Sunday Press*, 7 November 1965.

38 Mulvey, *A Cost-Benefit Study*, p. 2.

39 *Irish Times*, 6 November 1967, p. 7.

40 Mulvey, *A Cost-Benefit Study*, p. 2.

41 Author's personal communication with Charles Mulvey, 26 August 2021.

42 *The Higher Education Authority Report on University Reorganisation* (Dublin: The Stationery Office, 1972), p. 36.

43 O'Flanagan, 'The Immediate Past', p. 21.

44 RCSI/COU/42, 11 January 1973, p. 23.

45 *Irish Times*, 20 November 1972, p. 9.

46 *Journal of the Royal College of Surgeons in Ireland*, vol. 4, no. 4 (April 1969), p. 141.

47 O'Flanagan, 'The Immediate Past', p. 24–26.

48 O'Flanagan, 'The Immediate Past', p. 25.

49 South Africans of Indian origin – then synonymous with 'Asian' – were subject to the same apartheid laws as those of native origins. Indeed, eight decades earlier, M.K. Gandhi's experience of discrimination in South Africa considerably influenced his politicisation.

50 See *JRCSI* vol. 4, no. 3 (January 1969), p. 126.

51 Essack was later described as 'a graduate whose heart and mind are dedicated to this College so far from his home' (*JICPS*. vol. 10. no. 2 (October 1980), p. 89).

52 *Irish Medical Times*, 14 September 1984.

53 See, for example, *Evening Herald*, 5 March 1969. See also *JRCSI* vol. 4, no. 2 (October 1968), pp. 84–85.

54 O'Flanagan, 'The Immediate Past', p. 24.

55 RCSI/COU/42, 5 July 1973, p. 45.

56 *JICPS*, vol.1, no. 1 (July 1971), p. 3.

57 RCSI/COU/42, 10 May 1973, p. 34.

58 *Irish Times*, 2 February 1972, p. 6.

59 Quoted in Lyons, *Pride*, p. 270. See also Eoin O'Brien, 'Samuel Beckett at Saint-Lo – 'Humanity in Ruins', *JICPS*, vol. 19 (1990), pp. 137–45; and Phyllis Gaffney, *Healing Amid the Ruins: The Irish Hospital at St-Lô (1945–46)* (1999).

60 *Irish Times*, 29 June 1974, p. 13.

61 The Faculty celebrated its first four decades with a retrospective survey of its many achievements and personalities, *Faculty of Nursing & Midwifery 40th Anniversary History 1974–2014* (2014), by John Adams (*ad eundem* Fellow FoN&M 2013), Marie Carney (Dean of the FoN&M) and Thomas Kearns (Executive Director of the FoN&M).

62 These were in Orthodontics (Rodney Beresford Dockrell), Oral Surgery (Ian Arthur Findlay), Conservative Dentistry (Norman Patrick Butler) and Prosthetic Dentistry (W.A. Lawson).

63 For greater detail, see John B. Lee, *The Evolution of a Profession and of its Dental School in Dublin* (1992).

64 The last RCSI Dental Licentiate to process – alphabetically – out the door was Spencer Woolfe (Lic. 1975, Lic. Dent. 1976). In keeping with RCSI tradition, he followed in the footsteps of his father, Hyman (Lic. Dent. 1934), and brother Andrew (Francis Nolans Prize 1954, Lic. Dent. 1964 and – the last person to gain the dual qualification – Lic. 1966). My thanks to Drs Spencer and Andrew Woolf for their recollections.

65 *Irish Times*, 12 December 1974, p. 4.

66 The appointment process proceeded by increments, no doubt after the previous legal fiasco. The Planning Committee met five times before they spoke to Foley. His initial appointment in March 1971 only covered the drawing phase (RCSI/COU/40, 11 March 1971, p. 60); a subsequent contract was issued in April. An original partner in Buchan, Kane and Foley, Frank Foley was operating independently at the time of Michael Kane's first drawings, though the firm still carried his name; after Kane's death, he rejoined the firm. My thanks to Timothy Foley of Buchan, Kane and Foley for this information.

67 O'Flanagan, 'The Immediate Past,' p. 24.

68 This estimated figure is given in the *Irish Times*, 25 January 1974.

69 *Plan: the Architectural Magazine*, vol. 6, no. 9 (December 1975), pp. 5–14. See also Colin Brennan, 'The Royal College of Surgeons in Ireland: an architectural history 1805–1997', unpublished MA thesis, UCD, 1997, pp. 45–47. The observation about concrete always looking like concrete is Brennan's.

70 For another, more controversial, aspect of McGrath's fundraising, see Marie Coleman, *The Irish Sweep: A History of the Irish Hospitals Sweepstake, 1930–1987* (2009).

71 Ó Dálaigh expanded on his admiration for RCSI in a lecture entitled 'An Old Tradition in a New Mould' (*JICPS*, vol. 5, pp. 99–104 (1976)). The Court of Patrons had been set up some years previously, in 1968. After Ó Dálaigh, inductees included Alexander Lindsay Stewart of Ethicon Ltd (1975), Mohammed Essack (1980) and Senator Patrick McGrath (also 1980). A board recording later inductees hangs in 123 St Stephen's Green.

72 His books on the subject include *James Joyce & Medicine* (1975) and *'Thrust Syphilis Down to Hell' and Other Rejoyceana: Studies in the Borderlands of Literature* (1988).

73 See also, Stanley McCollum, 'The Royal College of Surgeons in Ireland: Search for a Degree', *JICPS*, vol. 17, no. 3 (July 1988), pp. 106–09.

74 See David Mitchell, 'The Irish Royal Colleges in the second half of the Nineteenth Century: An Ambivalent Relationship', *JICPS* vol. 13, no. 1 (January 1984), pp. 39–42.

75 Quoted in Widdess, p. 133.

76 *JICPS* vol. 4, no. 2 (1974), p. 72.

77 RCSI/COU/36, 14 November 1968, p. 155.

78 RCSI/COU/40, 7 October 1971, p. 71.

79 O'Flanagan, 'The Immediate Past', p. 26.

80 RCSI/COU/42, 14 December 1972, p. 21.

81 RCSI/COU/42, 11 January 1973, p. 24.

82 *Irish Times*, 30 April 1973, p. 13.

83 This quote is from RCSI/COU/42, 11 March 1976, p. 179; it is a reiteration of the Minister's opinion, declared in the Dáil, 22 January 1975. The meeting with McAuliffe Curtin took place in October 1975 (see O'Flanagan, p. 27). Not long after the Minister's decision, fresh legal counsel offered the redundant advice that the College could not, in fact, issue its own degrees.

84 My thanks to Prof MacGowan for this point. Also present was a recent arrival at RCSI, the new Academic Secretary, Joseph G. Grace.

85 The expression is O'Flanagan's, 'The Immediate Past', p. 27.

86 RCSI/COU/44, 19 January 1977, p. 220.

87 *JICPS*, vol. 6, no. 4 (April 1977), 'Editorial Comment: RCSI and UCD', p. 119. The editor was Eoin O'Brien (Lic. 1963).

88 In addition, RCSI students from the Class of 1977 were given the option of re-sitting their finals in Medicine and Surgery in order to receive the NUI degree they had so narrowly missed. Ten students availed of the offer.

89 Quoted in *JICPS*, vol. 8, no. 1 (July 1978), p. 27.

90 RCSI/COU/44, 8 May 1980, p. 401; 9 October 1980, p. 417. The house in South Frederick Street belonged to the New Ireland Assurance Company. The donation of the ceiling was orchestrated 'through the good offices of Senator Eoin Ryan and Mrs. Joan Duff' (p. 401).

91 See *Annual Report* 1981, p. 11; and Brennan, p. 50. Some later commentary attributes the fireplace to Pietro Bossi, but without citing evidence. Foley's advisor on these internal projects was Joan Duff – the wife of former PRCSI Frank Duff, but also eminently qualified in her own right: in 1978, she founded the Irish Museums Trust.

92 Notable here is the £120,000 raised by Colles Graves Foundation, New York – that is, donations from US-based graduates, parents and friends. Another £51,155 was raised by South African graduates, parents and friends. For a complete table, see *JICPS*, vol. 8, no. 4 (April 1979), p. 166.

93 RCSI/COU/44, 11 October 1979, p. 370.

94 RCSI/COU/45, 3 July 1980, p. 409. The final sale price was £121,040.

95 RCSI/COU/45, 12 November 1981, p. 579. For the estimated cost, see *JICPS* vol. 12, no. 3 (January 1983), p. 132.

96 O'Flanagan, p. 18.

97 RCSI/COU/44, 8 February 1979, p. 338.

98 RCSI also contributed to the Lord Mayor's fund for victims.

99 *JICPS* vol. 11, no. 2 (October 1981), p. 84.

100 *Irish Times*, 15 July 1981, p. 1.

101 Other notable Honorary Fellows in this era include: the Danish cardiothoracic surgeon and wartime resistance hero, Erik Husfeldt (1964); Sir Arthur Porritt (1964), a surgeon, sportsman (he won an Olympic bronze in the real-life *Chariots of Fire* race) and statesman; the Irish ophthalmologist Lionel Becher Somerville Large (1965); Ethicon's managing director, Leonard Bailey (1967); the innovative American vascular and cardiac surgeon Michael DeBakey (1967); the Guinness heir, Lord Moyne (1968), one of the original 'Bright Young Things', latterly an author and patron of the arts; Pietro Valdoni (1968), surgeon to the Pope; the Swedish-born, US-based Orvar Swenson (1969), author of the classic *Swenson's Pediatric Surgery*. In the 1970s, the list includes: the Nigerian plastic surgeon Horatio Orishejolomi Thomas (1970), the first African to receive the award; Owen Harding Wangensteen (1970), whose eponymous tube was credited with saving a million lives in his lifetime. Also honoured was George Dale Zuidema (1972) of Johns Hopkins (with which institution RCSI would enjoy a thirty-year exchange programme commencing in 1978); and Uganda-based Denis Parsons Burkitt (1973), already famous for his eponymous lymphoma (further fame was to follow with his advocacy of a high-fibre diet); and the American superstar surgeon Francis Daniels Moore (1973), who had appeared in his scrubs on the cover of *Time* a decade earlier. The first South African honoured was Jan Hendrik Louw (1974), best known for his work in congenital intestinal atresia (inspired by the death of his infant son from the condition, he reduced the mortality rate from 90 per cent to 10 per cent). Keen to show off the New Medical School, in 1976 RCSI awarded a record number of Honorary Fellowships, amongst whom were the first New Zealander, John Stallworthy, the Americans Francis Sooy and John Hartwell Harrison, and the Scot James Alexander Ross – the latter two took part in the first kidney transplants in their respective countries. Also honoured was the orthopaedic surgeon Sir Harry Platt, known for the 'Platt Report' (1959), which revolutionised the care of children in hospital by considering – largely for the first time – their emotional needs. (After Platt, children were allowed to keep their personal possessions and wear their own clothes, play was allowed, and parental access – previously limited to a few hours per week – was now considered of paramount importance.) The first Australian to be honoured was the colorectal specialist Sir Edward Hughes (1977), then President of the Royal Australasian College of Surgeons; Hughes' keen interest in road accident prevention led to the State of Victoria becoming the first jurisdic-

tion in the world to enact legislation for compulsory seatbelt use. The first Polish honoree was Witold Janusz Rudowski, who had studied medicine at a clandestine 'flying university' during the Nazi occupation; in the year he was conferred – 1978 – Soviet control prompted a resurgence of such underground education. Glasgow's Andrew Watt Kay (of the Kay augmented histamine test), Bristol's Ronald H.R. Belsey, known for his innovations in oesophageal surgery, and the Americans John W. Kirklin (whose heart-lung bypass machine facilitated perhaps one million cardiac operations in his lifetime) and Warren Cole (past-president of the American College of Surgeons) were the recipients of the 1979 awards. Continuing a tradition, Irish Presidents Cearbhall Ó Dálaigh (1975) and Patrick Hillery (1977) were also honoured, as were certain RCSI stalwarts: T.J. Gilmartin (1974), J.D.H. Widdess (1975) and Harold Joseph Browne (1976), described as 'one of the most popular, loved and trusted figures in Irish surgery... the ultimate Irish surgical sage' (O'Donnell, *Irish Surgeons and Surgery*, p. 304). The Anatomy Department's lecture theatre was named in Browne's honour in 2007.

102 Its official title was the *Outline of the Future Hospital System: Report of the Consultative Council on the General Hospital Services* (1968). The Chair of the Council that produced the report was UCD's Professor of Surgery, Patrick Alexis Fitzgerald (Hon FRCSI 1962). Other key contributors to the volume from RCSI were W.A.L. MacGowan, William O'Dwyer (Prof of Medicine 1975–85) and Eoin O'Malley (FRCSI 1947, PRCSI 1982–84).

103 Quoted in Mary E. Daly, 'The curse of the Irish Hospitals' Sweepstake: A hospital system, not a health system', in *Working Papers in History and Policy* No. 2 (2012).

104 RCSI/COU/44, 9 November 1978, p. 320. By contrast, the HEA was funding similar ventures in Galway (for UCG), and at the Mater (for UCD) and St James' (for Trinity). RCSI did not qualify due to its 'independent status' (*Irish Medical Times*, 11 May 1979).

105 RCSI/COU/46, 14 June 1984, p. 741.

106 RCSI/COU/46, 12 April 1984, p. 729.

107 For O'Brien's arguments, see his compilation, *The Charitable Infirmary Jervis Street, 1718–1987: A Farewell Tribute* (1987), pp. xvii–xviii.

108 These are indicative draft figures produced for the Council (RCSI/COU/42, 8 April 1976, p. 182; RCSI/COU/44, 13 October 1977, p. 257).

109 *Annual Report* 1981, p. 13.

110 RCSI/OH/2/1 (W.A.L. MacGowan).

111 See *JICPS* vol. 5, no. 3 (January 1976), p. 102; *IMT* 1 February 1980.

112 O'Donnell, *Irish Surgeons and Surgery*, p. 185. For all MacGowan's eminent achievements, his students were most likely more impressed by the fact that his nephew Shane was lead singer and chief songwriter with The Pogues.

113 Eighty-five students sat the exam in May 1983, but thereafter the Kuwaiti authorities decided to rotate the awarding body and Glasgow took over in 1984. RCPSG was already running Primary Fellowship examinations in Abu Dhabi and Tripoli. In recent years, relations between Kuwait and RCSI's Faculties of Dentistry and Radiology have been particularly strong.

114 *Annual Report* 1982, p. 13.

115 *Irish Medical Times*, 6 November 1981.

116 RCSI/COU/44, 22 April 1977, p. 230.

117 RCSI/COU/44, 11 October 1979, p. 370.

118 *Annual Report* 1981, p. 4.

119 *Irish Medical Times*, 20 August 1976.

120 The word is used in RCSI/COU/44, 9 November 1978, p. 318.

121 RCSI/COU/44, 8 November 1979, p. 374.

122 RCSI/COU/45, 2 July 1981, p. 572.

123 *Irish Medical Times*, 15 February 1980.

124 RCSI/OH/2/1 (W.A.L. MacGowan).

125 O'Donnell, *Irish Surgeons and Surgery*, p. 186.

126 The phrase is MacGowan's – see *Annual Report* 1981.

127 *JICPS* vol. 12, no. 2 (October 1982), p. 74.

128 *JICPS* vol. 9, no. 3 (January 1980), p. 101.

129 Such as a HP computer, an XY plotter, a reaction rate analyser and a flatbed recorder – see RCSI/COU/44, 12 May 1977, p. 239; 17 January 1980.

130 *JICPS* vol. 11, no. 3 (January 1982), p. 12. This article, entitled 'Medical Research – Means, Aims and Accomplishments', was O'Malley's address to the Biological Society in November 1981.

131 For LSD, see *JRCSI* vol. 6, no. 1 (July 1970), p. 35; for circadian rhythms, see Cliona Buckley, R.T.W.L. Conroy and G.C. Lindsay, 'Time Zone Transitions and Master Mariners', *JICPS* vol. 2, no. 4 (April 1973), pp. 109–12 and *Irish Times*, 22 January 1971, p. 5. Conroy was also the author, with J.N. Mills, of the groundbreaking *Human Circadian Rhythms* (1970).

132 *Irish Times*, 16 February 1974, p. 6.

133 See *JICPS* vol. 1, no. 1 (July 1971), p. 40.

134 Caroline de Costa, *The Women's Doc* (2021), p. 38; p. 55.

135 *Irish Times*, 26 April 1976, p. 5.

136 *Irish Times*, 30 April 1976, p. 11.

137 See *Daily Mirror*, 5 February 1985. Ironically, Hussey's vacated place was taken by the Chief Justice of Ireland.

138 *Irish Medical Times*, 23 July 1982.

139 As a portrait of an era – and, indeed, an 'all-male world' (p. 623) – O'Donnell's volume is particularly invaluable for its 'Afterword' of 'expunged phrases' (pp. 623–26).

140 My thanks to Vidhi Patel for this data, compiled as part of the 2023 Research Summer School.

141 *Irish Medical Times*, 8 June 1979.

142 These first began in 1984.

143 *Irish Times*, 3 March 1979.

144 *Irish Medical Times*, 22 April 1983.

145 *Irish Medical Times*, 15 April 1983.

146 *Irish Medical Times*, 29 October 1982.

147 In 1975, the Council wondered about making a bid on the hostel (RCSI/COU/42, 13 February 1975, p. 104); twenty-five years later, they did so.

148 *Annual Report* 1982, p. 2.

149 This figure is from the *Annual Report* 1983, p. 11; elsewhere – *JICPS* vol. 12, no. 3 (January 1983), p. 131 – the cost is given as £130,000.

150 *JICPS* vol. 12, no. 3 (January 1983), p. 127. As Medical Director of St Patrick's University Hospital, Lucey would become a well-known commentator on mental health issues in Ireland. Related at another level, RCSI was also represented (by Joseph Grace and Michael Horgan) on the Committee of Higher Education for Development and Co-operation (HEDCO) – see RCSI/COU/46, 6 March 1984, p. 723.

151 *Yearbook* 1974, p. 150.

152 *Annual Report* 1984, p. 58.

153 *Annual Report* 1982, p. 39.

154 *Annual Report* 1983, p. 41.

155 See RCSI/COU/44, 2 July 1977, p. 249; 18 January 1979, p. 335.

156 *JICPS* vol. 13, no. 1 (January 1984), p. 5.

157 O'Donnell, *Irish Surgeons and Surgery*, pp. 203–04.

158 See *Dictionary of Irish Biography* entry by Turlough O'Riordan (2013, revised 2021).

159 His wife, Una O'Higgins O'Malley, daughter of the assassinated government minister Kevin O'Higgins, founded the Glencree Centre for Peace and Reconciliation in 1974; in recent times, RCSI has favoured this venue for think-ins and away days.

160 *Irish Medical Times*, 4 February 1985.

161 The planting, by the new PRCSI, Victor Lane (FRCSI 1950, PRCSI 1984–86), took place on 13 December 1984.

162 *JICPS* vol. 13, no. 1 (January 1984), p. 7.

CHAPTER 8 NEW VENTURES, 1985-2010

1 RCSI/COU/47, 8 October 1987; *Annual Report* 1987, p. 13; *Annual Report* 1985, p. 38.

2 *Annual Report* 1988, p. 16.

3 RCSI/COU/46, 14 February 1985, p. 790.

4 RCSI/COU/46, 11 April 1985, p. 801.

5 *Annual Report* 1986, p. 65. Budgeted at £1.7 million, Millin House was delivered for £1.5 million. The architects were Brian O'Halloran and Associates, the contractors were Sisk & Co.

6 RCSI/COU/46, 12 June 1986, p. 903.

7 RCSI/COU/47, 3 July 1986, p. 902.

8 RCSI/COU/46, 8 November 1984, p. 765.

9 See *Annual Report* 1989, p. 63.

10 The central section, facing South King Street, is from 1888.

11 *Irish Times*, 13 September 1989. For An Taisce's complaint, see *Irish Times*, 29 August and 14 September 1988.

12 Through the planning phase, the Mercer Library was conceived of as a shared library space for both RCSI and RCPI. Also considered was the amalgamation of historical collections at Kildare Street, with only a nucleus of RCSI material staying at RCSI – but this did not come to pass (see RCSI/COU/47, 14 November 1985; 11 June 1987, p. 971; 2 July 1987, p. 986).

13 RCSI owned nos. 84 and 85, on the corner with Clonmel Street, and in October 1986 also acquired no. 83. The move to Mercer took place in September 1990.

14 *Irish Medical Times*, 1 January 1988, p. 8. Roads not taken before this included the location of the GP practice in Dolphin's Barn and the establishment of a Lectureship in Family Practice at a health centre in Coolock (RCSI/COU/47, 9 January 1986, p. 857).

15 Peter Harrington, 'A role for Irish general practice in the education of today's medical undergraduate', *JICPS* vol. 23, no. 2, 1994, p. 129.

16 These are words of the Dean of the Medical Faculty, Kevin O'Malley – see *Annual Report* 1987, p. 13.

17 *JICPS* vol. 20, no. 4, October 1991, p. 294.

18 See *JICPS* vol. 20, no. 4, October 1991, p. 296. In 1988 the Faculty of Nursing presented a cheque for £30,000; more followed.

19 Built by Michael McNamara & Co., the new residence cost £2.15 million.

20 *Irish Times RCSI Special Report*, 25 May 1994, p. 5.

21 See *Irish Times*, 12 September 1991, p. 6: 'Altogether, the project cost the college over £7 million, of which not a penny came from the State.' The correspondent, Frank McDonald, was not entirely impressed with the restoration decisions. Nearly thirty years later, McDonald was conferred with Honorary Fellowship (2019).

22 *Annual Report* 1988, p. 14.

23 *RCSIsmj*, vol. 1, no. 1 (2007), p. 8.

24 *JICPS* vol. 19, no. 3 (July 1990), p. 168.

25 The Bahraini connection, already of long standing, would result in the foundation of the RCSI-Medical University of Bahrain (2004).

26 This venture had been originally suggested to Kevin O'Malley by Godfrey Geh (Lic. 1965, Hon FRCSI 2020) in 1992.

27 This initiative had the mutual benefit of furnishing the new university with a proven medicine programme, and expanding RCSI's international undergraduate education model.

28 *JICPS* vol. 25, no. 3 (July 1996), p. 219.

29 *JICPS* vol. 17, no. 4 (October 1988), p. 219.

30 PARC also supported RCSI projects in Dublin, notably the Mercer Project. Its MD, David Hanly, was admitted to the RCSI Court of Patrons in 1997.

31 *JICPS* vol. 20, no. 2 (April 1991), p. 144.

32 *JICPS* vol. 25, no. 2 (April 1996), p. 150.

33 *Annual Report* 1994–95, p. 11.

34 See *JICPS* vol. 25, no. 2 (April 1996), p. 150.

35 RCSI/OH/2/1 (W.A.L. MacGowan).

36 *JICPS* vol. 25, no. 1 (January 1996), p. 62.

37 *JICPS* vol. 22, no. 3 (July 1993), p. 224.

38 *Irish Times*, 26 June 1996, p. 23; 9 October 1996, p. 2; 20 February 1998, p. 30.

39 *Annual Report* 1995–96, p. 12.

40 *Irish Times*, 22 May 1987.

41 See *RCSI News* no. 16 (August 1998), n.p. [p. 10].

42 The sale was reported in the *Irish Times*, 15 January 1997.

43 *Annual Report* 1995–96, p. 12.

44 *Irish Times*, 23 February 2000.

45 See *JICPS* vol. 20, no. 2 (April 1991), p. 141 – the list appeared in the *British Medical Journal*.

46 *Irish Times*, 18 October 1991.

47 *Irish Times*, 5 March 1996.

48 RCSI/COU/46, 8 March 1985, p. 793. Fees for 'developing' and 'developed' world students were £11,327 and £16,177, respectively.

49 *Irish Times*, 5 January 1997.

50 See RCSI/COU/47, 12 May 1988, p. 1038; 16 June 1988, p. 1044.

51 *Annual Report* 1995, p. 20.

52 *Annual Report* 1985, p. 24.

53 *Annual Report* 1991, p. 6.

54 Particular credit for this connection went to Prof Alan Johnson (Biochemistry).

55 *Annual Report* 1986, p. 13.

56 See O'Donnell, *Irish Surgeons and Surgery*, p. 187.

57 *Irish Times RCSI Special Report*, 25 May 1994, p. 3.

58 *Annual Report* 1999–2000, p. 10.

59 The inaugural appointees to these professorships were, respectively: Louis Collum, Michael Walsh, Max Ryan and Timothy O'Brien.

60 *JICPS* vol. 18, no. 4 (October 1989), p. 286.

61 *Irish Times*, 13 July 1998, p. 13.

62 Separately, RCSI received a £2 million personal donation from Sheikh Maktoom Bin Rashid Al-Maktoom, Prime Minister of the United Arab Emirates, to fund an Institute of Aging Research and Medicine of the Elderly to be based in the new facility (*JICPS* vol. 22, no. 2 (April 1993), p. 156), but this facility never came to fruition.

63 *JICPS* vol. 17, no. 3 (July 1988), p. 94.

64 The first *Annual Report* to use this title was 1999–2000;

however, it was in occasional use before this.

65 O'Donnell, *Irish Surgeons and Surgery*, p. 204.

66 *JICPS* vol. 18, no. 1 (January 1989), p. 65.

67 *JICPS* vol. 20, no. 4 (October 1991), p. 298.

68 See O'Donnell, *Irish Surgeons and Surgery*, pp. 22–23.

69 *JICPS* vol. 16, no. 1 (January 1987), p. 38.

70 O'Donnell, *Irish Surgeons and Surgery*, p. 62; *President's Report* 2001–02, p. 5.

71 *Irish Times*, 3 April 1997.

72 Kevin M. Cahill (ed.), *The Open Door: Health and Foreign Policy at the RCSI* (1999), p. 43.

73 Cahill, *The Open Door*, p. 94.

74 Cahill, *The Open Door*, p. 40.

75 RCSI/COU/47, 12 December 1985, p. 850.

76 *Annual Report* 1992, p. 11. After a long hiatus, another writer – the novelist Roddy Doyle – was conferred with the Honorary Fellowship in 2022. The doctor and novelist Abraham Verghese received an Honorary Doctorate from RCSI in 2014.

77 *JICPS* vol. 22, no. 4 (October 1993), p. 300.

78 *RCSI Alumni Magazine* (2017), p. 58.

79 *Annual Report* 1985, p. 7.

80 RCSI/COU/46, 10 April 1986, p. 887.

81 *Annual Report* 1991, p. 97.

82 *JICPS* vol. 25, no. 3 (July 1996), p. 230.

83 *Annual Report* 1996–98, p. 67.

84 *President's Report* 2001–02, p. 42.

85 *President's Report* 2002–03, p. 34.

86 Seanad Éireann debate – Wednesday, 12 February 2003, vol. 171, no. 7. Webpage: https://www.oireachtas.ie/en/debates/debate/seanad/2003-02-12/5/

87 Cameron, pp. 233–34.

88 The 2002 meeting was originally scheduled to take place in Jordan. Controversially, the venue was changed in the wake of the World Trade Center attacks, and some senior RCSI figures who disagreed with the decision did not travel to Hong Kong.

89 Eric O'Flynn, Krikor Erzingatsian, Declan Magee and the RCSI/COSECSA Collaboration (eds.), *Operating Together: 12 Years of Collaboration Between RCSI and COSECSA* (2019), p. 7.

90 *Operating Together*, p. 56.

91 In a valedictory editorial, Eoin O'Brien traced the forty-year history of the *JICPS*. His prediction – 'When the future history of the College comes to be written, the *JICPS* will prove to be an archive of inestimable value giving insight into the character of the two colleges that no minute book can give' – has been proved true. Twenty years on, his further warning – 'Where now will the details of the buildings, their statuary and portraiture, the physical development of the Colleges be recorded? Where will the pictorial records... be captured for all time? Where will the obituaries of presidents, professors, teachers and

porters be poignantly written?' (*JICPS* vol. 32, no. 1, January 2003, p. 4) – remains valid.

92 As RCSI had been planning the GEP course for some time, it declined a request from the HEA to wait until 2007 in order to coincide with three other universities' similar programmes. For this reason, RCSI's pioneering course had to wait until April 2007 to receive formal HEA approval.

93 This was delivered jointly with the Institute of Technology, Sligo.

94 Prof Nolan was Head of the Department of Chemistry and Physics from 1987; subsequently, this became the Department of Pharmaceutical and Medicinal Chemistry.

95 In October 2022, the Faculty would be renamed the Faculty of Radiologists & Radiation Oncologists, coinciding with the start of Dr Patricia Cunningham's tenure as the first female Dean.

96 Quoted in Lee (ed.), *Surgeons' Halls*, p. 154.

97 Quoted in Lee (ed.), *Surgeons' Halls*, p. 156.

98 *Annual Report* 2008–09, p. 13.

99 *Annual Report* 2008–09, p. 4.

100 Kavanagh was already considered a pioneer of wild game bird management in Ireland, notably for his work on the preservation of the grey partridge.

101 *President's Report* 2003–04, p. 18.

102 *President's Report* 2006–07, p. 13; p. 24.

103 *President's Report* 2006–07, p. 25

104 *President's Report* 2007–08, p. 27.

105 *President's Report* 2006–07, p. 24.

106 *President's Report* 2006–07, p. 23.

107 *Irish Times*, 10 March 2009.

108 This figure is quoted in both the *Irish Times* (10 March 2009) and the *RCSIsmj*, vol. 1, no. 1 (2008), p. 8.

109 In March 2019, the foundation stone for the RCSI Bahrain Health Oasis was laid by His Highness Sheikh Khalifa Bin Salman Al Khalifa, accompanied by Dara Calleary TD, Minister with responsibility for Labour Affairs at the Department of Enterprise, Trade and Employment. See also *President's Report* 2006–07, p. 14.

110 *Annual Report* 2009–10, p. 2.

111 As it happens, the decision to dissolve the NUI was reversed in 2011.

CHAPTER 9 UNIVERSITY STATUS, 2011-19

1 At the time of writing, the 2022–24 Council members are: Prof Laura Viani (President), Prof Deborah McNamara (Vice President), Mr James Geraghty, Prof Kevin Conlon, Mr David Moore, Prof K. Simon Cross, Prof Michael Kerin, Prof Thomas H. Lynch, Ms Margaret O'Donnell, Prof Camilla MA Carroll, Mr Sean Johnston, Mr Paddy Kenny, Prof Kilian Walsh, Mr John Caird, Ms Bridget Egan, Mr Keith Synnott,

Prof John Quinlan, Prof Paul Ridgway, Prof Ronan Cahill, Prof David Healy, Prof Calvin Coffey, The Hon. Mr Justice Peter Kelly and Roderick Ryan.

2 Since 2020, the make-up of the CAB has changed somewhat, being comprised of four Council members, six external members and two executive members (that is, the CEO and the Dean of the Medical Faculty).

3 At the time of writing, the SMT is: Prof Cathal Kelly (Vice Chancellor and Chief Executive/Registrar), Prof Hannah McGee (Deputy Vice Chancellor for Academic Affairs), Prof Fergal O'Brien (Deputy Vice Chancellor for Research and Innovation), Jennifer Cullinane (Director of Finance), Eunan Friel (Managing Director of Healthcare Management), Aine Gibbons (Director of Development, Alumni Relations, Fellows and Members), Barry Holmes (Director of Human Resources), Abi Kelly (Director of International Engagement and External Relations), Michael McGrail (Director of Corporate Strategy), Justin Ralph (Chief Technology Officer) and Kieran Ryan (Managing Director of Surgical Affairs).

4 *Annual Report* 2021–22, p. 86.

5 This was on 14 May 2014.

6 *Annual Report* 2016–17, p. 51. The quote is from Prof Arnold Hill (FRCSI 1992, Prof of Surgery, Head of the School of Medicine (this was a new role created in November 2013)).

7 *Annual Report* 2015–16, p. 39.

8 *Anatomy Room Gallery Catalogue* (2017), p. 2. Dr Khan (Medicine 2003, MRCSI 2008) appears in the upper left quadrant of the canvas.

9 *Anatomy Room Gallery Catalogue*, p. 4.

10 This was created by Dr Jane Burns, with Eric Clarke and Prof Richard Arnett.

11 The total external funding awarded to RCSI for the calendar year 2021 was €37.5 million, up from €31.5 million in 2020 (*Annual Report* 2021–22, p. 49).

12 *Annual Report* 2011–12, p. 49; *Annual Report* 2012–13, p. 4.

13 Building on a PhD partnership commenced in 2007, SPHeRE (led by Prof Anne Hickey) continues as the national doctoral training route of population and health systems research.

14 In 2021, Prof O'Brien was appointed Deputy Vice-Chancellor for Research and Innovation.

15 This is measured by the field-weighted citation index – see *Annual Report* 2019–20, p. 47.

16 SurgaColl Technologies was founded by Prof Fergal O'Brien (Anatomy and Regenerative Medicine).

17 *Annual Report* 2010–11, p. 7.

18 *Annual Report* 2017–18, p. 8.

19 My thanks to Justin Ralph, Chief Technology Officer, for his assistance with these notes.

20 In September 2014, the School of Nursing and Midwifery separated from the Faculty of Nursing and Midwifery to join the Faculty of Medicine and Health Sciences.

21 The inaugural Director of the Physician Associates programme was Prof Denni Woodmansee, succeeded by Prof Lisa Alexander in 2020.

22 In 2011, a similar, joint RCSI-UCD venture had been mooted for the other side of the country, at Terengganu, but this did not come to pass.

23 Appointed in 1986, Cunningham was the first full-time Professor of Anaesthesia in the Republic of Ireland. His predecessor, Prof Gilmartin, had been an Associate Professor.

24 *Irish Times*, 16 May 2011, p. 8.

25 See, for example, Eoin O'Brien's 'Letter to the Editor', *Irish Times*, 23 June, p. 17 ('I can do little other than protest to the council and fellows of RCSI, but I can express my concern in a more direct way to RCPI by resigning as a fellow').

26 *Irish Times*, 31 May 2011, p. 36.

27 *Irish Times*, 23 June 2011, p. 12.

28 Part of the RCPI response reads: 'The events of the past few months in Bahrain have been shocking. Unquestionably, this has damaged the international reputation of Bahrain and, sadly, has undermined the efforts towards modernization and reform, particularly in relation to healthcare that have been underway in Bahrain in recent years' (*Irish Times*, 25 June 2011, p. 15).

29 *Irish Times*, 25 June 2011, p. 15.

30 *Irish Times*, 15 May 2012, p. 17.

31 *Irish Times*, 16 Feb 2012, p. 7.

32 *Irish Times*, 26 March 2013, p. 7.

33 *Irish Medical Times*, 10 June 2013.

34 Since its establishment in 2018, the RCSI Art Committee has been chaired by Aíne Gibbons, Director of Development, Alumni Relations, Fellows and Members.

35 *EDI Strategy and Action Plan* 2018–22, p. 6.

36 *Annual Report* 2017–18, p. 20.

37 *Annual Report* 2015–16, p. 93.

38 The first incumbent in the role was Abi Kelly.

39 Education (Miscellaneous Provisions) Act 2015, p. 3.

40 Key advice was provided by Dr Don Thornhill, former Secretary General of the Department of Education and Science and Executive Chair of the HEA. Amongst those central to the process within RCSI were Adrian Devitt (Associate Director, Office of the CEO), and the Quality Enhancement Office, led by Prof David Croke (formerly Prof of Biochemistry) from 2010 to 2021.

41 This application was scrutinised by multiple parties on behalf of the Higher Education Authority, including the state agency QQI (Quality and Qualifications Ireland). Their examination covered a wide range of criteria, such as research record and programme provision; governance structures; student access requirements; prescribed student population composition and staff qualifications; financial viability; strong social and cultural links; international collaborations including joint research projects; and linkages supporting creativity and contribution to the promotion of the economic, cultural, social and scientific development of the State.

42 *Annual Report* 2019–20, p. 14.

CODA ON THE HORIZON, 2020 TO THE PRESENT

1 *Annual Report* 2019–20, p. 4.

2 This is the US Centre for Disease Control's (CDC) timeline and statistics.

3 Principally, this advice was from Prof Sam McConkey (International Health and Tropical Medicine) – see *Annual Report* 2019–20, p. 12. A Business Continuity Planning Group was also established.

4 These were the words of Justin Ralph, RCSI's Chief Technology Officer – see *Annual Report* 2019–20, p. 81.

5 *Irish Times*, 18 March 2020.

6 *RCSI – Reflecting on Our Covid-19 Experience* (March 2021), n.p. [p. 2].

7 The *Sunday Times* Good University Guide award noted in the previous chapter – University of the Year for Student Engagement – went to RCSI primarily for its efforts to negate the impact of the pandemic on its students. In 2022, the RCSI School of Medicine was also named joint winner of the 2022 ASPIRE to Excellence Award for Student Engagement, the first Irish medical school to receive this honour.

8 In Dublin, this was led by Philip Curtis (Director of Director of Student Recruitment, Admissions and Student Services) and Elizabeth Healy (Head of Student Recruitment), working in collaboration with Paul Nolan (Marketing).

9 See *Reflecting on Our Covid-19 Experience* for details of the 7,000-plus national and international media mentions in 2020.

10 RCSI's training of contact tracers was coordinated by Adrian Devitt (Strategy & Risk Management).

11 One early research paper (again, amongst many) that received widespread media attention was: Fogarty, H., Townsend, L., Ni Cheallaigh, C., Bergin, C., Martin-Loeches, I., Browne, P., Bacon, C.L., Gaule, R., Gillett, A., Byrne, M., Ryan, K., O'Connell, N., O'Sullivan, J.M., Conlon, N. and O'Donnell, J.S. (2020), 'COVID19 coagulopathy in Caucasian patients', *British Journal of Haematology*, vol. 189, no. 6, pp. 1044–49.

12 RCSI also conducted its own in-house screening and testing to ensure on-campus safety.

13 *Annual Report* 2020–21, p. 6.

14 *Annual Report* 2020–21, p. 6.

15 The award marked the centenary of Cameron's death.

16 This relationship had earlier been fostered by Prof John Waddington (Molecular and Cellular Therapeutics). Amongst Prof Waddington's many professional honours, in 2003 he was the first RCSI faculty-member of the modern era elected to the Royal Irish Academy (RIA), the country's leading body of experts in the sciences and humanities. The first two RCSI women to be likewise honoured (2022) were Prof Hannah McGee (Deputy Vice Chancellor for Academic Affairs) and Prof Mary Cannon (Psychiatry). Relatedly, Prof Noel Gerard McElvaney (MRIA, Prof of Medicine 1998–), won the HRB Impact Award in 2021.

17 This number is for articles published in 2021; the period 2017–21 counts 5,996 peer-reviewed publications (*Annual Report* 2021–22, p. 9; p. 44).

18 'Inthelia Therapeutics is developing novel treatments for sepsis; Vertigenius is focused on a digital health solution for patients with balance disorders; PrOBMet is developing targeted treatments for breast cancer brain metastatic patients; and Phyxiom is a health analytics platform to help patients with uncontrolled asthma and other chronic respiratory diseases' (*Annual Report* 2021–22, p. 14).

19 *Annual Report* 2021–22, passim. The collaboration with Perdana University is in a teach-out phase, with the last two remaining cohorts due to graduate in 2023 and 2024.

20 As with 26 York Street, the architects for Project Connect are Peter McGovern and Maria Mulcahy of Henry J. Lyons; the contractor is Bennett Construction; and the endeavour is overseen by RCSI SMT-member Michael McGrail (Director of Corporate Strategy).

Index

Facing page: 'Gold Leaf' by Billy Cahill, 2022.

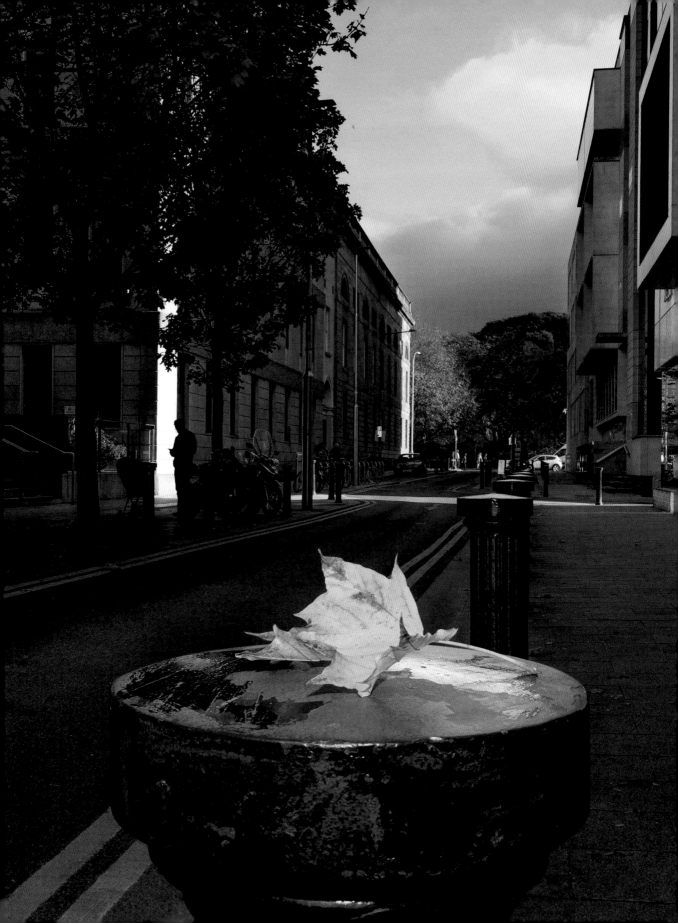